Vaccinations

Vaccinations

EDITED BY

GREGORY A. POLAND, MD, FIDSA, MACP, FRCP (LONDON)

Mary Lowell Leary Emeritus Professor of Medicine, Infectious Diseases, and Molecular
  Pharmacology and Experimental Therapeutics
Distinguished Investigator of the Mayo Clinic
Director, Mayo Vaccine Research Group Mayo Clinic
Rochester, MN, United States

ASSOCIATE EDITOR

JENNIFER A. WHITAKER, MD, MS

Assistant Professor of Medicine
Infectious Diseases
Mayo Clinic
Rochester, MN, United States

ELSEVIER

ELSEVIER

3251 Riverport Lane
St. Louis, Missouri 63043

Vaccinations   ISBN: 978-0-323-66210-9

Notices

Practitioners and researchers must always rely on their own experience and knowledge in evaluating and using any information, methods, compounds or experiments described herein. Because of rapid advances in the medical sciences, in particular, independent verification of diagnoses and drug dosages should be made. To the fullest extent of the law, no responsibility is assumed by Elsevier, authors, editors or contributors for any injury and/or damage to persons or property as a matter of products liability, negligence or otherwise, or from any use or operation of any methods, products, instructions, or ideas contained in the material herein.

Publisher: Dolores Meloni
Acquisition Editor: Robin R Carter
Editorial Project Manager: Pat Gonzalez
Production Project Manager: Poulouse Joseph
Cover Designer: Alan Studholme

Typeset by TNQ Technologies

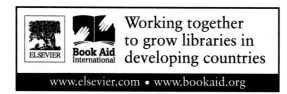

Working together
to grow libraries in
developing countries

www.elsevier.com • www.bookaid.org

List of Contributors

Tom T. Shimabukuro, MD, MPH, MBA
Deputy Director
Immunization Safety Office
Centers for Disease Control and Prevention
Atlanta, GA, United States

Jonathan Duffy, MD, MPH
Medical Officer
Immunization Safety Office
Centers for Disease Control and Prevention
Atlanta, GA, United States

John R. Su, MD, PhD, MPH
Medical Officer
Division of Healthcare Quality Promotion
CDC
Atlanta, GA, United States

Saad B. Omer, MBBS, MPH, PhD
Professor
Global Health, Epidemiology, and Pediatrics
Emory University, Schools of Public Health &
    Medicine & Emory Vaccine Center
Atlanta, GA, United States

Caroline M. Poland, LMHC, LCAC, CCTP, NCC
Director, Taylor University Counseling Center
Licensed Mental Health Counselor, Licensed Clinical
    Addictions Counselor
Taylor University
Upland, IN, United States

**Stefan Gravenstein, MD, MPH, MPH (hon), FACP,
    AGSF, FGSA**
Professor, Warren Alpert Medical School and Health
    Services Policy and Practice
School of Public Health Brown University
Associate Director, Center of Innovation for Long-Term
    Services and Supports
Providence Veterans Administration Medical Center
Clinical Director, Healthcentric Advisors
Providence, RI, United States

Anthony L. Cunningham, MBBS, MD
Centre for Virus Research
The Westmead Institute for Medical Research
University of Sydney
Sydney, NSW, Australia

Thomas C. Heineman, MD, PhD
Vice President
Clinical Development
Genocea Biosciences
Cambridge, MA, United States

Myron J. Levin, MD
Professor of Pediatrics and Medicine
University of Colorado School of Medicine
Aurora, CO, United States

**Gregory A. Poland, MD, FIDSA, MACP, FRCP
    (London)**
Mary Lowell Leary Emeritus Professor of Medicine,
    Infectious Diseases, and Molecular Pharmacology
    and Experimental Therapeutics
Distinguished Investigator of the Mayo Clinic
Director, Mayo Vaccine Research Group Mayo Clinic
Rochester, MN, United States

Inna G. Ovsyannikova, PhD
Professor of Medicine, Mayo Vaccine Research Group
Mayo Clinic
Rochester, MN, United States

Richard B. Kennedy, PhD
Professor of Medicine
Co-Director, Mayo Vaccine Research Group
Mayo Clinic
Rochester, MN, United States

Pritish K. Tosh, MD, FIDSA, FACP
Associate Professor of Medicine
Division of Infectious Diseases
Mayo Clinic
Rochester, MN, United States

Mark Loeb, MD, MSc, FRCPC
Departments of Pathology and Molecular Medicine
and Health Research Methods, Evidence, and
Impact (HEI)
McMaster University
Hamilton, ON, Canada

Lee H. Harrison, MD
Professor of Medicine
University of Pittsburgh
Pittsburgh, PA, United States

Daniel M. Altmann, PhD
Department of Medicine, Imperial College
London, United Kingdom

Jennifer A. Whitaker, MD, MS
Assistant Professor of Medicine
Infectious Diseases
Mayo Clinic
Rochester, MN, United States

Maria D. Mileno, MD
Associate Professor of Medicine
Division of Infectious Diseases
The Warren Alpert Medical School of Brown University
Providence, RI, United States

David J. Weber, MD, MPH
Professor of Medicine and Pediatrics, School of
Medicine
Professor of Epidemiology, Gillings School of Global
Public Health
Medical Director, UNC Hospitals' Departments of
Hospital Epidemiology and Occupational Health
Service
Associate Chief Medical Officer, UNC Health Care
Chapel Hill, NC, United States

Tamara Pilishvili, PhD, MPH
Epidemiologist
Respiratory Diseases Branch
Division of Bacterial Diseases
National Center for Immunizations and Respiratory
Diseases
Atlanta, GA, United States

Srinivas Acharya Nanduri, MD, MPH
Epidemiologist
Respiratory Diseases Branch
Centers for Disease Control and Prevention
Atlanta, GA, United States

Nancy M. Bennett, MD, MS
Professor of Medicine and Public Health Science
Director, Center for Community Health and
Prevention
Co-director, Clinical and Translational Science Institute
University of Rochester School of Medicine and
Dentistry
Rochester, NY, USA

Allison T. Chamberlain, MS, PhD
Assistant Professor
Department of Epidemiology
Rollins School of Public Health
Emory University
Atlanta, GA, United States

Elie A. Saade, MD, MPH
Assistant Professor of Medicine
Case Western Reserve University
Geriatric Medicine, Infectious Diseases and Infection
Control
University Hospitals Cleveland Medical Center
Researcher, Geriatric Research Education and Clinical
Center
Cleveland Veterans Affairs Medical Center
Cleveland, OH, United States

David H. Canaday, MD
Associate Director of Research, Geriatric Research,
Education and Clinical Center (GRECC)
Cleveland, VA, United States
Associate Professor, Division of Infectious Disease,
Case Western Reserve University
Cleveland, OH, United States

H. Edward Davidson, PharmD, MPH
Assistant Professor, Clinical Internal Medicine
Eastern Virginia Medical School
Partner, Insight Therapeutics, LLC
Norfolk, VA, United States

Lisa F. Han, MPH
Partner, Insight Therapeutics, LLC
Norfolk, VA, United States

Biao Wang, PhD
Vice President of Data Science, Oculys Health
Informatics
Waterloo, ON, Canada

Emily E. Sickbert-Bennett, MS, PhD
Department of Hospital Epidemiology
University of North Carolina Hospitals
Chapel Hill, NC, United States

Kenneth Valles, BS
Mayo Clinic School of Medicine, Medical Scientist
    Training Program
Mayo Clinic
Rochester, MN, United States

**Colleen Lau, MBBS (UWA), MPH&TM (JCU), PhD
    (UQ), FRACGP, FFTM (ACTM), FACTM**
NHMRC Fellow
Department of Global Health
Research School of Population Health
ANU College of Health & Medicine
The Australian National University
Canberra, ACT, Australia

John R. Lonks, MD
Associate Professor
Department of Medicine
Division of Infectious Diseases
The Warren Alpert Medical School of Brown University
The Miriam Hospital
Providence, RI, United States

Joseph Metmowlee Garland, MD
Assistant Professor of Medicine, Clinician Educator
Department of Medicine
Division of Infectious Diseases
The Miriam Hospital
Providence, RI, United States

Martha C. Sanchez, MD
Assistant Professor of Medicine
Division of Infectious Diseases
The Warren Alpert Medical School of Brown University
Providence, RI, United States

Gerard J. Nau, MD, PhD
Associate Professor of Medicine
Division of Infectious Diseases
The Warren Alpert Medical School of Brown University
Rhode Island Hospital
Providence, RI, United States

Jerome M. Larkin, MD
Associate Professor of Medicine
Division of Infectious Diseases
The Warren Alpert Medical School of Brown University
The Miriam Hospital
Providence, RI, United States

Preface

ADULT VACCINOLOGY IN THE 21ST CENTURY—CURRENT PRACTICE

The purpose of this book is to provide a concise update on the current practice of adult vaccinology in the 21st century. In particular, we have focused on the major issues faced by clinicians, public health officials, nurses, and others who recommend and deliver vaccines to adults. The field of vaccines is dynamic—new vaccines, new recommendations, new disease threats, and new issues frequently arise and require thoughtful answers. In this book we address these particular issues related to vaccine practice.

The reader will find chapters addressing vaccine safety and vaccine hesitancy, which are major issues that stymie attempts to fully protect those mostly at risk of serious—but vaccine-preventable—diseases. Given the historic demographic changes coming in the "graying of the globe," issues of immunosenescence and the need for strong older adult immunization programs have become increasingly evident. The reader will find an excellent chapter on vaccines for the elderly, as well as a chapter on zoster vaccines, which highlights one of the most recent vaccines approved in the United States.

New infectious diseases seem to threaten human health every year or two, and we have included a chapter on a topic of pressing public health importance: Zika infection and the considerable current attempts to develop a safe and effective vaccine. Influenza has been a continuing annual scourge punctuated by periodic significant antigenic drift and occasional viral shifts. This book includes a chapter that provides updates related to influenza vaccines for adult recipients. In regard to other vaccine-preventable diseases for which adults suffer disproportionate morbidity and mortality, Chapter 12 includes information about vaccines against pneumococcal infection, and Chapter 9 reviews vaccines for those who are immunocompromised.

To round out this book, we have provided practical and accessible information on vaccine immunology in adults, vaccines for adult travelers, and meningococcal vaccines. Finally, we have included a chapter directly relevant to you, the reader, on vaccines for healthcare providers. Research has repeatedly demonstrated that if healthcare providers are not immunized, they rarely become vaccine champions for those who entrust their care to the provider.

Our "compass" in planning this book has been to provide practical and actionable clinically relevant information on the practice of adult vaccinology. We trust we have been successful in this desire.

Gregory A. Poland, MD, FIDSA, MACP, FRCP (London)
Mary Lowell Leary Emeritus Professor of Medicine, Infectious Diseases, and Molecular Pharmacology and Experimental Therapeutics Distinguished Investigator of the Mayo Clinic Director, Mayo Vaccine Research Group Mayo Clinic Rochester, MN, United States

Jennifer A. Whitaker, MD, MS
Assistant Professor of Medicine Associate Program Director, Infectious Diseases Fellowship Mayo Clinic Rochester, MN, United States

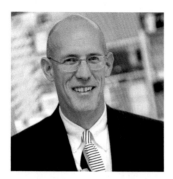

Gregory A. Poland

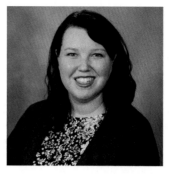

Jennifer A. Whitaker

Contents

CHAPTER 1

Vaccine Safety

JOHN R. SU, MD, PHD, MPH • JONATHAN DUFFY, MD, MPH •
TOM T. SHIMABUKURO, MD, MPH, MBA

INTRODUCTION

Safety means a condition free from risk or injury. Few things, if any, are completely risk free. All medical interventions and products, including vaccines, can have potential harms. The objective of vaccine safety science is to identify and quantify risks of vaccination, with the goal of preventing or reducing their occurrence. An adverse event following immunization (AEFI) is any untoward medical occurrence temporally associated with a vaccine or the process of administering a vaccine.[1] AEFIs might or might not be caused by a vaccine or the process of administering that vaccine. Some AEFIs are coincidental and actually due to other causes. An AEFI caused by a vaccine is called an "adverse reaction" in regulatory terminology; the terms "adverse effect" or "side effect" are sometimes used in other contexts to mean the same thing.[2] Determining if an AEFI is an adverse reaction can be difficult because most AEFIs that can occur after vaccination can also occur without any relation to vaccination. Such a determination requires evidence beyond temporal association with the vaccination.

Adverse reactions can conceptually be separated into a number of categories:[1]

1. Adverse reactions can be related to defects in vaccine quality (i.e., the vaccine was not manufactured according to specifications).
2. Adverse reactions can result from errors related to inappropriate vaccine handling, prescribing, or administration.
3. Adverse reactions can be anxiety-related reactions due to a patient's psychological response to vaccination rather than the vaccine itself.
4. Adverse reactions can also be related to inherent properties of the vaccine, such as the chemical or biological properties of the vaccine's antigens or other ingredients. However, not everyone receiving the vaccine will react to these inherent properties.

These types of reactions can occur in some patients and not others based on the individual person's susceptibility. For example, some people are allergic to a particular substance, even though the vast majority of people are not.

After an adverse reaction is identified, the risk of that reaction can be characterized by its probability and severity. Probability is the frequency with which an adverse reaction occurs and can range from rare to common. Severity is the clinical impact of the adverse reaction on the vaccine recipient and can range from mild to severe. Generally, mild reactions cause minimal or no impairment, are of short duration, and are self-limited. Severe reactions can require medical or surgical intervention or can result in permanent disability or death.

After risks are characterized by probability and severity, a benefit–risk assessment can be performed. Most currently available vaccines are preventive vaccines, which are meant to be given to persons to prevent disease (i.e., primary prevention); a therapeutic vaccine would be given to a person who already has a disease. For preventive vaccines, the benefit–risk assessment determines if the benefits of preventing the disease(s) targeted by the vaccine justify taking the risk of adverse reactions to the vaccine.

Patients and the public expect a high degree of safety with vaccines. The acceptable amount of risk associated with preventive vaccines is generally lower than that for other types of medical interventions. Persons who are already ill might accept more risk with interventions such as drugs or invasive procedures to alleviate or cure their active symptoms. In contrast, persons vaccinated for prevention might never be exposed to the agent targeted by the vaccine. Also, many vaccines for communicable diseases benefit both the vaccinated person and the community or society at large, by preventing the transmission of communicable diseases to other

Vaccinations. https://doi.org/10.1016/B978-0-323-55435-0.00001-X

1

persons and by contributing to overall immunity of the population to the disease prevented by the vaccine. Some jurisdictions therefore make certain vaccinations mandatory for activities such as school attendance, participation in daycare, or for certain types of healthcare employment. Many preventive vaccines are administered to a large proportion of the population, such as the routine vaccines administered to infants.[1]

Vaccines are prescription medical products regulated by the government. In the United States, the Food and Drug Administration (FDA) is the national regulatory agency that licenses and approves vaccines for use. The FDA requires testing to demonstrate the safety and efficacy of a vaccine before issuing a license. If an experimental candidate vaccine caused severe adverse reactions beyond an acceptable frequency during the research and development process, the vaccine would likely not be licensed. This regulatory approach results in licensed vaccines for which, typically, any common adverse reactions are mild and any severe adverse reactions are rare.

Once licensed, the vaccine-prescribing information document will list FDA-approved indications, as well as contraindications and precautions to vaccine administration. The FDA-approved indications are reasons to use the vaccine and the persons for whom the vaccine is approved (e.g., age range); recommendations for use from other organizations might differ from the FDA-approved indications (for example, some organizations might make recommendations based on clinical data that were not available at the time of FDA approval). For the vast majority of patients for whom a vaccine is indicated, the vaccine's benefits will outweigh the vaccine's risks. However, for a few patients, the risk might outweigh the benefits for a particular vaccine. A patient might have a contraindication, a condition that increases the likelihood of a serious adverse reaction to a particular vaccine (e.g., a severe allergy to gelatin, which is a component of some vaccines). A patient who has a contraindication to a vaccine should not receive that vaccine. Alternatively, a patient might have a precaution, a condition that could increase the likelihood or severity of an adverse reaction or reduce the vaccine's ability to produce immunity; such patients should only receive that vaccine after careful consideration by their healthcare provider. Other rare, severe adverse reactions have no known risk factors and cannot be predicted.

This chapter will present an overview of vaccine safety. First, examples of important adverse reactions will be described. Clinical considerations for the prevention and management of adverse reactions will be outlined, including populations with special considerations. Assessment and monitoring of vaccine safety will then be described. The safety of vaccines with compounds used to enhance immune response (adjuvants) and current vaccine safety concerns will be explored. Finally, approaches to the review of evidence and formulation of policy will be discussed. As this chapter will show, manufacturers that produce vaccines, government agencies that regulate and recommend vaccines, and healthcare providers who prescribe and administer vaccines all share responsibility for ensuring that vaccines are safe and used in a safe manner.

EXAMPLES OF ADVERSE REACTIONS
Common Adverse Reactions
Most adverse reactions to vaccination are mild and self-limited, for which the affected person does not seek medical care. Common reactions are usually detected and characterized during prelicensure clinical trials or early in postlicensure safety monitoring. One group of common reactions, collectively termed "injection-site reactions," includes signs and symptoms such as pain, pruritus, swelling, and erythema localized to the area near the injection site. Systemic reactions such as fever, myalgia, arthralgia, fatigue, headache, and malaise are also common adverse reactions with many vaccines. Local and generalized rashes can occur after administration of certain live attenuated viral vaccines, notably measles-containing vaccines, varicella (chickenpox), and herpes zoster (HZ) (shingles) vaccines.[3-5] Mild adverse reactions reflect an intact immune system reacting appropriately to the antigenic stimulus of a vaccine, are therefore expected, and generally do not represent clinically significant safety concerns.

Some common adverse reactions are specific to the type of vaccine and route of administration. For example, live attenuated influenza vaccine (LAIV) is administered intranasally, with resulting viral replication in the upper airway; nasal congestion frequently occurs after receipt of this vaccine.[6] Diarrhea and vomiting occur with greater frequency in children receiving live attenuated rotavirus vaccine (an oral vaccine indicated for the prevention of rotavirus gastroenteritis) than in control patients.[7] These reactions would not be expected after an injectable inactivated vaccine.

A key feature of these common, known, and expected adverse reactions is that they are clinically mild and resolve quickly on their own (e.g., hours to days). These reactions tend not to elicit major concern from patients, healthcare providers, or public health and regulatory officials.

Severe Adverse Reactions

Severe adverse reactions to vaccination are rare. Anaphylaxis is a severe, life-threatening allergic reaction that can occur after vaccination with any type of vaccine;[8] a list of vaccine components to which allergies might exist is available from the Centers for Disease Control and Prevention (CDC).[9] Anaphylaxis occurs with a frequency of about one to two cases per million doses administered of currently licensed vaccines,[10] with onset of symptoms usually immediately or shortly after vaccination. Effective treatments are available (e.g., intramuscular injection of epinephrine).

Guillain-Barré syndrome (GBS) is an acute demyelinating disease of peripheral nerves, believed to be of autoimmune etiology, associated with weakness and paralysis.[11] GBS has been a vaccine AEFI of concern since cases were observed in association with the 1976 "swine flu" vaccine.[12] An increased risk of GBS after the 2009 pH1N1 inactivated monovalent vaccines was observed in US studies[13-16] and in an international meta-analysis.[17] Data on an association between GBS and inactivated seasonal influenza vaccines have been variable and inconsistent across influenza seasons[8]; the risk of GBS appears to be small, on the order of one to two additional cases per million doses of vaccine administered. Notably, wild-type influenza virus disease is itself a risk factor for GBS and is more often associated with GBS than vaccination.[18]

Some rare adverse reactions to vaccination result from infection with a live attenuated vaccine strain virus. Live attenuated viruses in vaccines should replicate without causing severe illness, but in some persons (e.g., persons with underlying medical conditions) the vaccine strain virus can cause illness. The risk of disseminated vaccine strain varicella-zoster virus (VZV) disease can be greater in persons with immunocompromising conditions or who are severely immunosuppressed. Rarely, serious and sometimes fatal vaccine strain measles virus disease occurs among severely immunocompromised persons after combined measles, mumps, and rubella (MMR) vaccination.[5] According to vaccine recommendations for the United States, persons anticipating travel to areas where yellow fever (YF) is endemic should receive YF vaccine. Two rare, but severe and potentially fatal, adverse reactions can result from the YF vaccine strain virus. Yellow fever vaccine–associated viscerotropic disease (YEL-AVD) has signs and symptoms similar to wild-type YF disease (including multiorgan failure), occurs at a rate of 0.3 cases per 100,000 doses administered, and has a case fatality rate of about 46%. Yellow fever vaccine–associated neurologic disease, which includes multiple neurologic syndromes, occurs at a rate of 0.8 cases per 100,000 doses but is rarely fatal.[19]

Adverse Reactions Related to Vaccine Administration

Another category of adverse reactions are related to the act of injection rather than any inherent property of the vaccine or vaccine components. Vasovagal syncope (fainting) can occur after any medical procedure involving the use of needles, including a vaccine injection.[8] Post-vaccination vasovagal syncope is not uncommon, particularly among adolescents and young adults; some studies report an observed rate of about 1 per 1000 persons vaccinated (although the frequency might vary with age and other factors).[20] Shoulder injury related to vaccine administration (SIRVA) occurs after vaccine administration into or around the underlying structures of the shoulder joint (instead of the thick portion of the deltoid muscle). The resulting inflammatory reaction, such as deltoid bursitis or tendonitis/tendinopathy, damages these underlying structures.[8,21] Claims of SIRVA to the Vaccine Injury Compensation Program (VICP) have increased in recent years, and investigation into the epidemiology of these claims is underway.[22] Anxiety-related reactions can come to the attention of healthcare personnel and public health officials when they occur in clusters that affect multiple persons, often adolescents, who have contact with each other (e.g., where they are able to see or speak to each other) during situations where vaccinations are given to many persons in a common setting (e.g., school vaccination clinics).[1,23]

CLINICAL CONSIDERATIONS FOR VACCINE SAFETY

Healthcare providers should familiarize themselves with the prevention and management of adverse reactions. Providers should also understand the general approach to assessing if an AEFI was an adverse reaction (i.e., caused by a vaccine), including consideration of concurrent but potentially unrelated conditions, and how to report AEFIs suspected of being adverse reactions to public health and regulatory authorities.

Communicating With Patients About Vaccine Safety

Healthcare providers should be prepared to discuss with patients both the benefits and risks of vaccines. Federal law in the United States requires that, before administering any dose of vaccines specified by that law, providers must provide the vaccine information statement (VIS) for those vaccine(s) to the patient (or their guardian).[24] The VIS is a short document produced by the CDC that summarizes the most important information for each vaccine, including potential risks.[25] Providers should also give patients anticipatory guidance about the expected common adverse reactions of a particular vaccine, the duration and severity of those reactions, and treatments that can be self-administered if those reactions occur (e.g., cold compresses for uncomplicated injection-site reactions).

Deciding to Vaccinate

Patients might have a contraindication or a precaution to receiving a vaccine. As mentioned previously, a contraindication is a condition that increases the likelihood of a serious adverse reaction to a particular vaccine; a precaution is a condition that could increase the likelihood or severity of an adverse reaction or reduce the vaccine's ability to produce immunity. A contraindication common to most vaccines is a history of anaphylactic reaction to a previous dose of the same vaccine or any component of that vaccine. Some vaccines contain components to which patients might already know they are allergic because the components are encountered outside of vaccines. For example, MMR, varicella, and Japanese encephalitis vaccines contain gelatin, to which some people might be allergic. Some vaccines can contain small amounts of antibiotic used in the manufacturing process, such as the aminoglycoside antibiotic neomycin. Persons with a history of anaphylactic reaction to either gelatin-containing products or aminoglycoside antibiotics should be evaluated by an allergist before receiving vaccines containing these components, and the administration of such vaccines should be performed in facilities that can manage anaphylaxis if it should occur. Some vaccines come in vials or syringes containing natural rubber latex; use of these items should be avoided in persons with a history of an anaphylactic reaction to latex. Other vaccine components might rarely or only theoretically cause adverse reactions,[26] including yeast antigens (yeast are used in production of Hepatitis B and human papillomavirus [HPV] vaccines) and aldehydes (such as formaldehyde and glutaraldehyde) used to inactivate toxins or to act as a preservative.

Other contraindications include the use of live virus vaccines in persons with certain types of immunodeficiency or who are severely immunocompromised or severely immunosuppressed or are pregnant.[2] These special populations are discussed later in this chapter.

One precaution common to all vaccines is when the patient has a moderate or severe acute illness before vaccine administration. The objective here is to avoid a potential vaccine adverse reaction in a patient who is already ill, thereby avoiding confusion about whether symptoms were caused by the vaccine or the current illness. However, vaccinations are usually recommended with only mild illnesses.

Some contraindications and precautions are permanent conditions, whereas temporary conditions allow deferral of vaccination until the condition is no longer present.[1] A vaccine's prescribing information also describes specific populations who might have contraindications or precautions for the vaccine and interactions with other vaccines or drugs that should be reviewed and considered before deciding to vaccinate a patient. A questionnaire that screens for contraindications to vaccines can be a useful clinical tool to identify patients who should not receive a particular vaccine on a given day.[27]

Preventing Adverse Reactions Related to Vaccine Administration

Once the decision to vaccinate has been made, proper techniques and procedures should be used to prevent adverse reactions related to vaccine administration. Although usually associated with injectable vaccines, postvaccination syncope can also occur with intranasal vaccines. Which patient will experience syncope cannot be reliably predicted, and no proven strategies to prevent syncope exist. The Advisory Committee on Immunization Practices (ACIP) recommends that adolescents and adults be seated or lying down during vaccination and that patients be observed for 15 minutes after vaccination while remaining seated or lying down to decrease the risk of injury from syncope.[2] To prevent SIRVA or other injuries related to injection of a vaccine, proper injection technique should be used. The first step is confirming the proper route and site of administration, which is specific to each vaccine. The appropriate needle size should be selected based on factors such as the patient's age and body size. Instructions for proper injection technique are available from CDC.[28] Local measures (e.g., application of topical anesthetics) might help reduce pain of injected vaccines.[29]

When Prevention Strategies Do Not Exist

Some adverse reactions currently lack proven prevention strategies, such as injection-site reactions, myalgia, and fever. These symptoms can be treated symptomatically after they occur, if needed. Prophylactic measures such as analgesics or antipyretics are generally not recommended because not all patients will experience these symptoms (nor can such patients be reliably predicted). These drugs can suppress the immune response to the vaccine, and these drugs can have side effects themselves.[30,31]

Managing Severe Adverse Reactions

Healthcare providers should be prepared to recognize and manage rare but severe adverse reactions. Foremost are immediate-type hypersensitivity reactions, including anaphylaxis. In any setting where vaccines are administered, there should be an emergency plan in place to administer epinephrine and maintain airway patency. ACIP recommends that all vaccine providers be certified in cardiopulmonary resuscitation.[2]

Assessing Causality of an AEFI in an Individual Patient

When a patient experiences a clinically significant AEFI the provider should consider if the event was actually caused by the vaccine. Making this determination can be straightforward for certain types of AEFIs that are known to be caused by vaccines when they occur in the expected time frame. Examples include injection-site reactions, syncope, and anaphylaxis when no other inciting exposures can be identified. For other types of AEFIs, determining whether the vaccine caused the event can be more difficult because the event may have been caused by other factors that might only be identified after careful investigation (e.g., infection with *Campylobacter* spp. in a patient with GBS).[32]

The CDC's Clinical Immunization Safety Assessment (CISA) project developed an algorithm to assess causality of an AEFI in an individual patient,[33] and the World Health Organization developed an algorithm for use in lower resource settings. These algorithms are intended to guide the collection and interpretation of the necessary clinical data in a logical order and are useful for public health, research, and clinical purposes. These algorithms classify an AEFI's relationship to a vaccine into one of three possible categories based on the available evidence: (1) consistent with a causal relationship, (2) inconsistent with a causal relationship, or (3) indeterminate. Although clinicians are not expected to perform this formal assessment for every AEFI they encounter, they should understand the general concepts to better evaluate AEFIs in their patients and manage the outcomes.

The following are key steps in assessing causality:
- Confirm that the AEFI is diagnosed correctly.
- Determine if other possible causes for the event exist and if an alternative cause was present.

- Consider the onset of the AEFI in relation to the vaccination. The biological mechanism for a particular AEFI will dictate a plausible range of time during which that event can occur after vaccination. For example, anaphylaxis typically occurs within minutes to hours after vaccination, whereas a viral infection usually incubates days or weeks before symptoms develop. Events occurring before or after the plausible range of time for a particular event are more likely due to other causes.
- Locate evidence from clinical trials or epidemiologic studies to support or refute the existence of a causal association between the AEFI and the vaccine. However, population-level evidence that a vaccine can cause a particular event does not necessarily mean the vaccine caused the event in a specific patient.
- If indicated, conduct laboratory testing. In some situations, specific laboratory testing can confirm if vaccine caused the event (e.g., identification of a vaccine strain virus in an infected tissue sample). This type of testing may need to be performed by a state or federal public health laboratory or other reference laboratory. Guidelines for specimen collection and laboratory testing are available from CDC.[34]

In general, conclusive evidence of a causal relationship between a vaccine and a specific AEFI requires population-level evidence (e.g., randomized controlled trials, controlled epidemiologic studies). Case reports or case series rarely provide sufficient evidence of causality, except in specific circumstances, such as isolation of a vaccine strain virus from infected tissue or the recurrence of a condition with repeated exposure to the vaccine.[2] CDC's CISA project (described later in this chapter) is available for consultation for particularly challenging cases in the United States.[35]

Considerations for Giving Additional Doses After a Prior AEFI

Once a vaccine is suspected of causing an AEFI, the healthcare provider must consider whether or not to administer additional doses of the same (or other) vaccines in the future. Such consideration is of particular importance for allergic reactions. Identifying the specific vaccine component to which the patient is allergic might be warranted because some ingredients are used in multiple types of vaccines. Each vaccine's prescribing information lists its ingredients, and CDC maintains a summarized list of these ingredients.[36] In patients at high risk for a vaccine-preventable disease, vaccination with additional doses might be desirable despite a prior allergic reaction to the vaccine. These patients should be referred to an allergist, and vaccine administration might be preferred in the setting of the allergy clinic or facility with the availability of emergency equipment. An algorithm is available to guide the evaluation of patients with suspected allergic/hypersensitivity reactions to vaccines, and revaccination using special precautions might be possible for some patients.[37]

Reporting AEFIs

Clinically significant AEFIs suspected to be caused by a vaccine should be reported to the Vaccine Adverse Event Reporting System (VAERS) in the United States (or to a similar public health or regulatory monitoring system in other countries), to help contribute to a wider understanding of vaccine AEFIs. Healthcare providers are encouraged to report to VAERS on behalf of patients, though patients may submit a report themselves. VAERS is discussed in greater detail in the section titled "Vaccine safety assessment and monitoring."

SPECIAL POPULATIONS

When making vaccination decisions about certain persons or populations, such as pregnant women or immunocompromised patients, additional vaccine safety considerations exist.

Pregnant Women

Some vaccines are recommended for pregnant women, whereas pregnancy is a contraindication or precaution for other vaccines. General recommendations for vaccinating pregnant women are to avoid vaccination with live attenuated virus vaccines and to vaccinate with inactivated vaccines when indicated[28]

The only two vaccines currently recommended for pregnant women in the United States are inactivated influenza vaccine and combined tetanus, diphtheria, and acellular pertussis (Tdap) vaccines. Pregnant women are at risk for influenza and severe complications from influenza. Maternal antibodies induced by Tdap can prevent pertussis in the newborn. Postlicensure vaccine safety studies of maternal and fetal outcomes for both of these vaccines have been reassuring.[38–40]

The primary concern with the use of live virus vaccines in pregnant women is potential infection of the fetus or infant and subsequent negative outcomes because the wild-type strain of some vaccine-preventable viruses (e.g., rubella) is transmissible from the gestating mother to the unborn child. The only live virus vaccines with known adverse effects on unborn or nursing children are smallpox (i.e., vaccinia virus) and YF vaccines.[28] In utero infection with

vaccinia virus can lead to high rates of fetal loss; in utero infection with vaccine strain YF virus has also been documented, with a slightly increased risk of (mostly minor) skin malformations.[41,42] Despite the risk of fetal infection with YF vaccine virus, under specific conditions, a pregnant mother might still be given YF vaccine if exposure to YF virus is unavoidable.[19] Many other attenuated live virus vaccines, when inadvertently administered to gestating mothers, have had no observable adverse effects on the fetus. For example, wild-type rubella virus causes devastating congenital infection, but the attenuated strain in the MMR vaccine has not shown to have adverse effects on the fetus when inadvertently administered to the gestating mother.[43] Reviews of reported AEFIs among pregnant women in the United States after vaccination with LAIV vaccine and of data from a registry for VZV-containing vaccines during pregnancy also revealed no unexpected or concerning patterns in maternal or fetal outcomes.[39,44,45]

Inactivated vaccines (including toxoids such as diphtheria and tetanus toxoids) and subunit vaccines (such as inactivated influenza or hepatitis B vaccines) contain no viable bacteria or virus; the recommendations for their use during pregnancy depend on the vaccine and the risk for acquiring the natural infection.

The following table is a summation of current vaccine recommendations for pregnant women. A comprehensive discussion of recommendations for each vaccine in Table 1.1 is beyond the scope of this chapter; updated ACIP recommendations should be consulted for further details.

Breastfeeding Women

Smallpox vaccine (vaccinia) and YF vaccine are the only live virus vaccines that should be avoided while breastfeeding. Inactivated vaccines cannot transmit disease through breast milk; however, many inactivated vaccines do not have sufficient safety data and are therefore not recommended while a woman is breastfeeding. Specific guidance is available from CDC.[46]

Immunosuppressed and Immunocompromised Persons

Immunosuppressed persons have functional immune systems suppressed by medications, such as alkylating agents like methotrexate, or certain regimens of prednisone (e.g., up to 20 mg/day for $\geq$14 days[28]). Topical or inhaled steroids are not considered immunosuppressive. Immunocompromised persons lack a functional immune system (e.g., patients with cancer or chronic inflammatory conditions).[47,48] For purposes of this chapter, both groups will be referred to as "immunosuppressed."

TABLE 1.1
Vaccines and Guidance Regarding Pregnant Women

Routine or Travel	Vaccine	General Recommendation for Use in Pregnant Women
Routine	Hepatitis A	Base decision on risk versus benefit
	Hepatitis B	Recommended in some circumstances
	Human papillomavirus (HPV)	Not recommended
	Influenza, inactivated	Recommended
	Influenza, live attenuated	Contraindicated
	Combined measles, mumps, rubella (MMR)	Contraindicated
	Meningococcal (ACWY)	May be used if otherwise indicated
	Meningococcal (B)	Base decision on risk versus benefit
	13-Valent pneumococcal conjugate	No recommendation
	23-Valent pneumococcal polysaccharide	Inadequate data for specific recommendation
	Inactivated polio	May be used if needed
	Combined tetanus and diphtheria toxoid (Td)	Should be used if otherwise indicated (Tdap preferred)
	Combined tetanus and diphtheria toxoid and acellular pertussis (Tdap)	Recommended
	Varicella	Contraindicated
	Zoster, live attenuated	Contraindicated
	Zoster, inactivated	Inadequate data for specific recommendation[77]
Travel and other	Anthrax	Low risk of exposure: not recommended. High risk of exposure: may be used
	Tuberculosis (BCG)	Contraindicated
	Japanese encephalitis	Inadequate data for specific recommendation
	Rabies	May be used if otherwise indicated
	Typhoid	Inadequate data. Give Vi polysaccharide (an inactivated vaccine) if needed
	Smallpox	Preexposure: contraindicated Postexposure: recommended
	Yellow fever	May be used if benefit outweighs risk

Modified from "Guidelines for Vaccinating Pregnant Women" (https://www.cdc.gov/vaccines/pregnancy/hcp/guidelines.html) (last updated August 2016).

Immunosuppressed persons may be given inactivated vaccines. In some cases, the immunosuppressing condition itself is an indication for vaccination.[49] For example, patients with asplenia (either functional or anatomic [e.g., postsurgical]) should receive inactivated vaccines for meningococcus (e.g., meningococcal conjugate vaccine), pneumococcus (e.g., pneumococcal conjugate or polysaccharide vaccine), and *Haemophilus influenza* type b (Hib conjugate vaccines).[50,51] However, immunosuppressed persons can exhibit a reduced antibody response. Children with hypogammaglobulinemia have reduced antibody responses to diphtheria and tetanus toxoids, hepatitis B, and conjugate Hib vaccines and often are treated with replacement immunoglobulins.

Live virus vaccines are contraindicated for severely immunosuppressed persons because serious or fatal disseminated infections can occur. What specific criteria define "severely" immunosuppressed are not firmly established. One convention is CD4 T-cell count, where the term "immunocompromised" is specifically used; a count <500 cells/mm^3 is considered "immunocompromised" and <200 cells/mm^3 is considered "severely immunocompromised."[28,52] This convention is primarily used in the context of human immunodeficiency virus (HIV) infection and might have less utility among HIV-negative persons. The presence of invasive opportunistic infections in patients with a compatible medical history (e.g., disseminated fungal infections in organ transplant patients) can indicate a substantially immunosuppressed status.[53]

To mitigate the risk of disseminated infection, recipients of hematopoietic cell transplant (both autologous and allopathic) should wait 24 months before vaccinating with live virus vaccines (assuming immune competency has returned). More detailed guidance is available from CDC and the Infectious Diseases Society of America.[28,48]

HIV-Positive Persons

Generally, recommendations for HIV-positive persons are similar to recommendations for immunosuppressed persons.[54] HIV-positive persons may receive inactivated vaccines when indicated but can develop less robust antibody response after inactivated vaccines.[55–58] Provided the HIV-positive recipient is not severely immunocompromised, live virus vaccines may be safely administered. Given the risks posed by live virus vaccines (e.g., disseminated infection[59]), recommendations generally advise demonstrating an absence of protective antibody to measles virus, VZV, etc. before administering a live virus vaccine.[60]

Numerous analyses and reports found no increases in AEFIs after vaccination with measles virus, VZV, and YF vaccines among HIV-positive persons who were not severely immunocompromised.[61–65] Patients taking maraviroc (an antiretroviral drug administered to some HIV-positive persons) have a theoretical risk of YEL-AVD after receiving YF vaccine, but no cases have been reported as of this writing.[66,67] Because of insufficient safety data, the combined MMR and varicella vaccine (MMRV) remains contraindicated in HIV-positive persons.[60,68]

Despite some evidence about accelerating HIV progression and increases in viral load after vaccination among HIV-positive persons,[69,70] any such changes appear transient and without lasting impact.[71–73]

Persons With Autoimmune Conditions

Persons with autoimmune conditions such as rheumatoid arthritis and systemic lupus erythematosus are at increased risk for vaccine-preventable diseases[74,75] and should be vaccinated; general recommendations are to vaccinate with inactivated vaccines when indicated and defer live virus vaccines until immune function is sufficient. The American College of Rheumatology currently recommends vaccinating with live virus HZ vaccine at age ≥50 years before starting immunosuppressive therapy[76]; the recent approval of an inactivated HZ vaccine might lead to modification of this recommendation.[77]

Inactivated vaccines may be safely administered while a patient receives immunosuppressive therapy, but vaccine response can be blunted.[76] Vaccinating before treatment with B-cell (and presumably, T-cell) depleting medications such as rituximab[78] or vaccinating 6–12 months after discontinuing such medications[76] has been suggested.

Live virus vaccines may be administered concurrently with specific drugs such as methotrexate and/or low doses of prednisone; data on these drugs (and at what doses) are available.[28,76] Other medications should be discontinued before administering live virus vaccines, and how long to wait depends upon the specific medication(s).[28,76,79] For antitumor necrosis factor drugs and drugs blocking T-cell activation (e.g., abatacept) and IL-6 receptors (e.g., tocilizumab), some experts recommend ≥3 months before live virus vaccination. For drugs that selectively deplete B-cell (e.g., rituximab) and T-cell (e.g., alemtuzumab) populations, some experts suggest a wait of several months (e.g., 12 months for rituximab).[76]

Healthcare Workers and Household Contacts of Immunosuppressed Persons and Pregnant Women

Vaccination of healthy contacts reduces the chances of exposing immunosuppressed persons and pregnant women to vaccine-preventable disease and is highly recommended for any such contacts.[28] The only reports of transmission of vaccine strain live virus from recipients to immunosuppressed persons and pregnant women involve smallpox vaccine (vaccinia). Current recommendations are that recently vaccinated health-care workers require no restrictions on work activities.[80] However, healthcare workers in contact with immuno-compromised persons requiring isolation (e.g., bone marrow transplant) should not receive LAIV.[28]

VACCINE SAFETY ASSESSMENT AND MONITORING

Vaccine safety is evaluated throughout the research and development process before licensure; assessment also continues after a vaccine is licensed and recommended for use. This section will discuss the regulations and systems in place to assess vaccine safety from the early stages of vaccine development through widespread use (i.e., the postmarketing or postlicensure period).

Prelicensure Safety Assessment

Vaccines are regulated in the United States by the FDA, which also regulates drugs, devices, and other medical products. Similar functions are performed in other countries by their own national regulatory authorities. The decision to proceed with a first-in-human clinical trial of an experimental candidate vaccine depends on information gathered in preclinical studies, including animal testing. Clinical trials in humans proceed through three phases to gather the information required to apply for FDA licensure. In phase 1 clinical trials, the candidate vaccine is administered to a small number of typically healthy volunteers to gather basic safety information and to determine an optimal dose. In phase 2 trials, a few hundred persons generally receive the vaccine, to further assess immunogenicity and safety. In phase 3 trials, the primary goal is to assess the efficacy of the vaccine candidate for the indications sought in licensure. In addition, more vaccine safety data are gathered. The number of persons included in a phase 3 clinical trial depends on the endpoint under consideration and can range from several hundred to tens of thousands of persons. In a phase 3 trial in which a particular safety concern requires study, the number of participants needed will be determined based on the magnitude of the potential risk, with large numbers of participants required to detect small risks.

Upon successful completion of phase 3 clinical trials, the manufacturer must submit a Biologics License Application to the FDA. The FDA reviews the laboratory and clinical trial results to determine whether the vaccine is safe and efficacious for its intended use. The FDA also reviews the manufacturing process to ensure compliance with standards (i.e., current good manufacturing practices) and will continue to inspect manufacturing facilities after a vaccine is licensed. Vaccines are produced in lots, which are tested for consistency, purity, and potency before release. Lots are assigned a number that is printed on the vaccine packaging. Regulatory activities related to the manufacturing process are intended to prevent defects in vaccine quality. An historic event contributing to the development of some of these activities was the 1955 "Cutter incident," in which failure to fully inactivate live poliovirus during the production of inactivated polio vaccine led to paralysis of dozens of persons and the deaths of several others from poliovirus infection.[81] An example of FDA's authority to regulate vaccine production was the decision in 2004 to withhold nearly 50 million doses of influenza vaccine manufactured by the Chiron Corporation after inspections found evidence of bacterial contamination during the packaging process.[82]

Postlicensure Safety Assessment

Clinical safety assessments continue after a vaccine is licensed. Postlicensure vaccine safety activities build on and complement the safety information gained from prelicensure studies. Such assessments can identify and quantify rare AEFIs after larger numbers of people have received the vaccine, activities not typically possible with prelicensure clinical trials due to the relatively smaller number of people vaccinated. Postlicensure assessments can collect safety information from special populations who might have been excluded from prelicensure clinical trials, such as pregnant women or persons with chronic diseases. Postlicensure assessments can also monitor for changes in the occurrence of known adverse reactions.

Postlicensure safety assessments may be conducted by public health agencies, regulatory agencies, manufacturers, or academic researchers to investigate a particular question or concern. Postlicensure safety assessments are conducted by a variety of methods, depending on the question to be answered. Multiple methods are often used to complement each other.

Vaccine safety surveillance systems focus on identifying cases of AEFIs, using either a passive or active approach. Passive surveillance systems rely on spontaneous reports of AEFIs. Active surveillance systems use additional measures to search for and identify AEFIs.

Postlicensure studies might focus on testing a hypothesis or evaluating vaccine safety in a special population. These studies investigate a specific question. Observational epidemiologic studies investigate potential associations between a vaccine and one or more specific AEFIs, particularly rare events for which clinical trials would not be feasible or would not assess outcomes in a clinical practice environment (in contrast to the controlled conditions of a clinical trial). To conduct specific observational studies involving vaccines and maternal and child health, pregnancy exposure registries collect data on maternal and child outcomes for women who were vaccinated during pregnancy, intentionally or inadvertently (depending on the recommendations for a particular vaccine). The nonprofit Organization of Teratology Information Specialists is one group that specifically conducts pregnancy studies.[83] Some manufacturers operate pregnancy registries for their vaccines.

Postlicensure Safety Assessment Systems in the United States

In the United States, CDC and FDA operate several complementary systems to monitor and evaluate postlicensure vaccine safety.

The vaccine adverse event reporting system

VAERS is a national passive surveillance system operated jointly by the CDC and FDA.[84] VAERS is a specific system for vaccines, separate from other safety reporting systems such as FDA's MedWatch program (which collects reports for other types of regulated products such as drugs and medical devices). VAERS uses a standard form to collect individual case safety reports of AEFIs. VAERS accepts reports from anyone, including healthcare professionals, patients, parents, caregivers, and manufacturers. VAERS encourages the reporting of any clinically significant or unexpected AEFI occurring after the administration of any vaccine licensed in the United States, even if the person reporting is unsure of whether the vaccine caused the AEFI. Particular strengths of VAERS include its national scope and its ability to rapidly detect potential vaccine safety concerns, such as new, unusual, or rare AEFIs. VAERS does have limitations inherent to a passive reporting system, which include being subject to reporting bias, such as underreporting of mild or common AEFIs and increased reporting of events subject to heightened awareness. Reports may be incomplete or lacking in detail. VAERS does not include a comparison group (i.e., unvaccinated "controls") and generally cannot be used to determine if an AEFI was caused by the vaccine or was coincidental. Hypotheses generated from VAERS often require further investigation using other systems. More information on VAERS, including how to report AEFIs to VAERS, is available from CDC.[85]

The vaccine safety datalink (VSD)

The VSD was established in 1990 as a system to collaborate between the CDC and several integrated healthcare organizations.[86] The VSD has a population of over 9 million members enrolled in the healthcare organizations that is similar to the US population in respect to demographic characteristics. The VSD uses administrative databases to link patients' vaccination and other healthcare records to perform population-based active surveillance and epidemiologic research studies. The VSD can perform controlled observational studies to identify an association between a vaccine and specific AEFI and quantify the risk, if any. The VSD performs active, near–real-time sequential surveillance known as Rapid Cycle Analysis (RCA). RCA was introduced in 2005 as an innovative new surveillance method to monitor new vaccines when they are first introduced and for influenza vaccines each year.[87] The VSD has conducted numerous vaccine safety studies since 1990.[10]

CISA project

CDC also manages the CISA Project, a collaboration between CDC and seven medical research centers. CISA's activities fall into three main areas: (1) conducting clinical research, often focused on identifying risk factors for AEFIs, on strategies to prevent AEFIs, or on special populations that were not included in prelicensure clinical trials of vaccines; (2) providing expert evaluation of broader vaccine safety issues; and (3) providing a clinical case evaluation service for US healthcare providers when they have a specific vaccine safety concern about one of their patients residing in the United States.[35]

Postlicensure rapid immunization safety monitoring program

In 2009 the FDA established the postlicensure rapid immunization safety monitoring (PRISM) program for vaccines as part of FDA's broader Sentinel Initiative to create a surveillance system for postlicensure safety monitoring of various types of medical products.[88] PRISM uses medical billing claims data provided by several large health insurance companies to monitor the safety of vaccines and assess safety questions about specific vaccine products.

International Cooperation

International efforts also exist to share knowledge and information from different countries. When data on the same vaccine are available from multiple countries, pooling data or meta-analysis can be used to obtain more precise risk estimates, particularly for rare AEFIs. The Uppsala Monitoring Center in Uppsala, Sweden, which is the World Health Organization collaborating center for drug and vaccine safety monitoring, compiles AEFI case reports from multiple countries, including VAERS data from the United States.[89] The Brighton

Collaboration is a global research network, headquartered in Basel, Switzerland, that develops standardized research methods, such as AEFI case definitions for surveillance and research use, and has coordinated international studies.[90] The International Council for Harmonisation (ICH) in Geneva, Switzerland, is an international association that works to harmonize guidelines for global pharmaceutical development and regulation.[91] ICH created the Medical Dictionary for Regulatory Activities (MedDRA), a standardized terminology used to facilitate international sharing of regulatory information for medical products, including vaccines. The Council for International Organizations of Medical Sciences (CIOMS) is another international organization in Geneva, Switzerland, working to advance public health and has developed vaccine safety research and communication guidelines.[92]

Examples of Postlicensure Safety Assessments and Historical Impacts

The findings from postlicensure safety evaluations can reinforce existing practices or lead to changes in the way a vaccine is used, sometimes significantly impacting a vaccination program. In 1976 the United States implemented a national vaccination campaign in response to the novel A/New Jersey/76 (Hsw1N1) influenza virus that was thought to have pandemic potential and was referred to colloquially as "swine flu."[93] The vaccine for this virus was administered to over 40 million people before its use was suspended because cases of GBS, a demyelinating disorder, were reported among vaccinated persons. Subsequent reviews of the evidence concluded that the vaccine caused some cases of GBS.[94]

Another significant historical example of postlicensure safety monitoring ending the use of a vaccine in the United States involved the RotaShield vaccine. RotaShield was the first rotavirus vaccine licensed in the United States (1998) and was indicated for the prevention of rotavirus gastroenteritis in infants. Shortly after RotaShield's recommendation for use by the ACIP, VAERS received an unusually high number of reports of intussusception (a telescoping of the intestine within itself that can cause bowel obstruction) in children receiving RotaShield. These reports led to two epidemiologic studies that estimated the risk of intussusception at 10–20 additional cases per 100,000 infants vaccinated with RotaShield. The altered benefit–risk balance led ACIP to suspend its recommendation; the manufacturer voluntarily recalled Rotashield from the market shortly before ACIP withdrew its recommendation in November 1999.[95] Two newer rotavirus vaccines were licensed in 2006 and 2008. Each vaccine underwent

large prelicensure clinical trials that enrolled over 60,000 infants each and were powered to detect an intussusception risk of similar magnitude as with RotaShield.[96,97] Subsequent postlicensure epidemiologic studies estimated a risk of 1–5 additional cases of intussusception per 100,000 persons vaccinated. Policy makers considered this estimate an acceptable amount of risk when weighed against the vaccines' benefit of reducing the incidence of rotavirus gastroenteritis in infants.[7]

MONITORING VACCINE SAFETY DURING PUBLIC HEALTH RESPONSES

Routine postlicensure vaccine safety monitoring involves a continuous, regular, and standardized process under normal, nonurgent, and nonemergency situations. Monitoring vaccine safety during a public health response requires modification of normal surveillance procedures and, in some cases, rapid adjustment to maximize the capabilities of public health surveillance systems. Among the most important differences between routine monitoring and monitoring during a public health response are the intensity of effort, the pace of activities, and (depending on the vaccine) the breadth of outcomes on which surveillance focuses. Desirable attributes of a postlicensure vaccine safety monitoring system during a public health response include the following:

1. Surge capacity: the capability to rapidly scale up operations to handle increased workload. Surge capacity includes effectively and efficiently incorporating additional workforce to perform manual (human) tasks and incorporating and reconfiguring additional information technology (IT) infrastructure to accommodate increased volumes of data.

2. Speed: Rapidly processing, formatting, and analyzing large volumes of data through manual and automated procedures and IT. Speed also involves having in place standing protocols to facilitate operations during a public health response or emergency and continuously updated hardware and software for maximum processing speed.

3. Flexibility: the ability to rapidly adapt existing procedures, protocols, and systems to meet the specific needs of the public health response. Flexibility includes adapting other systems and databases not normally used for vaccine safety monitoring to meet additional requirements for specific types of responses.

4. Validated analytic methods: having tested and validated statistical methods available to rapidly

analyze large volumes of data, to detect potential safety signals (i.e., reports of AEFIs) in a timely manner.

5. Population coverage: maintaining surveillance over a sufficient portion of the population who have been or will be vaccinated to ensure the statistical power to detect rare AEFIs. The population under surveillance should also be diverse enough to allow generalizations to the overall population, including specified subgroups.

2009 H1N1 Influenza Pandemic

The large-scale US pandemic 2009 influenza A (H1N1) monovalent vaccination (pH1N1) program represents an example of vaccine safety monitoring during a national public health emergency. Although pH1N1 vaccines used in the United States were FDA-licensed products, the vaccine contained a novel influenza A antigen. Heightened public awareness around vaccine safety necessitated that CDC and FDA conduct timely and comprehensive safety surveillance to detect and respond to possible vaccine safety problems that might require programmatic or regulatory action.

To meet this challenge, CDC and FDA conducted enhanced passive surveillance in VAERS (including rapid report processing, follow-up of serious reports and reports of prespecified conditions of interest, and review of accompanying medical records when available) and data mining.[98] CDC also conducted active surveillance in the VSD using RCA, which was applied to the prospective monitoring of influenza vaccine for the first time in 2009 as part of the pH1N1 vaccination program.[99] In addition, FDA conducted active surveillance of pH1N1 vaccine safety in the Centers for Medicare & Medicaid Services database[100] and in its PRISM project.[101] Owing to heightened concern about GBS from experience during the 1976 "swine flu" vaccination program, CDC adapted its Emerging Infections Program's public health surveillance and research network to conduct additional surveillance for GBS after pH1N1 vaccination.[15] By early December 2009 the CDC's Morbidity and Mortality Weekly Report (MMWR) published pH1N1 vaccine safety data from VAERS and VSD, providing reassurance about the safety of pH1N1 vaccine.[102] Later, some monitoring systems detected a small, increased risk of GBS after inactivated pH1N1 vaccination; the magnitude of this risk was similar to the risk observed in some previous influenza seasons after inactivated seasonal influenza vaccine.[16]

Other parts of the US government participated in pH1N1 safety monitoring, including the Department of Defense, the Department of Veterans Affairs, and the Indian Health Service, using a variety of systems and analytic methods. In addition, the National Vaccine Program Office (NVPO) at the Department of Health and Human Services (HHS) created the National Vaccine Advisory Committee (NVAC) H1N1 Vaccine Safety Risk Assessment Working Group, comprising external experts tasked to regularly review pH1N1 vaccine safety data during the vaccination program, and to report their findings to the NVAC.[103] An estimated 80.8 million persons received pH1N1 vaccine.[104] The national effort to monitor pH1N1 vaccine safety during the 2009 H1N1 influenza pandemic demonstrated the capabilities of the US vaccine safety monitoring infrastructure to respond during a public health emergency and large-scale public vaccination program.

Smallpox Vaccination Program

The US civilian smallpox vaccination program implemented in 2003 is an example of a limited public health response targeting a specific population for vaccination, initiated to address concerns about the use of variola (smallpox) virus as a biological weapon of terrorism. In contrast to the large-scale, broad-based pH1N1 vaccination program during the 2009 H1N1 influenza pandemic (which involved participation of many US government, public health, and private sector entities), the smallpox vaccination program was narrower in scope, specifically targeting selected occupational groups. Persons recommended to receive smallpox vaccination included selected persons in direct contact with potential smallpox patients and persons administering preevent vaccinations. Recommendations for previously designated laboratory workers remained unchanged.[105] The US military implemented a separate smallpox vaccination program for its personnel.[106]

Smallpox vaccine is an active, replicating viral vaccine administered using a multiple puncture technique with a bifurcated needle. Because of rare, known, well-characterized, serious (and sometimes life-threatening) adverse reactions associated with this vaccine, intensive prevaccination screening for precautions and contraindications and postvaccination follow-up was conducted for vaccinated individuals. Features of the US civilian smallpox vaccination program included the following:

- programmatic oversight by the Joint Smallpox Vaccine Safety Working Group of the ACIP and the Armed Forces Epidemiological Board,[107]
- training and education for public health officials and medical personnel on smallpox vaccine safety and adverse reaction recognition, reporting, and treatment,

- a multifaceted approach to surveillance for AEs, including a comprehensive electronic database of all vaccinated persons,[108] telephone interviews, hospital-based surveillance,[109] a national pregnancy registry,[110] enhanced passive surveillance in VAERS (including a focus on prespecified conditions of interest, such as cardiac conditions),[111] and active surveillance.[112]

The safety profile of smallpox vaccine used in this program was similar to the profile for the same vaccine in the United States before 1977, with the exception of newly recognized cardiac AEFIs (i.e., myopericarditis and ischemic cardiac events).[111] These unexpected cardiac AEFIs were clinically investigated, revealing that myopericarditis was causally related to smallpox vaccination.[113] CDC subsequently issued revised screening and vaccination recommendations to minimize the risk of these types of reactions occurring in persons with preexisting cardiovascular risk factors.[114]

SAFETY OF ADJUVANTED VACCINES USED IN THE UNITED STATES

Adjuvants are compounds used to increase immune response to vaccines that might otherwise be poorly immunogenic; adjuvants are typically used in inactivated vaccines composed of highly purified proteins. Adjuvants not only increase antibody response but can also promote specific and nonspecific immune responses.[115-117]

Aluminum salts (potassium aluminum sulfate ["alum"], aluminum hydroxide, and aluminum phosphate) have been used as adjuvants for decades, in part because of their observed safety and low frequency of adverse reactions.[115] Exposure to aluminum from aluminum-adjuvanted vaccines is low; the highest aluminum content is in the combination diphtheria and tetanus toxoids, acellular pertussis, inactivated polio, and hepatitis B vaccine (Pediarix), with a maximal content of 0.85 mg.[116] Aluminum salts are highly insoluble and are thus expected to be absorbed slowly over time.[117] Consistent with this expectation, kinetic studies in rabbits show slow absorption of aluminum from intramuscular injections of aluminum salts.[118] Taking these observations into account, Mitkus et al. determined that absorption of aluminum from vaccines during the first year of life (arguably when persons will experience the heaviest exposure to aluminum from vaccines) is well below established safety limits for aluminum exposure.[119]

Aluminum salts were the only type of adjuvant used in a US licensed vaccine until 2009, when Cervarix was approved. Cervarix is a vaccine against HPV serotypes 16 and 18 containing AS04, which is composed of monophosphoryl lipid A (MPL) and alum. MPL in combination with aluminum salts not only promotes an antibody response but also a Th1 helper T-cell response as well.[120]

Two FDA-approved influenza vaccines now use another class of adjuvant known as oil-in-water emulsion adjuvants. The oil, squalene, is a lipid generated through a number of metabolic pathways that can be derived from sources such as shark liver and recombinant strains of yeast. The adjuvant effect of squalene appears mediated by recruitment of antigen-presenting cells and upregulation of cytokines and chemokines.[121] MF59 and AS03 are adjuvants proprietary to different manufacturers that contain squalene. AS03 also includes alpha-tocopherol, another immunostimulatory compound.[122] The only vaccine containing MF59 licensed in the United States is an adjuvanted influenza vaccine (FLUAD, a seasonal influenza vaccine indicated for use in persons aged 65 years and older). Before approval in the United States, FLUAD was already in use in 38 other countries,[123] with no greater frequency of serious AEFIs compared to nonadjuvanted inactivated influenza vaccines,[124-126] though injection-site reactions are more common. An influenza A (H5N1) prepandemic/pandemic influenza vaccine is available for emergency use and contains AS03 but is not a commercially available product for the general public in the United States.[127]

Vaccines containing two other new adjuvants were licensed by the FDA in 2017. Shingrix, an inactivated vaccine containing AS01$_B$ (MPL and a liposomal formulation of a saponin, QS21) has been recommended for use to prevent HZ.[77] MPL promotes a Th1 helper T-cell response via stimulation of antigen-presenting cells through the Toll-like receptor 4 pathway; the mechanism of QS21 is not yet clearly elucidated but might involve activation of the innate immune system.[128] Evidence suggests that MPL and QS21 work synergistically to effect a vaccine response.[128] Preclinical studies observed no increased occurrence of AEFIs with AS01$_B$ compared with placebo.[129] HEPLISAV-B, a vaccine containing immunostimulatory cytosine phosphoguanine (CpG) oligonucleotides (CpG 1018) is indicated to prevent hepatitis B.[130] CpG 1018 contains unmethylated CpG motifs and acts as a Toll-9 receptor agonist.[121] One clinical trial showed an increased risk of acute myocardial infarction and/or death after HEPLISAV-B compared with another vaccine. The FDA concluded that the evidence did not support a causal relationship between the vaccine and these events, but postmarketing safety studies are planned to examine this issue further.[131]

SELECTED VACCINE SAFETY CONCERNS

A number of common vaccine safety concerns are discussed on the CDC website: https://www.cdc.gov/vaccinesafety/concerns/index.html. In particular, some historical concerns are addressed at https://www.cdc.gov/vaccinesafety/concerns/concerns-history.html. In the following sections, a few of these concerns are briefly reviewed.

Autism Spectrum Disorders

Concerns about vaccines causing autism spectrum disorders (ASDs) in young children stem from a paper that was retracted for its unsound science, including violation of ethics protocols, conflicts of interest, and other irregularities.[132,133] Nonetheless, concerns about the possible association of vaccines with ASDs persist, with hypotheses related to the combined MMR vaccine, thimerosal in vaccines, and multiple vaccinations.[134] Multiple epidemiologic studies have failed to show any relationship between vaccines and ASDs.[135,136]

Thimerosal

In the United States, thimerosal, an ethylmercury-based preservative, has been used in multidose vials of inactivated vaccines for many years. Despite this long history of safe use with no evidence of untoward health outcomes,[137] thimerosal was removed from routinely recommended childhood vaccines used in the United States beginning in 1999 and completed by 2001 (with the exception of some formulations of influenza vaccine), as part of an effort to reduce children's overall exposure to mercury.[137] To date, no evidence links thimerosal to clinically important adverse health outcomes[8]; specifically, epidemiologic evidence convincingly argues against thimerosal causing ASDs.[138]

2009 Pandemic Influenza Vaccine with AS03 Adjuvant and Narcolepsy

The global emergence of a novel strain of influenza A in 2009 (pH1N1) led to a number of vaccines for this pandemic strain. In 2010 reports described an increased risk of narcolepsy with cataplexy in some European countries that used Pandemrix, most strikingly in Finland and Sweden.[139] Pandemrix was an inactivated pH1N1 vaccine containing the adjuvant AS03. Other inactivated pH1N1 vaccines were used during the 2009 influenza pandemic, including another AS03-adjuvanted vaccine (Arepanrix),[140,141] as well as

MF59-adjuvanted vaccines and nonadjuvanted vaccines,[141–143] with no increased risk of narcolepsy observed. Narcolepsy with cataplexy is strongly associated with human leukocyte antigen HLA DQB1*0602, suggesting an autoimmune reaction could deplete hypothalamic neurons producing hypocretin (a neuropeptide promoting wakefulness); however, no specific biologic mechanism has been established to support this hypothesis to date.[144–146]

The underlying reasons for an increased risk of narcolepsy among some populations remain elusive, as do the reasons for the observed association with Pandemrix. However, interest in the topic remains active and includes studies with longer term follow-up in countries outside of northern Europe.

Health Concerns Related to HPV Vaccine

Concerns about safety are a contributing factor to the relatively low vaccine coverage with HPV vaccine in the United States.[147] HPV vaccine has been alleged to be associated with a wide variety of autoimmune and neurologic diseases; however, recent large epidemiologic studies found no such associations.[148] Public concerns nonetheless remain for two particular disorders: (1) postural orthostatic tachycardia syndrome (POTS) and (2) complex regional pain syndrome (CRPS). POTS is an unusually large, sustained increase in heart rate when moving from a supine position (e.g., lying down) to an upright posture (e.g., sitting or standing). Symptoms of POTS include fatigue, headache, chest pain, shortness of breath, and syncope. CRPS is a chronic pain disorder that typically occurs after acute trauma to an extremity, symptoms of which include continued exaggerated pain, abnormalities in skin color/temperature, perspiration, and muscle weakness. Efforts to date have not found evidence of possible causal associations of these conditions with HPV vaccine,[149,150] but evaluating such associations is challenging. POTS and CRPS are rare, are diagnosed based on complex clinical criteria,[151,152] and share nonspecific symptoms with many other medical conditions.

Concerns About the Number and Frequency of Vaccines

During the first 2 years of life, children receive up to 26 doses of vaccines for 14 diseases.[51] Some parents are concerned that this vaccination schedule is "too many, too soon," possibly overwhelming the child's developing immune system, weakening the immune system or causing developmental disorders. To date, no evidence supports the allegation of "too many, too soon"; studies demonstrate that vaccines elicit a similar immune response whether given separately or concurrently.[153] Studies also demonstrate that the number of vaccines or vaccine antigens is not associated with ASDs or other developmental disorders.[135,154]

HOW VACCINE SAFETY EVIDENCE IS REVIEWED AND TURNED INTO POLICY

Postlicensure vaccine safety surveillance data help inform policy decisions related to vaccination programs and recommendations, regulatory action, and decisions affecting compensation for vaccine-associated injuries. A number of organizations participate in this process.

The ACIP is an external advisory committee that provides advice to CDC on vaccine recommendations in the US civilian population.[155] ACIP recommendations and guidelines, once reviewed and adopted by CDC, are published in the MMWR as CDC recommendations on vaccine use in the United States.[156] Vaccine safety data are routinely presented at ACIP meetings (which are open to the public), to inform discussions on the benefit–risk balance of vaccination and to guide the ACIP in its policy recommendations to CDC. If postlicensure vaccine safety data reveal a new safety concern indicating that the benefit–risk balance of a specific vaccine might be different than previously assumed, ACIP could take action, which might involve public health communication to inform the healthcare provider community and the public. One recent example is the case of febrile seizures in young children after simultaneous administration of inactivated influenza vaccine and 13-valent pneumococcal conjugate vaccination.[157] ACIP might also modify its recommendations, as when an increased risk of febrile seizures was identified after MMRV vaccination compared to MMR and varicella vaccines administered separately in young children.[158] In extreme cases, ACIP can withdraw a recommendation, such as when the increased risk of intussusception after the Rotashield rotavirus vaccine was considered unacceptably high.[95]

FDA's external advisory committees include the Vaccines and Related Biological Products Advisory Committe[159] and the Pediatric Advisory Committee, which might review safety data and provide advice to FDA.[160] Data from prelicensure and postlicensure vaccine safety monitoring and from FDA postlicensure commitments (studies that FDA requests a manufacturer to perform) can result in changes to a vaccine's prescribing information. The changes often involve communications about additional adverse reactions or language communicating risk of AEFIs after vaccination.[161] Postlicensure vaccine safety data might also result in updates to the label sections for contraindications or "warnings and precautions," which provide guidance to healthcare providers on which patients should not receive or should consider postponing vaccination. An example of a label change was the addition of language describing the risk of Kawasaki disease after RotaTeq rotavirus vaccine that was evaluated in a postlicensure epidemiologic study.[162]

The NVPO coordinates the collaboration of vaccine and immunization activities among several federal agencies (including CDC, FDA, and the National Institutes of Health). NVPO's objectives are to maximize the prevention of human disease through immunization and to minimize AEFIs while identifying and bridging gaps in federal vaccine and immunization activities.[163] Part of these pursuits include the National Vaccine Plan, which sets objectives for the use of vaccination to prevent disease and provides strategies to achieve them.

The National Academy of Medicine (NAM), previously known as IOM, is an independent organization of subject matter experts from diverse fields that can provide guidance to the United States and the international community to address critical issues in health, medicine, and related policy. NAM and its reports have informed policy decisions about vaccination. At the request of HHS, NAM has reviewed evidence for specific vaccines, vaccine types, and health outcomes to inform recommendations for changes that affect compensation for vaccine injuries (described in the following section). NAM's 2012 report[8] provided much of the evidence base for the 2017 Vaccine Injury Table (VIT) update.

HHS has also requested NAM review the evidence for specific vaccine safety topics of interest to the public health and healthcare provider communities and the general public. These reviews and the resulting NAM reports have informed policy discussions and decisions and have provided strategic guidance on areas of focus for future research. NAM reports succinctly and comprehensively reviewed a large body of scientific evidence on autism, MMR vaccine, and thimerosal, concluding that neither MMR vaccination nor thimerosal in childhood vaccines caused autism;[138,164] these reports reassured healthcare providers and the public and facilitated public health messaging regarding vaccine safety and autism. A 2013 NAM report on the safety of the childhood immunization schedule found that the evidence generally supports the safety of the schedule but recommended conducting observational studies further assessing the safety of the childhood immunization schedule as a whole,[165] which led to proposals for additional research.[166]

COMPENSATION FOR VACCINE INJURIES

A patient who has a medically significant adverse reaction to a vaccine might be eligible for financial compensation. The US National Childhood Vaccine Injury Act of 1986 was passed in response to marketplace concerns about manufacturer liability, vaccine supply and prices, and public concern about vaccine safety.[167] This law provides substantial protection and indemnity for vaccine manufacturers and healthcare providers who administer vaccines from legal and financial liability for injuries associated with vaccination. One result of the act was the establishment of the National VICP. VICP is a US government-managed, no-fault alternative to the civil tort system for adjudicating claims of vaccine-related injuries and for providing financial compensation for such injuries.[168] VICP covers vaccines routinely recommended by CDC for use in children. Adults who receive these vaccines are also covered under VICP. For example, because influenza, HPV, pneumococcal conjugate, and other routinely recommended childhood vaccines are also recommended for adults, these vaccines are covered under VICP regardless of the vaccine recipient's age. Individuals seeking financial compensation for alleged vaccine-related injuries must seek recourse by filing a claim with and proceeding through the VICP process first before pursuing legal options in the civil tort system. Final decisions on compensation are made or approved (in the case of settlements) by special masters who are appointed by the court.[168]

The VIT is a listing of vaccines, conditions, and qualifications that guide the administration of VICP. The VICP periodically updates the VIT when new vaccine safety data become available from surveillance and research. The VICP, in coordination with its external advisory committee, the Advisory Commission on Childhood Vaccines, issues recommendations to the Secretary of HHS for changes to the VIT, which then become official policy through the federal rulemaking process. An example is the 2017 VIT update, which occurred after a comprehensive review of vaccine safety data by HRSA and CDC scientists, including the 158 vaccine-AEFI causality conclusions from the 2012 IOM report, *Adverse Effects of Vaccines: Evidence and Causality*.[8] Notable VIT changes included the addition of SIRVA after any injectable vaccine and GBS after inactivated seasonal influenza vaccines.[21]

The Countermeasures Injury Compensation Program (CICP), also administered by HRSA, is the US government program for compensating individuals for injuries related to vaccines, drugs, and other medical countermeasures used in response to public health

emergencies and security threats, such as during influenza pandemics or bioterrorism attacks.[169] Two important differences between CICP and VICP exist: (1) CICP covers vaccines and other medical countermeasures, such as antivirals and antibiotics, whereas VICP only covers vaccines routinely recommended by CDC for use in children; and (2) CICP is an administrative program where final decisions are made by HHS, whereas VICP is a legal program in which decisions are made through a legal process (i.e., the courts).

CONCLUSION

The safety of vaccines is important to public health officials, regulators, clinicians, and the general public. Vaccine safety is extensively evaluated before licensure and continues to be monitored and assessed after a vaccine is licensed. Clinicians play an important role in postlicensure procedures and should be aware of the latest vaccine safety information. The following authoritative resources are updated when new information becomes available: (1) the FDA-approved prescribing information included with a vaccine's packaging material, (2) the VIS produced by CDC, and (3) ACIP recommendations published by CDC (available on the CDC website).

Patients often regard clinicians as their most trusted source of vaccine information, and despite potential hesitations about vaccines, they often follow their clinician's recommendations. Clinicians who understand the many steps taken to evaluate vaccine safety can better discuss with patients the benefits and risks of vaccines and reassure both patients and the general public about the safety of vaccines.

DISCLAIMER

The findings and conclusions in this chapter are those of the authors and do not necessarily represent the official position of the Centers for Disease Control and Prevention.

REFERENCES

1. CIOMS/WHO. *Definition and Application of Terms for Vaccine Pharmacovigilance: Report of CIOMS/WHO Working Group on Vaccine Pharmacovigilance*; 2010. Available from: http://www.who.int/vaccine_safety/initiative/tools/CIOMS_report_WG_vaccine.pdf.
2. Kroger A, Duchin J, Vazquez M. *General Best Practice Guidelines for Immunization*. Best Practices Guidance of the Advisory Committee on Immunization Practices (ACIP); 2014. Available from: www.cdc.gov/vaccines/hcp/acip-recs/general-recs/downloads/general-recs.pdf.

3. Harpaz R, Ortega-Sanchez IR, Seward JF. Advisory committee on immunization practices centers for disease control and prevention. Prevention of herpes zoster: recommendations of the advisory committee on immunization practices (ACIP). *MMWR Recomm Rep*. 2008; 57(RR-5):1–30;quiz CE2-4 18528318.
4. Marin M, Guris D, Chaves SS, et al. Prevention of varicella: recommendations of the advisory committee on immunization practices (ACIP). *MMWR Recomm Rep*. 2007;56(RR-4):1–40. PubMed PMID: 17585291.
5. McLean HQ, Fiebelkorn AP, Temte JL, Wallace GS, Centers for Disease Control and Prevention. Prevention of measles, rubella, congenital rubella syndrome, and mumps, 2013: summary recommendations of the Advisory Committee on Immunization Practices (ACIP). *MMWR Recomm Rep*. 2013;62(RR-04):1–34. PubMed PMID: 23760231.
6. Harper SA, Fukuda K, Cox NJ, Bridges CB, Advisory Committee on Immunization Practices. Using live, attenuated influenza vaccine for prevention and control of influenza: supplemental recommendations of the Advisory Committee on Immunization Practices (ACIP). *MMWR Recomm Rep*. 2003;52(RR-13):1–8. PubMed PMID: 14557799.
7. Cortese MM, Parashar UD, Centers for Disease Control and Prevention. Prevention of rotavirus gastroenteritis among infants and children: recommendations of the Advisory Committee on Immunization Practices (ACIP). *MMWR Recomm Rep*. 2009;58(RR-2):1–25. PubMed PMID: 19194371.
8. Institute of Medicine. *Adverse Effects of Vaccines: Evidence and Causality*. Washington, DC: The National Academies Press; 2012.
9. Centers for Disease Control and Prevention. *Ingredients of Vaccines—Fact Sheet*; 2011. Available from: https://www.cdc.gov/vaccines/vac-gen/additives.htm.
10. McNeil MM, Weintraub ES, Duffy J, et al. Risk of anaphylaxis after vaccination in children and adults. *J Allergy Clin Immunol*. 2016;137(3):868–878. https://doi.org/10.1016/j.jaci.2015.07.048. PubMed PMID:26452420; PubMed Central PMCID: PMCPMC 4783279.
11. Yuki N, Hartung HP. Guillain-Barre syndrome. *N Engl J Med*. 2012;366(24):2294–2304. https://doi.org/10.1056/NEJMra1114525. PubMed PMID: 22694000.
12. Schonberger LB, Bregman DJ, Sullivan-Bolyai JZ, et al. Guillain-barre syndrome following vaccination in the national influenza immunization program, United States, 1976–1977. *Am J Epidemiol*. 1979;110(2):105–123. PubMed PMID: 463869.
13. Greene SK, Rett M, Weintraub ES, et al. Risk of confirmed Guillain-Barre syndrome following receipt of monovalent inactivated influenza A (H1N1) and seasonal influenza vaccines in the Vaccine Safety Datalink Project, 2009-2010. *Am J Epidemiol*. 2012;175(11): 1100–1109. https://doi.org/10.1093/aje/kws195. PubMed PMID: 22582210.
14. Tokars JI, Lewis P, DeStefano F, et al. The risk of Guillain-Barre syndrome associated with influenza A (H1N1) 2009 monovalent vaccine and 2009-2010 seasonal influenza vaccines: results from self-controlled analyses. *Pharmacoepidemiol Drug Saf*. 2012;21(5):546–552. https://doi.org/10.1002/pds. 3220. PubMed PMID: 22407672.
15. Wise ME, Viray M, Sejvar JJ, et al. Guillain-Barre syndrome during the 2009-2010 H1N1 influenza vaccination campaign: population-based surveillance among 45 million Americans. *Am J Epidemiol*. 2012;175(11): 1110–1119. https://doi.org/10.1093/aje/kws196. PubMed PMID:22582209; PubMed Central PMCID: PMCPMC 3888111.
16. Salmon DA, Proschan M, Forshee R, et al. Association between Guillain-Barre syndrome and influenza A (H1N1) 2009 monovalent inactivated vaccines in the USA: a meta-analysis. *Lancet*. 2013;381(9876):1461–1468. https://doi.org/10.1016/S0140-6736(12)62189-8. PubMed PMID: 23498095.
17. Dodd CN, Romio SA, Black S, et al. International collaboration to assess the risk of Guillain Barre Syndrome following Influenza A (H1N1) 2009 monovalent vaccines. *Vaccine*. 2013;31(40):4448–4458. https://doi.org/10.1016/j.vaccine.2013.06.032. PubMed PMID: 23770307.
18. Vellozzi C, Iqbal S, Broder K. Guillain-Barre syndrome, influenza, and influenza vaccination: the epidemiologic evidence. *Clin Infect Dis*. 2014;58(8):1149–1155. https://doi.org/10.1093/cid/ciu005. PubMed PMID: 24415636.
19. Gershman M, Staples JE. *Yellow Fever. CDC Yellow Book 2018: Health Information for International Travel*. New York: Oxford University Press; 2017.
20. Duffy J, Johnsen P, Ferris M, et al. Safety of a meningococcal group B vaccine used in response to two university outbreaks. *J Am Coll Health*; 2017:1–8. https://doi.org/10.1080/07448481.2017.1312418. PubMed PMID: 28362241.
21. Health Resources and Services Administration. *Vaccine Injury Table*; 2017. Available from: https://www.hrsa.gov/vaccinecompensation/vaccineinjurytable.pdf.
22. Nair N. *Update on SIRVA*. Washington, DC: National Vaccine Adivsory Committee Meeting; June 6, 2017.
23. World Health Organization. *Weekly Epidemiological Record*. vol. 91. 2016:21–32.
24. Title 42—The Public Health and Welfare. Government Publishing Office. Available from: https://www.gpo.gov/fdsys/pkg/USCODE-2010-title42/pdf/USCODE-2010-title42-chap6A-subchapXIX-part2-subpartc-sec300aa-26.pdf.
25. Centers for Disease Control and Prevention. *Vaccine Information Statements (VISs)*; 2017. Available from: https://www.cdc.gov/vaccines/hcp/vis/current-vis.html.
26. Kelso JM. Update on vaccination guidelines for allergic children. *Expert Rev Vaccines*. 2009;8(11):1541–1546. https://doi.org/10.1586/erv.09.107. PubMed PMID: 19863246.

27. Immunization Action Coalition. *Screening Checklists*; 2017. Available from: http://www.immunize.org/handouts/screening-vaccines.asp.

28. Centers for Disease Control and Prevention. General recommendations on immunization. In: Hamborsky JKA, Wolfe S, eds. *Epidemiology and Prevention of Vaccine-preventable Diseases*. 13th ed. Washington, DC: Public Health Foundation; 2015.

29. Meissner HC. ID Snapshot: how to reduce pain during vaccination. *AAP News*; March 3, 2016. http://www.aappublications.org/news/2016/03/03/VaccinePain030316.

30. Bancos S, Bernard MP, Topham DJ, Phipps RP. Ibuprofen and other widely used non-steroidal anti-inflammatory drugs inhibit antibody production in human cells. *Cell Immunol*. 2009;258(1):18−28. https://doi.org/10.1016/j.cellimm.2009.03.007. PubMed PMID:19345936; PubMed Central PMCID: PMCPMC 2693360.

31. Das RR, Panigrahi I, Naik SS. The effect of prophylactic antipyretic administration on post-vaccination adverse reactions and antibody response in children: a systematic review. *PLoS One*. 2014;9(9):e106629. https://doi.org/10.1371/journal.pone.0106629. PubMed PMID: 25180516; PubMed Central PMCID: PMCPMC4152293.

32. Wijdicks EF, Klein CJ. Guillain-barre syndrome. *Mayo Clin Proc*. 2017;92(3):467−479. https://doi.org/10.1016/j.mayocp.2016.12.002. PubMed PMID: 28259232.

33. Halsey NA, Edwards KM, Dekker CL, et al. Algorithm to assess causality after individual adverse events following immunizations. *Vaccine*. 2012;30(39):5791−5798. https://doi.org/10.1016/j.vaccine.2012.04.005. PubMed PMID: 22507656.

34. Soush S, Beall B, McGee L, et al. Chapter 22: Laboratory support for surveillance of vaccine-preventable diseases. In: *Manual for the Surveillance of Vaccine-preventable Diseases*. Atlanta, GA: Centers for Disease Control and Prevention; 2015.

35. Centers for Disease Control and Prevention. *Clinical Immunization Safety Assessment (CISA) Project*; 2015. Available from: https://www.cdc.gov/vaccinesafety/ensuringsafety/monitoring/cisa/index.html.

36. Centers for Disease Control and Prevention. Appendix B: Vaccines. In: Hamborsky JKA, Wolfe S, eds. *Epidemiology and Prevention of Vaccine-preventable Diseases*. 13th ed. Washington, DC: Public Health Foundation; 2015.

37. Wood RA, Berger M, Dreskin SC, et al. An algorithm for treatment of patients with hypersensitivity reactions after vaccines. *Pediatrics*. 2008;122(3):e771−e777. https://doi.org/10.1542/peds.2008-1002. PubMed PMID: 18762513.

38. McMillan M, Clarke M, Parrella A, Fell DB, Amirthalingam G, Marshall HS. Safety of tetanus, diphtheria, and pertussis vaccination during pregnancy: a systematic review. *Obstet Gynecol*. 2017;129(3):560−573. https://doi.org/10.1097/AOG.0000000000001888. PubMed PMID: 28178054.

39. Moro PL, Broder K, Zheteyeva Y, et al. Adverse events in pregnant women following administration of trivalent inactivated influenza vaccine and live attenuated influenza vaccine in the Vaccine Adverse Event Reporting System, 1990-2009. *Am J Obstet Gynecol*. 2011;204(2):146.e1-7. https://doi.org/10.1016/j.ajog.2010.08.050. PubMed PMID: 20965490.

40. Moro PL, Cragan J, Tepper N, et al. Enhanced surveillance of tetanus toxoid, reduced diphtheria toxoid, and acellular pertussis (Tdap) vaccines in pregnancy in the Vaccine Adverse Event Reporting System (VAERS), 2011-2015. *Vaccine*. 2016;34(20):2349−2353. https://doi.org/10.1016/j.vaccine.2016.03.049. PubMed PMID: 27013434.

41. Tsai TF, Paul R, Lynberg MC, Letson GW. Congenital yellow fever virus infection after immunization in pregnancy. *J Infect Dis*. 1993;168(6):1520−1523. PubMed PMID: 8245539.

42. Centers for Disease Control and Prevention. *Yellow Fever. CDC Yellow Book 2018: Health Information for International Travel*. New York: Oxford University Press; 2017.

43. Preblud SR. Some current issues relating to rubella vaccine. *JAMA*. 1985;254(2):253−256. PubMed PMID: 3999370.

44. Moro P, Baumblatt J, Lewis P, Cragan J, Tepper N, Cano M. Surveillance of adverse events after seasonal influenza vaccination in pregnant women and their infants in the vaccine adverse event reporting system, july 2010-may 2016. *Drug Saf*. 2017;40(2):145−152. https://doi.org/10.1007/s40264-016-0482-1. PubMed PMID: 27988883.

45. Marin M, Willis ED, Marko A, et al. Closure of varicella-zoster virus-containing vaccines pregnancy registry— United States, 2013. *MMWR Morb Mortal Wkly Rep*. 2014;63(33):732−733. PubMed PMID: 25144545.

46. Centers for Disease Control and Prevention. *Vaccinations*; 2015. Available from: https://www.cdc.gov/breastfeeding/recommendations/vaccinations.htm.

47. Keiser PB, Nutman TB. Strongyloides stercoralis in the immunocompromised population. *Clin Microbiol Rev*. 2004;17(1):208−217. PubMed PMID:14726461; PubMed Central PMCID: PMCPMC321465.

48. Rubin LG, Levin MJ, Ljungman P, et al. 2013 IDSA clinical practice guideline for vaccination of the immunocompromised host. *Clin Infect Dis*. 2014;58(3):309−318. https://doi.org/10.1093/cid/cit816. PubMed PMID: 24421306.

49. Lopez A, Mariette X, Bachelez H, et al. Vaccination recommendations for the adult immunosuppressed patient: a systematic review and comprehensive field synopsis. *J Autoimmun*. 2017;80:10−27. https://doi.org/10.1016/j.jaut.2017.03.011. PubMed PMID: 28381345.

50. Kim DK, Bridges CB, Harriman KH, Advisory Committee on Immunization Practices AAIWG. Advisory committee on immunization practices recommended immunization schedule for adults aged 19 years or older−United States, 2016. *MMWR Morb Mortal Wkly Rep*. 2016;65(4):88−90. https://doi.org/10.15585/mmwr.mm6504a5. PubMed PMID: 26845417.

51. Robinson CL, Advisory Committee on Immunization Practices ACAIWG. Advisory committee on immunization

practices recommended immunization schedules for persons aged 0 through 18 years—United States, 2016. *MMWR Morb Mortal Wkly Rep*. 2016;65(4):86–87. https://doi.org/10.15585/mmwr.mm6504a4. PubMed PMID: 26845283.

52. World Health Organization. *Clinical Guidelines: Antiretroviral Therapy. Consolidated Guidelines on the Use of Antiretroviral Drugs for Treating and Preventing HIV Infection*. 2nd ed. Geneva, Switzerland: WHO Press; 2016:71–190.

53. Burke VE, Lopez FA. Approach to skin and soft tissue infections in non-HIV immunocompromised hosts. *Curr Opin Infect Dis*. 2017;30(4):354–363. https://doi.org/10.1097/QCO.0000000000000378. PubMed PMID: 28542092.

54. Centers for Disease Control and Prevention. *HIV Infection and Adult Vaccination*; 2017. Available from: https://www.cdc.gov/vaccines/adults/rec-vac/health-conditions/hiv.html.

55. Amendola A, Tanzi E, Zappa A, et al. Safety and immunogenicity of 23-valent pneumococcal polysaccharide vaccine in HIV-1 infected former drug users. *Vaccine*. 2002;20(31–32):3720–3724. PubMed PMID: 12399200.

56. Kim HN, Harrington RD, Crane HM, Dhanireddy S, Dellit TH, Spach DH. Hepatitis B vaccination in HIV-infected adults: current evidence, recommendations and practical considerations. *Int J STD AIDS*. 2009;20(9):595–600. https://doi.org/10.1258/ijsa.2009.009126. PubMed PMID: 19710329.

57. Szczawinska-Poplonyk A, Breborowicz A, Samara H, Ossowska L, Dworacki G. Impaired antigen-specific immune response to vaccines in children with antibody production defects. *Clin Vaccine Immunol*. 2015;22(8):875–882. https://doi.org/10.1128/CVI.00148-15. PubMed PMID 26018535; PubMed Central PMCID: PMCPMC4519726.

58. Vigano A, Zuccotti GV, Pacei M, et al. Humoral and cellular response to influenza vaccine in HIV-infected children with full viroimmunologic response to antiretroviral therapy. *J Acquir Immune Defic Syndr*. 2008;48(3):289–296. https://doi.org/10.1097/QAI.0b013e3181632cda. PubMed PMID: 18545155.

59. Leung J, Siegel S, Jones JF, et al. Fatal varicella due to the vaccine-strain varicella-zoster virus. *Hum Vaccin Immunother*. 2014;10(1):146–149. https://doi.org/10.4161/hv.26200. PubMed PMID: 23982221; PubMed Central PMCID: PMCPMC4181020.

60. Crum-Cianflone NF, Wallace MR. Vaccination in HIV-infected adults. *AIDS Patient Care STDS*. 2014;28(8):397–410. https://doi.org/10.1089/apc.2014.0121. PubMed PMID: 25029589; PubMed Central PMCID: PMCPMC4117268.

61. Levin MJ, Gershon AA, Weinberg A, et al. Immunization of HIV-infected children with varicella vaccine. *J Pediatr*. 2001;139(2):305–310. https://doi.org/10.1067/mpd.2001.115972. PubMed PMID: 11487761.

62. Scott P, Moss WJ, Gilani Z, Low N. Measles vaccination in HIV-infected children: systematic review and meta-analysis of safety and immunogenicity. *J Infect Dis*. 2011;204(suppl 1):S164–S178. https://doi.org/10.1093/infdis/jir071. PubMed PMID: 21666158.

63. Shafran SD. Live attenuated herpes zoster vaccine for HIV-infected adults. *HIV Med*. 2016;17(4):305–310. https://doi.org/10.1111/hiv.12311. PubMed PMID: 26315285.

64. Sprauer MA, Markowitz LE, Nicholson JK, et al. Response of human immunodeficiency virus-infected adults to measles-rubella vaccination. *J Acquir Immune Defic Syndr*. 1993;6(9):1013–1016. PubMed PMID: 8340890.

65. Veit O, Niedrig M, Chapuis-Taillard C, et al. Immunogenicity and safety of yellow fever vaccination for 102 HIV-infected patients. *Clin Infect Dis*. 2009;48(5):659–666. https://doi.org/10.1086/597006. PubMed PMID: 19191654.

66. Pulendran B, Miller J, Querec TD, et al. Case of yellow fever vaccine–associated viscerotropic disease with prolonged viremia, robust adaptive immune responses, and polymorphisms in CCR5 and RANTES genes. *J Infect Dis*. 2008;198(4):500–507. https://doi.org/10.1086/590187. PubMed PMID:18598196; PubMed Central PMCID: PMCPMC3734802 18598196.

67. Roukens AH, Visser LG, Kroon FP. A note of caution on yellow fever vaccination during maraviroc treatment: a hypothesis on a potential dangerous interaction. *AIDS*. 2009;23(4):542–543. https://doi.org/10.1097/QAD.0b013e328323aeb4. PubMed PMID: 19165082.

68. Marin M, Broder KR, Temte JL, et al. Use of combination measles, mumps, rubella, and varicella vaccine: recommendations of the Advisory Committee on Immunization Practices (ACIP). *MMWR Recomm Rep*. 2010;59(RR-3):1–12. PubMed PMID: 20448530.

69. Brichacek B, Swindells S, Janoff EN, Pirruccello S, Stevenson M. Increased plasma human immunodeficiency virus type 1 burden following antigenic challenge with pneumococcal vaccine. *J Infect Dis*. 1996;174(6):1191–1199. PubMed PMID: 8940208.

70. Stanley SK, Ostrowski MA, Justement JS, et al. Effect of immunization with a common recall antigen on viral expression in patients infected with human immunodeficiency virus type 1. *N Engl J Med*. 1996;334(19):1222–1230. https://doi.org/10.1056/NEJM199605093341903. PubMed PMID: 8606717.

71. Castro P, Plana M, Gonzalez R, et al. Influence of a vaccination schedule on viral load rebound and immune responses in successfully treated HIV-infected patients. *AIDS Res Hum Retroviruses*. 2009;25(12):1249–1259. https://doi.org/10.1089/aid.2009.0015. PubMed PMID: 19943787.

72. Stermole BM, Grandits GA, Roediger MP, et al. Long-term safety and serologic response to measles, mumps, and rubella vaccination in HIV-1 infected adults. *Vaccine*. 2011;29(16):2874–2880. https://doi.org/10.1016/j.vaccine.2011.02.013. PubMed PMID: 21352938; PubMed Central PMCID: PMCPMC3073409.

73. Sullivan PS, Hanson DL, Dworkin MS, et al. Effect of influenza vaccination on disease progression among

HIV-infected persons. *AIDS*. 2000;14(17):2781–2785. PubMed PMID: 11125897.

74. Manzi S, Kuller LH, Kutzer J, et al. Herpes zoster in systemic lupus erythematosus. *J Rheumatol*. 1995;22(7): 1254–1258. PubMed PMID: 7562754.

75. Naveau C, Houssiau FA. Pneumococcal sepsis in patients with systemic lupus erythematosus. *Lupus*. 2005;14(11): 903–906. https://doi.org/10.1191/0961203305lu2242xx. PubMed PMID: 16335583.

76. Buhler S, Eperon G, Ribi C, et al. Vaccination recommendations for adult patients with autoimmune inflammatory rheumatic diseases. *Swiss Med Wkly*. 2015;145: w14159. https://doi.org/10.4414/smw.2015.14159. PubMed PMID: 26218860.

77. Dooling KL, Guo A, Patel M, et al. Recommendations of the advisory committee on immunization practices for use of herpes zoster vaccines. *MMWR Morb Mortal Wkly Rep*. 2018;67(3):103–108.

78. van Assen S, Elkayam O, Agmon-Levin N, et al. Vaccination in adult patients with auto-immune inflammatory rheumatic diseases: a systematic literature review for the European League against Rheumatism evidence-based recommendations for vaccination in adult patients with auto-immune inflammatory rheumatic diseases. *Autoimmun Rev*. 2011;10(6):341–352. https://doi.org/10.1016/j.autrev.2010.12.003. PubMed PMID: 21182987.

79. Singh JA, Saag KG, Bridges Jr SL, et al. 2015 American College of Rheumatology guideline for the treatment of rheumatoid arthritis. *Arthritis Care Res Hob*. 2016;68(1): 1–25. https://doi.org/10.1002/acr.22783. PubMed PMID: 26545825.

80. Advisory Committee on Immunization Practices. Centers for disease control and prevention. Immunization of health-care personnel: recommendations of the advisory committee on immunization practices (ACIP). *MMWR Recomm Rep*. 2011;60(RR-7):1–45. PubMed PMID: 22108587.

81. Nathanson N, Langmuir AD. The cutter incident. Poliomyelitis following formaldehyde- inactivated poliovirus vaccination in the United States during the spring of 1955. II. Relationship of poliomyelitis to cutter vaccine. *Am J Hyg*. 1963;78:29–60. PubMed PMID: 14043545.

82. Centers for Disease Control and Prevention. Updated interim influenza vaccination recommendations—2004-05 influenza season. *MMWR Morb Mortal Wkly Rep*. 2004;53(50):1183–1184. PubMed PMID: 15614237.

83. Organization of Teratology Information Specialists. *MotherToBaby: Medications & More during Pregnancy & Breastfeeding: Ask the Experts*; 2017. Available from: https://mothertobaby.org/.

84. Shimabukuro TT, Nguyen M, Martin D, DeStefano F. Safety monitoring in the vaccine adverse event reporting system (VAERS). *Vaccine*. 2015;33(36):4398–4405. https://doi.org/10.1016/j.vaccine.2015.07.035. PubMed PMID: 26209838; PubMed Central PMCID: PMCPMC4632204.

85. Centers for Disease Control and Prevention. *Vaccine Adverse Event Reporting System (VAERS)*; 2017. Available from: https://www.cdc.gov/vaccinesafety/ensuringsafety/monitoring/vaers/index.html.

86. McNeil MM, Gee J, Weintraub ES, et al. The vaccine safety datalink: successes and challenges monitoring vaccine safety. *Vaccine*. 2014;32(42):5390–5398. https://doi.org/10.1016/j.vaccine.2014.07.073. PubMed PMID: 25108215.

87. Lieu TA, Kulldorff M, Davis RL, et al. Real-time vaccine safety surveillance for the early detection of adverse events. *Med Care*. 2007;45(10 suppl 2):S89–S95. https://doi.org/10.1097/MLR.0b013e3180616c0a. PubMed PMID: 17909389.

88. Shoaibi A. *Prism Identifies Vaccine Safety Issues*; 2017. Available from: https://blogs.fda.gov/fdavoice/index.php/2017/04/prism-identifies-vaccine-safety-issues/.

89. Letourneau M, Wells G, Walop W, Duclos P. Improving global monitoring of vaccine safety: a quantitative analysis of adverse event reports in the WHO adverse reactions database. *Vaccine*. 2008;26(9):1185–1194. https://doi.org/10.1016/j.vaccine.2007.12.033. PubMed PMID: 18243428.

90. Brighton Collaboration. Available from: https://www.brightoncollaboration.org/about-us/structure.html; 2017.

91. International Council for Harmonisation of Technical Requirements for Pharmaceuticals for Human Use. *Welcome to the ICH Official Website*; 2017. Available from: http://www.ich.org/home.html.

92. Council for International Organizations of Medical Sciences. Adverse Events Following Immunization. Definition and Application of Terms of Vaccine Pharmacovigilance (report of CIOMS/WHO Working Group on Vaccine Pharmacovigilance); 2012:39–53.

93. Gaydos JC, Top Jr FH, Hodder RA, Russell PK. Swine influenza a outbreak, Fort Dix, New Jersey, 1976. *Emerg Infect Dis*. 2006;12(1):23–28. https://doi.org/10.3201/eid1201.050965. PubMed PMID: 16494712; PubMed Central PMCID: PMCPMC3291397.

94. Sencer DJ, Millar JD. Reflections on the 1976 swine flu vaccination program. *Emerg Infect Dis*. 2006; 12(1):29–33. https://doi.org/10.3201/eid1201.051007. PubMed PMID: 16494713; PubMed Central PMCID: PMCPMC3291400.

95. Centers for Disease Control and Prevention. Withdrawal of rotavirus vaccine recommendation. *MMWR Morb Mortal Wkly Rep*. 1999;48(43):1007. PubMed PMID: 10577495.

96. GlaxoSmithKline. *Product Insert: ROTARIX (Rotavirus Vaccine, Live, Oral) Oral Suspension*; 2008. Available from: https://www.gsksource.com/pharma/content/dam/GlaxoSmithKline/US/en/Prescribing_Information/Rotarix/pdf/ROTARIX-PI-PIL.PDF.

97. Merck. *Product Insert: RotaTeq (Rotavirus Vaccine, Live, Oral, Pentavalent) Oral Solution*; 2006. Available from: https://www.merck.com/product/usa/pi_circulars/r/rotateq/rotateq_pi.pdf.

98. Vellozzi C, Broder KR, Haber P, et al. Adverse events following influenza A (H1N1) 2009 monovalent vaccines reported to the vaccine adverse event reporting system, United States, October 1, 2009-January 31, 2010. *Vaccine.* 2010;28(45):7248−7255. https://doi.org/10.1016/j.vaccine.2010.09.021. PubMed PMID: 20850534.

99. Lee GM, Greene SK, Weintraub ES, et al. H1N1 and seasonal influenza vaccine safety in the vaccine safety datalink project. *Am J Prev Med.* 2011;41(2):121−128. https://doi.org/10.1016/j.amepre.2011.04.004. PubMed PMID: 21767718.

100. Burwen DR, Sandhu SK, MaCurdy TE, et al. Surveillance for Guillain-Barre syndrome after influenza vaccination among the Medicare population, 2009-2010. *Am J Public Health.* 2012;102(10):1921−1927. https://doi.org/10.2105/AJPH.2011.300510. PubMed PMID: 22970693; PubMed Central PMCID: PMCPMC3490645.

101. Nguyen M, Ball R, Midthun K, Lieu TA. The Food and drug administration's post-licensure rapid immunization safety monitoring program: strengthening the federal vaccine safety enterprise. *Pharmacoepidemiol Drug Saf.* 2012;21(suppl 1):291−297. https://doi.org/10.1002/pds.2323. PubMed PMID: 22262619.

102. Centers for Disease Control and Prevention. Safety of influenza A (H1N1) 2009 monovalent vaccines - United States, October 1-November 24, 2009. *MMWR Morb Mortal Wkly Rep.* 2009;58(48):1351−1356. PubMed PMID: 20010511.

103. National Vaccine Advisory Committee. *National Vaccine Advisory Committee (NVAC) H1N1 Vaccine Safety Risk Assessment Working Group (VSRAWG)*; 2012. Available from: https://www.hhs.gov/sites/default/files/nvpo/nvac/reports/vsrawg_report_january_2012.pdf.

104. Centers for Disease Control and Prevention. *Final Estimates for 2009−10 Seasonal Influenza and Influenza a (H1N1) 2009 Monovalent Vaccination Coverage—United States, August 2009 through May, 2010*; 2011. Available from: https://www.cdc.gov/flu/fluvaxview/coverage_0910estimates.htm.

105. Wharton M, Strikas RA, Harpaz R, et al. Recommendations for using smallpox vaccine in a pre-event vaccination program. Supplemental recommendations of the advisory committee on immunization practices (ACIP) and the healthcare infection control practices advisory committee (HICPAC). *MMWR Recomm Rep.* 2003;52(RR-7):1−16. PubMed PMID: 12710832.

106. Grabenstein JD, Winkenwerder Jr W. US military smallpox vaccination program experience. *JAMA.* 2003;289(24):3278−3282. https://doi.org/10.1001/jama.289.24.3278. PubMed PMID: 12824209.

107. Neff J, Modlin J, Birkhead GS, et al. Monitoring the safety of a smallpox vaccination program in the United States: report of the joint Smallpox Vaccine Safety Working Group of the advisory committee on immunization practices and the Armed Forces Epidemiological Board. *Clin Infect Dis.* 2008;46(suppl 3):S258−S270. https://doi.org/10.1086/524749. PubMed PMID: 18284367.

108. Centers for Disease Control and Prevention. Smallpox vaccine adverse events monitoring and response system for the first stage of the smallpox vaccination program. *MMWR Morb Mortal Wkly Rep.* 2003;52(5):88−89. PubMed PMID: 12588007.

109. Klevens RM, Kupronis BA, Lawton R, et al. Monitoring health care workers after smallpox vaccination: findings from the Hospital Smallpox Vaccination-Monitoring System. *Am J Infect Control.* 2005;33(6):315−319. PubMed PMID: 16110599.

110. Ryan MA, Seward JF. Smallpox vaccine in pregnancy registry T. Pregnancy, birth, and infant health outcomes from the national smallpox vaccine in pregnancy registry, 2003-2006. *Clin Infect Dis.* 2008;46(suppl 3):S221−S226. https://doi.org/10.1086/524744. PubMed PMID: 18284362.

111. Casey CG, Iskander JK, Roper MH, et al. Adverse events associated with smallpox vaccination in the United States, January-October 2003. *JAMA.* 2005;294(21):2734−2743. https://doi.org/10.1001/jama.294.21.2734. PubMed PMID: 16333009.

112. Thomas TN, Reef S, Neff L, Sniadack MM, Mootrey GT. A review of the smallpox vaccine adverse events active surveillance system. *Clin Infect Dis.* 2008;46(suppl 3):S212−S220. https://doi.org/10.1086/524742. PubMed PMID: 18284361.

113. Morgan J, Roper MH, Sperling L, et al. Myocarditis, pericarditis, and dilated cardiomyopathy after smallpox vaccination among civilians in the United States, January-October 2003. *Clin Infect Dis.* 2008;46(suppl 3):S242−S250. https://doi.org/10.1086/524747. PubMed PMID: 18284365.

114. Centers for Disease Control and Prevention. Supplemental recommendations on adverse events following smallpox vaccine in the pre-event vaccination program: recommendations of the Advisory Committee on Immunization Practices. *MMWR Morb Mortal Wkly Rep.* 2003;52(13):282−284. PubMed PMID: 12729078.

115. Gupta RK, Siber GR. Adjuvants for human vaccines—current status, problems and future prospects. *Vaccine.* 1995;13(14):1263−1276. PubMed PMID: 8585280.

116. GlaxoSmithKline Biologicals. *Highlights of Prescribing Information (Pediarix)*; 2016. Available from: https://www.gsksource.com/pharma/content/dam/GlaxoSmithKline/US/en/Prescribing_Information/Pediarix/pdf/PEDIARIX.PDF.

117. Weisser K, Stubler S, Matheis W, Huisinga W. Towards toxicokinetic modelling of aluminium exposure from adjuvants in medicinal products. *Regul Toxicol Pharmacol*; 2017. https://doi.org/10.1016/j.yrtph.2017.02.018. PubMed PMID: 28237896.

118. Flarend RE, Hem SL, White JL, et al. In vivo absorption of aluminium-containing vaccine adjuvants using 26Al. *Vaccine.* 1997;15(12−13):1314−1318. PubMed PMID: 9302736.

119. Mitkus RJ, King DB, Hess MA, Forshee RA, Walderhaug MO. Updated aluminum pharmacokinetics following infant exposures through diet and vaccination. *Vaccine*. 2011;29(51):9538–9543. https://doi.org/10.1016/j.vaccine.2011.09.124. PubMed PMID: 22001122.

120. Coffman RL, Sher A, Seder RA. Vaccine adjuvants: putting innate immunity to work. *Immunity*. 2010;33(4):492–503. https://doi.org/10.1016/j.immuni.2010.10.002. PubMed PMID: 21029960; PubMed Central PMCID: PMCPMC3420356.

121. Shah RR, Hassett KJ, Brito LA. Overview of vaccine adjuvants: introduction, history, and current status. *Methods Mol Biol*. 2017;1494:1–13. https://doi.org/10.1007/978-1-4939-6445-1_1. PubMed PMID: 27718182.

122. Haensler J. Manufacture of oil-in-water emulsion adjuvants. *Methods Mol Biol*. 2017;1494:165–180. https://doi.org/10.1007/978-1-4939-6445-1_12. PubMed PMID: 27718193.

123. Centers for Disease Control and Prevention. *FLUAD™ Flu Vaccine With Adjuvant*; 2016. Available from: https://www.cdc.gov/flu/protect/vaccine/adjuvant.htm.

124. Frey S, Poland G, Percell S, Podda A. Comparison of the safety, tolerability, and immunogenicity of a MF59-adjuvanted influenza vaccine and a non-adjuvanted influenza vaccine in non-elderly adults. *Vaccine*. 2003;21(27–30):4234–4237. PubMed PMID: 14505903.

125. Sindoni D, La Fauci V, Squeri R, et al. Comparison between a conventional subunit vaccine and the MF59-adjuvanted subunit influenza vaccine in the elderly: an evaluation of the safety, tolerability and immunogenicity. *J Prev Med Hyg*. 2009;50(2):121–126. PubMed PMID: 20099444.

126. Vesikari T, Groth N, Karvonen A, Borkowski A, Pellegrini M. MF59-adjuvanted influenza vaccine (FLUAD) in children: safety and immunogenicity following a second year seasonal vaccination. *Vaccine*. 2009;27(45):6291–6295. https://doi.org/10.1016/j.vaccine.2009.02.004. PubMed PMID: 19840662.

127. U.S. Food and Drug Administration. *Common Ingredients in U.S. Licensed Vaccines*; 2014. Available from: https://www.fda.gov/biologicsbloodvaccines/safetyavailability/vaccinesafety/ucm187810.htm.

128. Didierlaurent AM, Laupeze B, Di Pasquale A, Hergli N, Collignon C, Garcon N. Adjuvant system AS01: helping to overcome the challenges of modern vaccines. *Expert Rev Vaccines*. 2017;16(1):55–63. https://doi.org/10.1080/14760584.2016.1213632. PubMed PMID: 27448771.

129. Chlibek R, Bayas JM, Collins H, et al. Safety and immunogenicity of an AS01-adjuvanted varicella-zoster virus subunit candidate vaccine against herpes zoster in adults ≥50 years of age. *J Infect Dis*. 2013;208(12):1953–1961. https://doi.org/10.1093/infdis/jit365. PubMed PMID: 23904292.

130. Corporation DT. *Product Insert: HEPLISAV-B [Hepatitis B Vaccine (Recombinant), Adjuvanted] Solution for Intramuscular Injection 2017*; December 19, 2017. Available from: https://www.fda.gov/downloads/BiologicsBloodVaccines/Vaccines/ApprovedProducts/UCM584762.pdf.

131. Lowes R. *Heplisav-b Vaccine for Hep B Finally Wins FDA Approval*. Medscape Public Health; 2017.

132. Retraction—Ileal-lymphoid-nodular hyperplasia, non-specific colitis, and pervasive developmental disorder in children. *Lancet*. 2010;375(9713):445. https://doi.org/10.1016/S0140-6736(10)60175-4. PubMed PMID: 20137807.

133. Dyer C. Wakefield was dishonest and irresponsible over MMR research, says GMC. *BMJ*. 2010;340:c593. https://doi.org/10.1136/bmj.c593. PubMed PMID: 20118180.

134. Gerber JS, Offit PA. Vaccines and autism: a tale of shifting hypotheses. *Clin Infect Dis*. 2009;48(4):456–461. https://doi.org/10.1086/596476. PubMed PMID: 19128068; PubMed Central PMCID: PMCPMC2908388.

135. DeStefano F, Price CS, Weintraub ES. Increasing exposure to antibody-stimulating proteins and polysaccharides in vaccines is not associated with risk of autism. *J Pediatr*. 2013;163(2):561–567. https://doi.org/10.1016/j.jpeds.2013.02.001. PubMed PMID: 23545349.

136. Modabbernia A, Velthorst E, Reichenberg A. Environmental risk factors for autism: an evidence-based review of systematic reviews and meta-analyses. *Mol Autism*. 2017;8:13. https://doi.org/10.1186/s13229-017-0121-4. PubMed PMID: 28331572; PubMed Central PMCID: PMCPMC5356236.

137. Offit PA. Thimerosal and vaccines—a cautionary tale. *N Engl J Med*. 2007;357(13):1278–1279. https://doi.org/10.1056/NEJMp078187. PubMed PMID: 17898096.

138. Institute of Medicine. *Immunization Safety Review: Vaccines and Autism*. Washington, DC: The National Academies Press; 2004.

139. Eurosurveillance editorial t. European Medicines Agency updates on the review of Pandemrix and reports of narcolepsy. *Euro Surveill*. 2010;15(38). PubMed PMID: 20929650.

140. Montplaisir J, Petit D, Quinn MJ, et al. Risk of narcolepsy associated with inactivated adjuvanted (AS03) A/H1N1 (2009) pandemic influenza vaccine in Quebec. *PLoS One*. 2014;9(9):e108489. https://doi.org/10.1371/journal.pone.0108489. PubMed PMID: 25264897; PubMed Central PMCID: PMCPMC4180737.

141. Weibel D, Sturkenboom M, Black S, et al. Narcolepsy and adjuvanted pandemic influenza A (H1N1) 2009 vaccines - Multi-country assessment. *Vaccine*. 2018; 3(suppl 1). [Epub ahead of print].

142. Duffy J, Weintraub E, Vellozzi C, DeStefano F, Vaccine Safety Datalink. Narcolepsy and influenza A(H1N1) pandemic 2009 vaccination in the United States.

Neurology. 2014;83(20):1823—1830. https://doi.org/10.1212/WNL.0000000000000987. PubMed PMID: 25320099.

143. Kim WJ, Lee SD, Lee E, et al. Incidence of narcolepsy before and after MF59-adjuvanted influenza A(H1N1)pdm09 vaccination in South Korean soldiers. *Vaccine.* 2015;33(38):4868—4872. https://doi.org/10.1016/j.vaccine.2015.07.055. PubMed PMID: 26238720.

144. Kornum BR, Burgdorf KS, Holm A, Ullum H, Jennum P, Knudsen S. Absence of autoreactive CD4+ T-cells targeting HLA-DQA1*01:02/DQB1*06:02 restricted hypocretin/orexin epitopes in narcolepsy type 1 when detected by EliSpot. *J Neuroimmunol.* 2017;309:7—11. https://doi.org/10.1016/j.jneuroim.2017.05.001. PubMed PMID: 28601291.

145. Planty C, Mallett CP, Yim K, et al. Evaluation of the potential effects of AS03-adjuvanted A(H1N1)pdm09 vaccine administration on the central nervous system of non-primed and A(H1N1)pdm09-primed cotton rats. *Hum Vaccin Immunother.* 2017;13(1):90—102. https://doi.org/10.1080/21645515.2016.1227518. PubMed PMID: 27629482; PubMed Central PMCID: PMCPMC5287305.

146. Thebault S, Waters P, Snape MD, et al. Neuronal antibodies in children with or without narcolepsy following H1N1-AS03 vaccination. *PLoS One.* 2015;10(6):e0129555. https://doi.org/10.1371/journal.pone.0129555. PubMed PMID: 26090827; PubMed Central PMCID: PMCPMC4474558.

147. Pathela P, Jamison K, Papadouka V, et al. Measuring adolescent human papillomavirus vaccine coverage: a match of sexually transmitted disease clinic and immunization registry data. *J Adolesc Health.* 2016;59(6):710—715. https://doi.org/10.1016/j.jadohealth.2016.07.021. PubMed PMID: 27671357.

148. Gee J, Weinbaum C, Sukumaran L, Markowitz LE. Quadrivalent HPV vaccine safety review and safety monitoring plans for nine-valent HPV vaccine in the United States. *Hum Vaccin Immunother.* 2016;12(6):1406—1417. https://doi.org/10.1080/21645515.2016.1168952. PubMed PMID: 27029786; PubMed Central PMCID: PMCPMC4964727.

149. European Medicines Agency. *Review Concludes Evidence Does Not Support That HPV Vaccines Cause CRPS or POTS;* 2015. Available from: http://www.ema.europa.eu/ema/index.jsp?curl=pages/news_and_events/news/2015/11/news_detail_002429.jsp&mid=WC0b01ac058004d5c1.

150. World Health Organization. *Global Advisory Committee on Vaccine Safety Statement on Safety of HPV Vaccines;* 2015. Available from: http://www.who.int/vaccine_safety/committee/GACVS_HPV_statement_17Dec2015.pdf.

151. Harden RN, Bruehl S, Perez RS, et al. Validation of proposed diagnostic criteria (the "budapest criteria") for complex regional pain syndrome. *Pain.* 2010;150(2):268—274. https://doi.org/10.1016/j.pain.2010.04.030. PubMed PMID: 20493633; PubMed Central PMCID: PMCPMC2914601.

152. Raj SR. Postural tachycardia syndrome (POTS). *Circulation.* 2013;127(23):2336—2342. https://doi.org/10.1161/CIRCULATIONAHA.112.144501. PubMed PMID: 23753844; PubMed Central PMCID: PMCPMC3756553.

153. Offit PA, Quarles J, Gerber MA, et al. Addressing parents' concerns: do multiple vaccines overwhelm or weaken the infant's immune system? *Pediatrics.* 2002;109(1):124—129. PubMed PMID: 11773551.

154. Fombonne E, Zakarian R, Bennett A, Meng L, McLean-Heywood D. Pervasive developmental disorders in Montreal, Quebec, Canada: prevalence and links with immunizations. *Pediatrics.* 2006;118(1):e139—e150. https://doi.org/10.1542/peds.2005-2993. PubMed PMID: 16818529.

155. Smith JC. The structure, role, and procedures of the U.S. Advisory Committee on Immunization Practices (ACIP). *Vaccine.* 2010;28(suppl 1):A68—A75. https://doi.org/10.1016/j.vaccine.2010.02.037. PubMed PMID: 20413002.

156. Smith JC, Snider DE, Pickering LK, Advisory Committee on Immunization Practices. Immunization policy development in the United States: the role of the advisory committee on immunization practices. *Ann Intern Med.* 2009;150(1):45—49. PubMed PMID: 19124820.

157. Centers for Disease Control and Prevention. Prevention and control of influenza with vaccines: recommendations of the Advisory Committee on Immunization Practices (ACIP)—United States, 2012-13 influenza season. *MMWR Morb Mortal Wkly Rep.* 2012;61(32):613—618. PubMed PMID: 22895385.

158. Centers for Disease Control and Prevention, Advisory Committee on Immunization Practices. Update: recommendations from the advisory committee on immunization practices (ACIP) regarding administration of combination MMRV vaccine. *MMWR Morb Mortal Wkly Rep.* 2008;57(10):258—260. PubMed PMID: 18340332.

159. U.S. Food and Drug Administration. Charter of the Vaccines and Related Biological Products Advisory Committee. Available from: https://www.fda.gov/AdvisoryCommittees/CommitteesMeetingMaterials/BloodVaccinesandOtherBiologics/VaccinesandRelatedBiologicalProductsAdvisoryCommittee/ucm129571.htm.

160. Cope JU, Rosenthal GL, Weinel P, Odegaard A, Murphy DM. FDA safety reviews on drugs, biologics, and vaccines: 2007-2013. *Pediatrics.* 2015;136(6):1125—1131. https://doi.org/10.1542/peds.2015-0469. PubMed PMID: 26598453.

161. U.S. Food and Drug Administration. *Center for Drug Evaluation and Research (CDER), Center for Biologics Evaluation and Research (CBER). Guidance for Industry: Safety Labeling Changes—Implementation of Section 505(o)(4) of the FD&C Act;* 2013. Available from: https://www.fda.gov/downloads/drugs/guidancecomplianceregulatoryinformation/guidances/ucm250783.pdf.

162. U.S. Food and Drug Administration. Information Pertaining to Labeling Revision for RotaTeq. Available from: https://www.fda.gov/BiologicsBloodVaccines/Vaccines/ApprovedProducts/ucm142393.htm.

163. U.S. Department of Health and Human Services. *About the National Vaccine Program Office (NVPO)*; 2017. Available from: https://www.hhs.gov/nvpo/about/index.html.

164. Institute of Medicine. *Immunization Safety Review: Measles-mumps-rubella Vaccine and Autism*. Washington, DC: The National Academies Press; 2001.

165. Institute of Medicine. *The Childhood Immunization Schedule and Safety: Stakeholder Concerns, Scientific Evidence, and Future Studies*. Washington, DC: The National Academies Press; 2013.

166. Glanz JM, Newcomer SR, Jackson ML, et al. White Paper on studying the safety of the childhood immunization schedule in the Vaccine Safety Datalink. *Vaccine*. 2016; 34(suppl 1):A1–A29. https://doi.org/10.1016/j.vaccine.2015.10.082. PubMed PMID: 26830300.

167. Institute of Medicine. *Priorities for the National Vaccine Plan. Appendix C, 1986 National Childhood Vaccine Injury Act (Public Law 99-660)*. Washington, DC: The National Academies Press; 2010.

168. Cook KM, Evans G. The national vaccine injury compensation program. *Pediatrics*. 2011;127(suppl 1):S74–S77. https://doi.org/10.1542/peds.2010-1722K. PubMed PMID: 21502255.

169. Centers for Disease Control and Prevention. Announcements: countermeasures injury compensation program. *MMWR Morb Mortal Wkly Rep*. 2010;59(25):780.

CHAPTER 2

Interpersonal Communication Approaches to Increase Adult Vaccine Acceptance

SAAD B. OMER, MBBS, PHD • CAROLINE M. POLAND, LMHC, LCAC, CCTP, NCC • ALLISON T. CHAMBERLAIN, MS, PHD

Background, Vaccines have been an extremely effective tool for reducing morbidity and mortality globally. However, until recently the primary focus of immunization programs has been on childhood vaccination. In recent years there have been promising developments in adult vaccinations, with an increasing emphasis on pregnant and elderly populations. Success in the development of adult vaccines and recommendations for increasing vaccinations of adult populations have not been matched by uptake of adult vaccines. Childhood vaccination coverage is high overall, whereas adult vaccination coverage has lagged substantially.

There are several reasons for the suboptimal uptake of adult vaccines. First, unlike many childhood vaccines that are routine—and in many circumstances required for participation in social activities (e.g., public school attendance)—adult vaccines are unaccompanied by such mandates. Because adult vaccination is largely voluntary, adults need other compelling reasons to vaccinate. These reasons can include a desire to stay healthy (or avoid illness) or to protect the health of others by vaccinating oneself. Second, there are both supply-side and demand-side challenges. Supply-side challenges are logistical factors that can serve as access barriers to adult vaccines. A good example is not stocking vaccines in adult primary care practices. Demand-side challenges are those that reduce or fail to stimulate patient demand or acceptance for the vaccines. An example of a demand-side barrier is a provider who is ineffective in conveying the importance of adult vaccines to patients. Given the traditional focus on the promotion of childhood vaccines, providers who deal with adult populations have not had substantial training in vaccine promotion strategies.

In this chapter we compile several evidence-informed, demand-side interventions to increase vaccination rates. Although a significant proportion of the evidence discussed in this chapter comes from childhood vaccination, it is also relevant to adult populations. Moreover, although there are potentially useful systemic interventions, the primary focus of this chapter is on interpersonal strategies—although these principles can also be adapted to systems-level and mass communication interventions.

GENERAL CONSIDERATIONS FOR INTERPERSONAL COMMUNICATIONS INTERVENTIONS

There are several common misconceptions regarding vaccines—and adult vaccines are no exception. For example, many adults report false beliefs such as influenza vaccine gives recipients "the flu," natural infection is better than vaccination, and vaccines administered during pregnancy can result in adverse birth outcomes such as preterm birth. An understandable response to encountering these misconceptions is to correct them. However, there are risks associated with attempts to correct misinformation.

Since the 1950s, psychologists have known about the so-called boomerang effect. In this phenomenon people receiving information contrary to their preexisting beliefs not only discard new information but also become even more supportive of their original views.[1] This effect has been replicated in the context of vaccines as well.

In a randomized controlled trial involving more than 1700 parents with children less than 17 years old, researchers evaluated what messaging strategies

Vaccinations. https://doi.org/10.1016/B978-0-323-55435-0.00002-1

work best in attempting to debunk the myth that the Measles, Mumps, and Rubella (MMR) vaccine causes autism.[2] In the stratified analysis of parents by their baseline attitudes toward vaccination, among those parents with the least favorable attitudes toward vaccination, attempting to correct their misperceptions about a link between MMR vaccination and autism actually resulted in a significant *decrease* in their intention of vaccinating another child with MMR vaccine. Among parents with more favorable attitudes toward vaccination, there was no change in intention to vaccinate. Interestingly this effect on intention to vaccinate was observed while parents' scores on factual knowledge about vaccines increased, suggesting that deeply held misperceptions may not be overcome by simply providing more factual information.

Another thing to remember when crafting vaccine-related messages is that humans are excellent linguists but are poor "statisticians" in that our assessment of event probability is not intuitive. For example, most children, from an early age, can differentiate between feelings such as sad and bored, whereas many people cannot viscerally distinguish between probabilities of substantially different magnitudes.

One study conducted among 369 mothers of children aged below 5 years revealed some interesting findings regarding awareness of the statistical probabilities of risk, disease severity, and the power of regret.[3] The study, among other things, presented women with absolute numbers showing that the risk of an unvaccinated child contracting a disease is substantially higher than the risk of having a vaccine-associated adverse event. However, presentation of these probabilities did not matter in terms of increasing vaccine acceptance. What mattered more was the perceived severity of the disease or adverse event. If a mother perceived the disease as more severe than the adverse event, she would tend to vaccinate. Additionally, when it came to the influence of regret, women anticipated significantly greater regret from a decision not to vaccinate than a decision to vaccinate. Although similar findings have not been observed in every study—for example, a study conducted among 684 parents after the 2009–2010 H1N1 influenza pandemic revealed that factors such as familial influence and self-efficacy were more influential in pandemic vaccine acceptance than perceptions of disease risk and severity—the power that understanding disease severity can have within the context of discussions about vaccine-associated adverse events is noteworthy. The implication is that in vaccine-related conversations with patients particularly concerned about potential harms caused by vaccines, there should be a higher focus on the severity of disease rather than the frequency or probability of such an event.

INTRODUCTION TO APPROACHES TO PATIENT-PROVIDER COMMUNICATION

The communication approaches discussed in this chapter are derived from a variety of disciplines including behavioral economics and clinical and social psychology. Because of this interdisciplinary focus, the elements we focus on extend beyond simple provision of factual information to patients. Research shows that vaccination reluctance or refusal results from more than a simple lack of knowledge. It can be rooted in deeply held beliefs and can be greatly influenced by family members, friends, or peers. It can also be influenced by the way clinical conversations about vaccinations are approached.

Although most individuals encountered in a clinical setting will be accepting the recommended vaccines, some may have questions. Those who have questions are likely to lie somewhere between vaccine refuser and outright acceptor, with very few individuals completely refusing all vaccines. When a healthcare provider encounters an individual (or parent) who is hesitant about receiving vaccines (or administering vaccines to her child), whether she has just a few specific questions or seems reluctant overall, how the healthcare provider discusses vaccines is as important as what the provider says. People who are questioning the decision to vaccinate will not only listen to what is said but pay close attention to how the topic is approached, the manner in which advice is offered, and the confidence with which the healthcare provider speaks about the specific vaccine topic. These aspects are incorporated in subsequent sections.

The three approaches discussed in this chapter are presumptive communication, motivational interviewing, and a cognitive style–based intervention (Table 2.1). Just as therapeutic approaches often need to be adapted to the clinical situation, vaccine communication often needs to be adapted to the population being targeted for vaccination and the individual being encouraged to receive the vaccine.

PRESUMPTIVE COMMUNICATION

One particular technique that has been used effectively in patient-provider communication about vaccination is the presumptive communication approach.[4] In this method the healthcare provider presumes the patient will choose to vaccinate, using both verbal and

TABLE 2.1
A Summary of Communication Approaches Discussed in This Chapter

Approach Name	Description of the Approach	Resource Requirement	Potential Application
Presumptive communication	In this approach the provider presumes the patient will choose to vaccinate using both verbal and nonverbal cues to steer the patient toward a decision to vaccinate. The most powerful feature of this approach is that it sets vaccination as the default choice for the patient.	Minimal resource requirement. Healthcare providers need to be familiar with this approach. It is important that everyone in the clinic, not just the provider, conveys vaccination as the default option.	This could be the approach to start vaccine conversations with many patients. Depending on how the patient responds, the healthcare provider can switch other approaches, such as motivational interviewing.
Motivational interviewing	In this approach patients begin to voice the reasons for change while helping them to develop an intrinsic motivation. This allows the patient to develop an increased sense of agency and to be a healthy "expert in his/her own life".	Healthcare provider education on the four parts of MI (OARS).	For patients who are struggling to see reasons for change (i.e., vaccine acceptance) or for patients who have a lower level of agency or confidence in self to make decisions.
Preferred cognitive styles	Through an understanding of a patient's internal world and thought processes, the healthcare provider can help them move toward accepting vaccines. Through learning the specific strategies associated with each of the cognitive styles, a healthcare provider can "speak the same language" as the patient in a more effective way, using communication strategies that increase the likelihood for change to occur.	Healthcare provider education on the types of cognitive styles and the communication styles that best fit each style.	This is helpful for all patients, especially those who have a preferred cognitive style unlike the analytical, fact driven style in which a lot of health communication is delivered.

nonverbal cues to steer the patient toward a decision to vaccinate. As such, the most powerful feature of this approach is that it sets vaccination as the default choice for the patient. By presuming vaccination will occur, it requires the patient make a conscious decision to decline vaccination rather than to accept vaccination. This strategy of aligning decision-making defaults with the desired decisional outcome is also a cornerstone of behavioral economics, a growing field of inquiry exploring how human psychology explains economic decision-making.

The most direct way to illustrate this approach is through its relatively simple verbal architecture, the effectiveness of which is based entirely on how vaccines are presented to the patient (Fig. 2.1). An approach most extensively researched by Opel et al. revealed that instead of asking a patient whether or not he or she would want to receive a vaccine, simply changing the "ask" to an "announcement" substantially increased vaccine acceptance (Douglas J).[5] For example, instead of asking a patient, "Would you like to receive a flu vaccine today?" stating "It's time to receive a flu vaccine," can increase vaccine acceptance. This simple change alters the choice architecture of the vaccination decision itself, presenting vaccination as the norm or default choice. By engaging the patient in this manner, the

Framing
Presume Vaccination

Making vaccination the default choice for your patients should frame your entire approach.

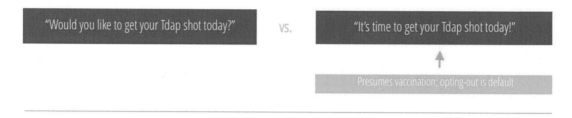

FIG. 2.1 Framing vaccine communications messages.

healthcare provider can more effectively shift the decision-making balance in favor of vaccination rather than away from it. Although research has shown this presumptive approach to be effective in improving willingness to vaccine, one area to address in future research is how providers feel about using this approach.

It is important to note that although the success of the presumptive approach is rooted in its inherent ability to immediately convey a preference or a norm to a patient, it does not and should not preclude a patient from seeking further advice or guidance from his provider in regard to vaccine questions. The verbal architecture of the presumptive approach should not come across so strong so as to be viewed as coercive, paternalistic, or bullyish. With that said, there is a fine line between an effective use of the presumptive approach and an overbearing use of the approach. Although more research is necessary to definitively declare when switching from a more presumptive stance to a more participatory stance is warranted, a good rule of thumb is to normalize the presumptive strategy as the way to initiate a vaccine conversation across all visits in which a vaccine is anticipated. By using this approach routinely to initiate the discussion, the provider immediately conveys his or her professional opinion of the topic (i.e., that vaccination is

the right choice) in a way that is both definitive, yet comfortably normal. It is then up to the patient to challenge the status quo, which if they choose to do so should be addressed in a respectful and professional manner.

The presumptive approach can be further bolstered by structural or cultural changes to how vaccines are managed within a clinic. For example, establishing standing orders that enable nurses or medical assistants to administer routine vaccines before a provider's prescription of the vaccine enables the staff to operationalize the theme that vaccination is the norm in the practice. Standing orders have been shown to markedly increase vaccination rates[6,7], and this is due primarily to their ability to remove the need for a provider's prescription.

Clinic staff members often play just as important a role in interacting with patients as the provider does, and making the staff aware of this fact is essential. Involving the staff themselves can also substantially bolster a practice's portrayal that vaccination is the norm. It can also gain their buy-in to a cultural shift in the way vaccines are managed and promoted to patients. Teaching the staff how and when to use the presumptive approach themselves can also empower them to effect change in the patients they serve.

MOTIVATIONAL INTERVIEWING

Motivational interviewing (MI) is another technique that can be used in patient-provider communication as it is a patient-centered approach. The goal of this approach is to allow the patient to begin to voice reasons for change (even ones in which they may not initially agree). William Miller, one of the creators of the MI approach, wrote the following about the approach: "Special attention was focused on evoking and strengthening the client's own verbalized motivations for change… Pushing or arguing against resistance seemed particularly counterproductive in that it evoked further defense of the status quo. A guiding principle of MI was to have the client, rather than the counselor, voice the arguments for change." (Ref. 8 p. 528).

Encouraging the patient to voice arguments for change leads the patient to develop more openness to the idea than before, making way for behavior change that ideally would remain sustained. When people voice reasons for an action or behavior, even one they are in opposition to, research shows that their attitudes and behaviors begin to shift in the direction they are voicing. This change and the development of a new perspective is a process and should not be expected to occur immediately. An added benefit of engaging in the MI process in one area of health (i.e., vaccinations) is that the intrinsic motivation that has been strengthened and can be applied to other areas as well (i.e., smoking cessation or exercise adherence). Within this patient-centered style of communication, the patient's goals can be briefly explored, and change can be discussed and processed within his or her personal goal or value framework (Ref. 9 p. 1024). MI has been shown to be useful across a broad range of behaviors and concerns.

Expressing empathy and helping the patient develop intrinsic motivation is done through OARS communication: open-ended questions, affirmations, reflective listening, and summary statements (Table 2.2). These four communication components include the patient in the decision-making process, leading to a collaborative process between the provider and the patient.

Through the empathy expressed with MI, it is possible for the healthcare provider to relate to the patient's worldview and engage in a patient-centered approach. These techniques allow the healthcare provider, in a brief clinical encounter, to assess what drives the patient's underlying values that influence his or her decisions about vaccines. As the patient is treated as the expert in his or her own life and the healthcare

provider responds with openness and empathy, a safe environment is provided for the patient to express these values about his or her health. It is critical for the healthcare provider to try to identify values that both the patient and provider share and with which they both agree. Taking an example from childhood vaccine promotion, a hesitant mother of young children might identify a value as "I want to do my best to protect my child, which is why I'm hesitant to let my child receive a vaccine." The healthcare provider might respond by saying "A value of mine is also helping to protect your child. It sounds like we overlap in that." That allows the patient and provider to feel they are "on the same team" and working toward the same goal or value. Defenses that may have been in place previously slowly drop when mutual ground and values are identified. Relating to the patient's worldview, especially through the process of MI, should remain a priority for the provider.

In MI the healthcare provider allows the patient to be the expert in his or her own life, and the healthcare provider is taking the "one-down stance" to the patient. Taking a "one-down stance" means that the provider takes on the stance of a curious learner to the life and thought processes of the patient. It allows the patient to be in control, and doing so communicates empathy and respect for the patient. Instead of taking on a position of power or lecturing, the provider steps down and allows a conversation to occur. A critical piece in this process of respect building is for the healthcare provider to seek permission to share information with the patient.

Although MI can be beneficial, patients may continue to refuse vaccines. When vaccine refusal has been documented in the patient's chart, it is important to go back to this conversation in future visits (again engaging in a respectful and not forceful or lecturing process). In revisiting this topic, it is important for the healthcare provider to continue engaging with the patients with them as the expert in his or her life. If this is a new patient to the healthcare provider, it might be helpful to start by saying "In looking over your chart, I noticed that you have rejected this vaccine in the past. Can you tell me more about that?" With a returning patient to the healthcare provider, ways to engage in that conversation may go as follows: "I recall last time you were here you were hesitant about ___ vaccine. I'd like to circle back to that and hear where you're at today? Are there any additional thoughts, questions, or concerns you have about that vaccine?"

TABLE 2.2
Summary of Motivational Interviewing Techniques Applied to Vaccine-Related Communications

	What the Purpose is of This Component	How to Do This/Examples of Statements or Questions	Additional Helpful Notes
Open-ended questions	This keeps conversation flowing with the patient doing most of the talking. This builds a trusting relationship and allows the healthcare provider to gain an understanding of patient values, beliefs, etc.	• What questions might you have today? • What are your current hesitations with receiving this vaccine? • How can I be of help to you today?	Avoid why questions here (reframe to a what or how question) as why questions can sound accusatory.
Affirmations	With affirmations, the healthcare provider points out strengths they see in the patient or ways that the patient has already made a good decision for themselves. This not only shows that the healthcare provider is present in the conversation but also is crucial to the trust-building process. This also helps build up the patient's self-efficacy.	• (to a nervous patient) "I know it can be hard to make a doctor's appointment, and I'm glad that you decided to take care of yourself by coming in today." • "I can see that you're putting effort into taking care of yourself by working out regularly."	This requires very attentive listening.
Reflective listening	By reflecting back what the healthcare provider is hearing to the patient, the patient has an opportunity to externally look at his or her beliefs and words allowing him/her to consider different decisions or behavioral changes.	• Simply repeat back what the patient just stated • "You're feeling concerned/confused because ____" • Repeat back what the client was saying but in an exaggerated manner (so are you saying that there are no instances in which ____	This tends to be the most difficult communication component within MI.
Summary statements	Allows the healthcare provider to pull together what has been discussed and make sure that the healthcare provider and patient are on the same page of understanding.	• "So far we've talked about ____" • "Previously you had mentioned ____ concern about vaccination, and just now we discussed ____" • "We've discussed your concerns, and you sound a little more sure about your decision to receive a vaccine today."	

COGNITIVE STYLE–BASED INTERVIEWING

MI overlaps nicely with many other communication styles and therapeutic models, including the Preferred Cognitive Styles and Health Decision Making Model (PCSDM). This model, created by one of the authors (Poland) of this chapter, was first published about in 2011.[10] A foundational idea of the PCSDM is that individuals do not make decisions in the same manner, and therefore to treat patients in a singular and formulaic way will lead to poor results, especially in vaccine acceptance. The PCSDM model acknowledges that an understanding of a patient's internal world and thought processes are critical in helping them move toward accepting vaccines. Underlying the model is the well-documented finding that individuals have different cognitive biases and use various heuristics while making decisions, especially under conditions of uncertainty.[11] It is critical for healthcare providers to not only understand these various cognitive biases and styles but also to understand how to best talk with and communicate information according to that patient's preferred cognitive style. A cognitive style is a basic thinking style that each person generally adheres to. It impacts how the individual both perceives and processes information, particularly under conditions of uncertainty.[12] The concept is basic—understand the preferred method by which someone processes information and makes decisions and mimic that process in designing your education specifically for that patient. While many providers, because of their training, may use cognitive styles that are very analytic, educating a patient should first involve determining his or her preferred cognitive style (Ref. 13 p. 347).

In similar ways to MI, the healthcare provider is seeking to understand the patient's internal world, tailoring communication to that patient and allowing them to be an expert in his or her own life and his or her own styles of decision-making. Each individual

has a primary cognitive style that they use while making various types of decisions but may also use other styles to help in processing information. As mentioned previously, most often information is presented within the health field by the healthcare provider in a very analytical way, focusing on facts and data (an example of this is the Vaccine Information Sheets). That is because healthcare providers themselves, generally by virtue of their predisposition toward science, as well as their training and professionalization, are more comfortable with this analytical style. Although this strategy is seen as the "correct way" for an analytical-style healthcare provider, it can be counterproductive to someone who is using a fear-based or denialist cognitive style. A

TABLE 2.3
Summary of Cognitive Styles and the Best Approaches for Each Style

Cognitive Style	Main Effect	Verbal Expression	Approach
Denialist	Disbelieves accepted scientific facts, despite overwhelming evidence. Prone to believe conspiracy theories	"I don't care what the data show, I don't believe the vaccine is safe"	Provide consistent messaging repeatedly over time from trustworthy sources, provide educational materials, solicit questions, avoid "hard sell" approach, use motivational interviewing approaches
Innumerate	Cannot understand or has difficulty manipulating numbers, probabilities, or risks	"One-in-a-million risk sounds high, for sure I'll be the 1 in a million that has a side effect, I'll avoid the vaccine"	Provide nonmathematical information, analogies, or comparators using a more holistic "right brain" or emotive approach
Fear-based	Decision-making based on fears	"I heard vaccines are harmful and I'm not going to get them"	Understand source of fear, provide consistent positive approach, show risks in comparison to other daily risks, demonstrate risks of not receiving vaccines, use social norming approaches
Heuristic	Often appeals to availability heuristic (what I can recall equates with how commonly it occurs)	"I remember GBS happened in 1977 after flu vaccines, that must be common, and therefore I'm not getting a flu vaccine"	Point out inconsistencies and fallacy of heuristic thinking, provide educational materials, appeal to other heuristics
Bandwagoning	Primarily influenced by what others are doing or saying	"If others are refusing the vaccine there must be something to it, I'm going to skip getting the vaccine"	Understand primary influencers, point out logical inconsistencies, use social-norming and self-efficacy approaches
Analytical	Left brain thinking, facts are paramount	"I want to see the data so I can make a decision"	Provide data requested, review analytically with patient

This table was originally published in Poland CM, Poland GA. Vaccine education spectrum disorder: the importance of incorporating psychological and cognitive models into vaccine education. *Vaccine*. 2011;29(37);6145–6148. https://doi.org/10.1016/j.vaccine.2011.07.131.

patient's cognitive style acts as a lens through which they receive information.

In illustrating the PCSDM model, the authors of the model have discussed the more common cognitive styles: denialist, innumerate, fear-based, heuristic, bandwagoning, and analytical (Table 2.3).

Layered over the PCSDM (as well as previously discussed approaches such as MI) is the idea of belief-dependent realism. Humans tend to believe that they are rational beings, making wise and appropriate decisions. However, people "form beliefs for a variety of subjective, personal, emotional, and psychological reasons in the context of environments created by family, friends, colleagues, culture, and society at large; after forming beliefs, we then defend, justify, and rationalize them with a host of intellectual reasons, cogent arguments, and rational explanations. *Beliefs come first, explanations for beliefs follow.*" (Ref. 14 p. 5) Preferred cognitive styles play out in the process of belief-dependent realism, creating a lens from which our beliefs impact how we view data, stories, and information. The PCSDM, layered with MI techniques, allow for a process in which the lens slowly begins to change, allowing explanations to begin to form beliefs.

MESSAGE CONTENT

In addition to overall vaccine communication approaches, the content of the message itself is important (Fig. 2.2). Discussions with vaccine-hesitant individuals should not only focus on side effects of vaccines; consequences of vaccine-preventable diseases should be front and center in such discussions. Individuals are not often familiar with how dangerous some of these diseases can be for themselves and their loved ones. Instead, they may be more familiar and more fearful of well-publicized reports of rare adverse events occurring after vaccination—events that in most cases, may not have been causally related to the vaccination itself. Therefore it is important to emphasize that diseases such as pneumococcal pneumonia, influenza, pertussis, and tetanus have not been eradicated and do pose great threats to those who are most vulnerable.

When pivoting to the disease, there is a fine line between informing a patient and intimidating or scaring a patient. As mentioned previously, research has shown that emphasizing the severity of the disease can be effective in overcoming concerns over serious but extremely rare adverse events associated with vaccination. But when emphasizing disease severity, a provider can all too easily frighten patients with daunting stories of illness or death. Providers therefore must straddle this line carefully because the purpose is not to scare patients into getting vaccinated. Rather the goal is to shift the focus of the conversation, in a very matter-of-fact manner, from myths about the vaccine to facts about the disease. Once an individual has been given information about how serious vaccine-preventable diseases can be, then they should be eager to hear about what they can do to protect themselves.[15] It is vital at this

Content
Guiding Principles

Be knowledgeable about the severity of the diseases

Be able to provide 1 or 2 easy facts for patients to remember

Be informative, but not scary

Avoid statistics: Humans are bad statisticians, but good linguists

Focus on the facts you want to communicate

FIG. 2.2 Guiding principles for vaccination messaging content.

point in the conversation to provide the patient with the fact that vaccination is the single best way to get protected from these risks. This concept is based in what is called the extended parallel processing model.

This model is a theoretical framework developed to improve the effectiveness of risk communications and to understand human behavior when confronted with risks. It is a model that has been studied extensively among healthcare workers and emergency responders, such as firefighters, to gauge their willingness to respond after a large-scale disaster. Research applying this model to practice has shown that a person is more willing to respond to an unknown risk when they perceive the threat to be great, and they have a solid understanding of what they can do to protect themselves from that threat. In other words, they know what self-efficacious actions they can do to protect themselves from that risk and that the actions they take are effective. Translating these concepts then to vaccine acceptance means that individuals with the greatest understanding of disease risk and the greatest awareness that the act of vaccinating will protect them from that risk will be more likely to vaccinate than those who do not know about disease risks or view vaccination as the best way to protect themselves.

While most vaccine messages are focused on protecting the patient himself/herself, highlighting the risk of disease and benefits of vaccines for the patient's loved ones can be helpful (community/"herd" immunity–based appeals may only be effective in collectivistic societies).[16] For example, in the case of pregnant women, bringing up the ability of a vaccine administered during pregnancy to protect her newborn against diseases such as influenza and pertussis could be useful. Similarly, for the elderly it is appropriate to talk about potential indirect protection for their grandchildren.

CORRECTING MYTHS

Sometimes there is no choice but to tackle the misconception directly. In these cases the following steps modified from the "Debunking Handbook" are useful to remember: First, clearly state that what the individual believes is a myth and avoid repeating the myth.[17] Although this approach may risk evoking defensiveness on the part of the patient, this strategy is important because it makes your view on this issue clear to the patient (Table 2.4). Second, explain in a succinct and understandable way why the myth is not true.

Too much information may inadvertently reinforce the myth, whereas a few straightforward facts may be helpful in decreasing misperception. Then finally, and

TABLE 2.4
Steps for Addressing a Vaccine-Related Myth Directly

Step	Influenza Vaccine Causes the Flu Myth: Provider Responses
1. Clearly state, in a matter-of-fact way, that the patient's assertion is a myth	"Sounds like staying healthy is a primary concern for you, and that is very important. But I must reiterate that *influenza vaccines do not cause the flu*. That is a myth."
2. State why the myth is not true	"Flu shots, like the type that you get in your arm, are made entirely from killed, or inactivated flu virus. That means that the virus particles in the shot are not able to make you sick."
3. Replace the myth with the best alternative explanation	"What the flu shot does do is activate your immune system to help your body build its defenses against flu. When this happens, you may feel achy, almost like you do when you are getting sick. These symptoms are usually mild, and it is important to remember that this is just your body reacting to the vaccine to help build your immunity."

Based on the principles outlined in: Cook J, Lewandowsky S. *The Debunking Handbook.* St. Lucia, Australia: University of Queensland; 2011.

most importantly, replace the myth with the next best alternative explanation. The reason why this is critical is because if the healthcare provider has been successful in debunking the myth for the individual, a kind of information void has been created in her mind. When that happens, the patient will have a desire to fill that void with another plausible explanation for whatever association the myth was explaining. This is a healthcare provider's opportunity then to clearly and confidently share an easy fact with the patient. In fact, this is a good opportunity to pivot to discussing disease severity.

CONCLUSION

In recent years, the evidence base relevant to vaccine acceptance interventions has expanded, and several evidence-informed approaches have emerged. Of these, presumptive communication is a promising approach to use when starting vaccine-related conversations in a clinical setting (and in mass communication campaigns). For some individuals, MI and PCSDM provide options for more intensive engagement to address vaccine-related concerns. Irrespective of the approach, the message content should highlight the disease rather than just rebutting the myths. In situations in which it is unavoidable to rebut the myth, there are principles that focus on rebutting the myth instead of arguing against it. Most importantly it is useful to continue the conversation with vaccine-hesitant individuals. Persuasion approaches might not be effective the first time; however, discontinuing the relationship with vaccine-hesitant individuals ends the conversation and is a lost opportunity to persuade the patient through subsequent interaction. Finally, vaccine acceptance and communication science is an active area of research with an ever-expanding evidence base. Therefore those interested in and/or responsible for addressing vaccine hesitancy need to stay abreast of latest developments in this field.

ACKNOWLEDGMENTS

Some of the content was adapted from the VaxChat CME module for Obstetricians developed by Drs. Chamberlain and Omer with input from the P3+ study team. The VaxChat module was developed with support from NIH grant R01AI110482 (MPIs Saad Omer and Daniel Salmon).

REFERENCES

1. Hovland CI, Janis IL, Kelley HH. *Communication and Persuasion: Psychological Studies of Opinion Change*. New Haven Yale University Press; 1953.
2. Nyhan B, Reifler J, Richey S, Freed GL. Effective messages in vaccine promotion: a randomized trial. *Pediatrics*. 2014; 133(4):e835–e842. https://doi.org/10.1542/peds.2013-2365.
3. Sadique MZ, Devlin N, Edmunds WJ, Parkin D. The effect of perceived risks on the demand for vaccination: results from a discrete choice experiment. *PLoS One*. 2013;8(2): e54149. https://doi.org/10.1371/journal.pone.0054149.
4. Opel DJ, Omer SB. Measles, mandates, and making vaccination the default option. *JAMA Pediatr*. 2015;169(4): 303–304. https://doi.org/10.1001/jamapediatrics.2015.0291.
5. Opel DJ, Heritage J, Taylor JA, et al. The architecture of provider-parent vaccine discussions at health supervision visits. *Pediatrics*. 2013;132(6):1037–1046.
6. Ogburn T, Espey EL, Contreras V, Arroyo P. Impact of clinic interventions on the rate of influenza vaccination in pregnant women. *J Reprod Med*. 2007;52(9):753–756.
7. Yonas MA, Nowalk MP, Zimmerman RK, Ahmed F, Albert SM. Examining structural and clinical factors associated with implementation of standing orders for adult immunization. *J Healthc Qual*. 2012;34(3):34–42. https://doi.org/10.1111/j.1945-1474.2011.00144.x.
8. Miller WR, Rose GS. Toward a theory of motivational interviewing. *Am Psychol*. 2009;64(6):527–537. https://doi.org/10.1037/a0016830.
9. Borrelli B, Riekert KA, Weinstein A, Rathier L. Brief motivational interviewing as a clinical strategy to promote asthma medication adherence. *J Allergy Clin Immunol*. 2007;120(5): 1023–1030. https://doi.org/10.1016/j.jaci.2007.08.017.
10. Poland CM, Poland GA. Vaccine education spectrum disorder: the importance of incorporating psychological and cognitive models into vaccine education. *Vaccine*. 2011; 29(37):6145–6148. https://doi.org/10.1016/j.vaccine.2011.07.131.
11. Kahneman D. *Thinking, Fast and Slow*. 1st ed. New York: Farrar, Straus and Giroux; 2011.
12. Harder JT, Czyzewski A, Sherwood AL. Student self-efficacy in a chosen business career path: the influence of cognitive style. *Coll Student J*. 2015;49(3):341–354.
13. Poland GA, Poland CM, Jacobson RM, Opel DJ, Marcuse EK. Political, ethical, social, and psychological aspects of vaccinology. In: Milligan GN, Barrett ADT, eds. *Vaccinology: An Essential Guide*. Chichester, West Sussex: John Wiley and Sons, Inc; 2015:335–357.
14. Shermer M. *The Believing Brain: From Ghosts and Gods to Politics and Conspiracies — How We Construct Beliefs and Reinforce Them as Truths New York*. New York: Henry Holt and Company, LLC; 2011.
15. Omer SB, Amin AB, Limaye RJ. Communicating about vaccines in a fact-resistant world. *JAMA Pediatr*. 2017; 171(10):929–930. https://doi.org/10.1001/jamapediatrics.2017.2219.
16. Bohm R, Betsch C, Korn L, Holtmann C. Exploring and promoting prosocial vaccination: a cross-cultural experiment on vaccination of health care personnel. *Biomed Res Int*. 2016;2016:6870984. https://doi.org/10.1155/2016/6870984.
17. Cook J, Lewandowsky S. *The Debunking Handbook*. St. Lucia, Australia: University of Queensland; 2011.

CHAPTER 3

Special Considerations for Vaccines and the Elderly

ELIE SAADE, MD, MPH • DAVID H. CANADAY, MD •
H. EDWARD DAVIDSON, PHARMD, MPH • LISA F. HAN, MPH •
STEFAN GRAVENSTEIN, MD, MPH, MPH (HON), FACP, AGSF, FGSA

INTRODUCTION

The epidemiology, clinical manifestation, and the ability for vaccines to prevent or alter the course of infection changes as people age, with older adults typically having milder initial presentation, more severe consequences, and declining vaccine effectiveness. When we refer to "older," we often arbitrarily mean age 50, 65, 75, or 80 years and older, depending on the parameters set by the given study. In all cases, these generalized observations still hold true with age-related risk.

In addition to age, a second factor affecting disease expression and vaccine effectiveness is the increasing likelihood of having health conditions and their treatments that further modulate immune response and thereby response to vaccines, symptom presentation, pathogen clearance, and pace of recovery. Additional factors for older adults relate to exposure risk such as from caregivers, family, and others living in close quarters (e.g., institutionalized settings), along with issues related to resources, diet, and hygiene.

Vaccines offer one of the few proven ways to directly modulate infection risk, including the risk in older adults. Vaccines can also indirectly affect infection risks that are not direct sequelae of the vaccine-specific infection. For example, an individual who avoids influenza infection will also have reduced risk for staphylococcus and aspiration pneumonia, a potential downstream benefit of influenza vaccination. In the hospital setting, older adults are often at high risk for aspiration pneumonia, for a variety of reasons, including certain neurologic disorders such as dementia, stroke, and Parkinson's disease. Similarly, those with chronic obstructive pulmonary disease are at high risk for acute bronchitis. Both the severity and risk for these outcomes could be modified by influenza and pneumococcal

vaccination. Furthermore, lower infection rates and fewer antibiotic prescriptions resulting from vaccination could potentially have effects on the flora related to indwelling urinary catheters and urinary tract infections. The same potential reduction in antibiotic exposure should attenuate the elevated risk older individuals have for *Clostridium difficile* and its complications.[1]

Gerontologists argue that increased inflammaging is a feature of aging and have coined the term "inflammaging," which occurs alongside the declining immune regulation and its consequences, immunosenescence. The beneficial impact of inflammation in younger populations becomes detrimental with aging due to factors such as macrophage dysregulation, reduction of innate immunity regulation, and so forth. Together, these then produce what we consider the low-level chronic inflammatory status typically seen in elderly individuals.[2] Inflammaging affects both the primary infectious clinical syndrome and the secondary consequences such as a prothrombotic milieu that is created by the active infection.

Among infections that disproportionately affect older adults, the VPDs are of particular public health concern, especially given both the relative cost-effectiveness of vaccines currently recommended for this age group and the low vaccine uptake. Using data from peer-reviewed literature and government disease-surveillance programs, McLaughlin et al. estimated that the annual cost for VPD in the United States (US) in 2013 was $26.5 billion for adults aged 50 years and older, including $15.3 billion for those aged 65 years and older.[3] These costs are likely to increase with the aging of the population and do not fully account for some indirect vaccine benefits noted previously. Clearly there are geriatrics-specific issues related to vaccines that can have a significant impact on morbidity, mortality, and cost, and these are the subject of this review.

AGE, A SOCIODEMOGRAPHIC RISK FOR GETTING DISEASE

There is a wide variation in vaccination coverage influenced by social, demographic, and economic factors.[4] Using global distribution of influenza vaccine doses as a proxy for vaccination coverage rates, the International Federation of Pharmaceutical Manufacturers and Associations estimated that only 23 countries had a sufficient vaccine supply in 2015 to achieve a vaccination rate superior to 75% in their elderly population. We will largely restrict our discussion to US health-related factors because of the scope of this review. In the US, where the seasonal vaccination coverage in the elderly for the 2015–16 season was estimated at 63%, health-related behavior is affected by aspects of knowledge, attitude, beliefs, and practices including sociodemographic determinants, perception of disease severity, and awareness of vaccine recommendations. According to the Centers for Disease Control and Prevention (CDC) National Health Interview Survey, which collects information from a nationally representative sample of noninstitutionalized US civilian population, socioeconomic differences in vaccination coverage persist in all age groups, including old adults. Higher coverage is observed for whites than for most other groups, including in institutionalized settings.[5] An increase in vaccination uptake among whites in recent years contributes to a widening of the differences compared to prior years. For example, influenza vaccination coverage among whites aged ≥ 65 years (75.1%) is higher than that for blacks (64.3%) and Hispanics (64.1%); even though the trend is similar to younger adults, the disparity is wider in the older group. A similar phenomenon is seen for pneumococcal vaccination (68.1%, 50.2%, and 41.7% in elderly whites, blacks, and Hispanics, respectively) and herpes zoster (HZ) vaccination in persons aged ≥ 60 years (34.6%, 13.6%, and 16% in elderly whites, blacks, and Hispanics, respectively).[5]

Other socioeconomic and sociodemographic factors contribute to differential immunization uptake.[6–9] Vaccination coverage is lower among adults without health insurance, even after adjusting for confounding factors, and lowering the financial barriers to receiving vaccines increases vaccine uptake.[10] In addition, foreign-born elderly persons and, among those, individuals without US citizenship are less likely than others to be vaccinated.[11,12] Some studies show that elderly adults who are married or are living with others have a higher vaccine acceptance and uptake rate; however, those who are caregivers of children or old or sick people may, conversely, have a lower probability of being vaccinated.[6]

Higher education level and health-related literacy may have a positive influence on vaccination acceptance. Vaccination rates tend to be higher in those with better economic status, although some studies show either no difference or an inverse relationship. Place of residence may determine ease of vaccine access, but studies about differences between urban and rural settings have yielded variable results. Patients who are enrolled with the Veterans Affairs (VA) system have a higher rate of vaccination, likely related to a multifaceted intervention that includes patient reminders, standing orders, free-standing vaccination clinics, and clinician incentives. Nursing homes with standing order policies for annual influenza vaccination have higher rates with less racial disparity than those without such policies.[6–9,13,14]

AGE, CLINICAL PRESENTATION, AND VACCINE PREVENTABLE DISEASE

As people age, their presentation and outcomes for the three leading VPDs changes. The best available data relate to hospitalization and mortality risk, but there are also clinical data, especially for influenza, on the relationship of prior vaccination and the risk for acquiring disease, clinical presentation, and disease severity. In all cases, vaccines appear to attenuate risk for developing disease but also its clinical symptoms on presentation when vaccines fail to prevent the targeted disease.

Age and Clinical Presentation of Influenza

The risk for influenza and pneumonia-related morbidity and mortality increases with age, for many interrelated reasons, and the clinical presentation differs. Influenza typically presents with respiratory symptoms that include any combination of localizing symptoms of sniffling, coryza, sneezing, wheezing, sore throat, coughing, dyspnea, watery eyes, nausea, vomiting and diarrhea, and systemic symptoms of myalgia, malaise, and fever. Aside from malaise, these symptoms are largely milder in older adults (Table 3.1)

We and others have reported that presenting symptoms change and are attenuated when infection occurs despite vaccination[17,18] (Fig. 3.1). In addition the

TABLE 3.1
Changing Clinical Symptoms of Influenza With Age[15,16]

Sign/Symptom	Children	Adults	Elderly
Cough (nonproductive)	++	++++	+++
Fever	+++	+++	+
Myalgia	+	+	+
Headache	++	++	+
Malaise	+	+	+++
Sore throat	+	++	+
Rhinitis/nasal congestion	++	++	+
Abdominal pain/diarrhea	+	−	+
Nausea/vomiting	++	−	+

+, least frequent; ++++, most frequent; −, not found.

symptoms can be clinically indistinguishable between various respiratory viral infections in both community-dwelling and institutionalized elderly.[19,20]

Early recognition of influenza or influenza-like illness (ILI) prompt treatment initiation, and prophylaxis measures are key to successful outbreak control in long-term care (LTC). Although presentation of ILI varies even in younger individuals, clinical presentation usually includes one or more symptoms (e.g., abrupt onset of fever, chills, myalgias, and headache along with sore throat and cough) but may be subtler or even absent in older adults, complicating early recognition. They may instead have a blunted febrile response to infection and exhibit mainly a decline in functional status and other clinical indicators (Fig. 3.2), such as new or increasing confusion, incontinence, falling, deteriorating mobility, reduced food intake, or failure to cooperate with the staff.[21–23]

Vaccine preventable disability

Influenza illness negatively affects the ability of elderly individuals to independently perform the basic activities of daily living (ADLs), such as dressing, eating, toileting, personal hygiene, and ambulation; unintentional weight loss, infections, and pressure ulcers have also been associated with functional decline. In a retrospective longitudinal study, Gozalo et al. found that nursing home (NH) quality as measured by ADL decline, weight loss, pressure ulcers, and

infections is significantly and negatively impacted coincidentally and proportional to local influenza severity, suggesting that seasonal influenza has a major negative impact on the quality of life for the surviving NH elderly population.[21] Elderly patients who are hospitalized face the prospect of a higher level of care at discharge, and a minority of patients experience catastrophic disability and loss of independence. McElhaney et al. report that among older adults, the effects of influenza infection may extend beyond the acute period, with subsequent decrease in independence and functioning, increased frailty, disability, care requirements, and costs. Frailty, a state of increased vulnerability to adverse outcomes relative to others of the same age, may also contribute to the decline in vaccine effectiveness.[24] Andrew et al. analyzed data from the Serious Outcomes Surveillance Network of Public Health Agency of Canada, Canadian Institutes of Health Research Influenza Research Network, to estimate the impact of frailty on vaccine effectiveness estimates; using prospectively collected data for laboratory-confirmed cases, they report vaccine effectiveness (VE) of trivalent influenza vaccine (IV) in people aged ≥65 years hospitalized during the 2011−12 influenza season using a case-control design.[25] They found that VE was strikingly different across frailty levels, with the nonfrail patients having better VE than the prefrail and frail groups. This is in line with other studies examining the interaction of frailty status and influenza vaccination and suggests that frailty needs to be considered as a confounding factor in influenza vaccine studies and potentially with other immunizations as well.

In addition to contributing to the more difficult-to-measure functional impairment in frail elders noted previously, influenza is associated with adverse cardiovascular (CV) outcomes. Currently, estimates indicate that influenza, ILI, and respiratory tract infections increase the risk of myocardial infarction (odds ratio [OR], 2.01; 95% confidence interval [CI], 1.47−2.76), and this risk is highest among those older adults with known CV diseases.[26–28] Kwong et al. reported that the incidence ratio of admission for myocardial infarction in the 7 days after acute influenza during the risk interval as compared with the control interval was 6.05-fold (95% CI, 3.86−9.50) over the control interval.[29] The report from Smeeth et al., however, suggests the risk for first and subsequent myocardial infarction or stroke after systemic respiratory tract infection is larger and extends long after the event, potentially for months.[30] Furthermore and perhaps mechanistically

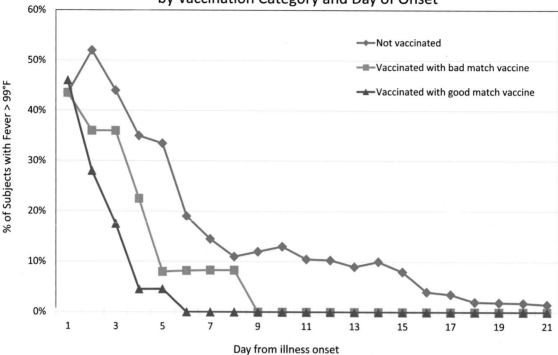

Proportion of Individuals with Fever from Flu, by Vaccination Category and Day of Onset

FIG. 3.1 Fever from infection such as influenza is attenuated with age and vaccines, including when the vaccine is not a good match to the circulating influenza strain. In this study, about 500 nursing home residents of average age over 65 years were followed up prospectively with twice weekly face-to-face visits by study staff to assess for new clinical signs and symptoms suggestive of a change in condition, including mild respiratory symptoms or behavior. When such a change was detected, both nasopharyngeal and throat swabs were collected for subsequent culture and PCR testing, and the face-to-face visits were increased to daily until symptoms had resolved for at least 48 h. The graph presents the data from the entire subset whose laboratory test confirmed influenza and grouped by the population that had received no vaccine or that relative to the circulating A/H3N2 virus, a good-match vaccine, or a poorly matched vaccine. All of those with laboratory-confirmed influenza are represented here, but the majority failed to mount a significant increase in oral temperature (>37.2°C or 99°F), and those who had not received any vaccine took the longest to return to clinical baseline. The influenza attack rate was similar between the unvaccinated and poorly matched vaccine recipients but about a quarter as frequent for the recipients of the well-matched vaccine.[17]

related, there is evidence that coinfection with the 1918 pandemic influenza virus and *S. pneumoniae* activates coagulation pathways and can lead to widespread pulmonary thrombosis.[31]

What makes the clinical presentation of influenza in older adults different and why are they more vulnerable to these outcomes? We can categorize these causes and effects on altered presentation into four groups, relating to changing physiology, the accumulation of underlying conditions, altered cytokine response to infections, and underlying adaptive and senescent immunity (Table 3.2).

There are several features of aging that reduce viral clearance. From a pulmonary standpoint, the declining number of ciliated cells and of cilia per cell in the mucociliary escalator reduces coughing, cough productivity, and viral clearance.[19] Kyphosis, often seen in older adults, and pulmonary aging affect the functional residual capacity and reduce the amount of air expelled forcefully within one second (forced expiratory volume in one second [FEV1]), affecting pulmonary viral clearance, if not also efficiency of carbon dioxide elimination and oxygenation. Secretions, including saliva production, decline with age and often specifically

Influenza Negatively Affects Functional Status in Nursing Home Residents

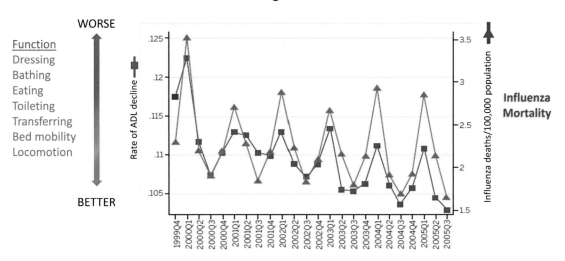

Quarterly pattern of the rate of decline of activities of daily living [ADL (■)] vs influenza city-level mortality (▲) for long-stay (>90 days) nursing home residents in 122 CDC-monitored cities in the US, 1999-2005.

FIG. 3.2 Influenza severity at the city level statistically tracks very closely with degree of increasing functional impairment among nursing home residents living nearby. This figure shows the quarterly pattern of the rate of decline of activities of daily (eating, bathing, dressing, toileting, transferring, bed mobility, locomotion) on a 28-point scale, in which more points equate to greater functional dependence, over a span of 6 years.[21]

relate to medication use, particularly those with anticholinergic properties.[33,34]

A second area of change with age is reduced cardiac response to hypoxia, which means the perception of dyspnea may be delayed. Similarly, the declining cardiac reserve with age and potentially reduced sensitivity to hypoxia may delay clinical presentation and increase the severity at the time of presentation.[35]

There are many immunologic factors that change with aging and prominently contribute to alterations in clinical presentation. The reduced and delayed increase in proinflammatory cytokines contributes to the reduction and delay of symptoms at influenza onset. Furthermore, the return to baseline for immunologic mediators, especially Tumor Necrosis Factor (TNF)-alpha, takes longer in older adults, and translates to slower symptomatic recovery. This may be related to the heightened risk of thrombotic diseases in older adults after acute infectious illness.

There are several aspects of multimorbidity with advancing age that affect how older people present with illness: (1) impact on immune response by the disease itself; (2) selected medications used for chronic disease, such as statins; and (3) the influence of the disease in altering clinical presentation.[36] Many diseases affect immunologic hardiness, whether directly through response to infection or indirectly by attenuating vaccine-induced protective effects.[37] These include chronic kidney disease, endocrine disease (including diabetes), connective tissue diseases, and various malignancies. All are conditions that tend to increase in prevalence with age. Furthermore, medications for malignancies and connective tissue diseases themselves may blunt immune responsiveness to infection and vaccination.[38] As people age, they also have an increasing likelihood of taking medications that might affect both immunity and production of secretions.[34] These collectively affect presentation and complications.

Age and Presentation of *Streptococcus Pneumoniae*

Streptococcus pneumoniae is a common human colonizer found in the oropharynx of close to 10% of adults and more than 30% of children, without any signs of disease; there are no other known reservoirs. Nasopharyngeal colonization is the key event preceding infection and disease, as well as cross-transmission. Most of the

TABLE 3.2
Biologic Changes With Age and Their Effect on Clinical Presentation and Outcomes[17,19,32]

Biologic Change With Age	Clinical Effect
Impaired mucociliary function in respiratory tract	Reduced cough and less efficient viral clearance and mucus clearance
Decreased respiratory muscle strength and protective mucus level and reduced lung compliance	Reduced functional residual capacity and FEV1, decreased pulmonary virus clearance, and reduced carbon dioxide elimination and oxygenation efficiency
Reduced cardiac response to hypoxia	Delayed dyspnea perception and potentially increased severity at time of presentation
Delayed increase in inflammatory cytokines (IL-6, TNF-alpha, IL-8, IL-1) with infection	Delayed clinical onset of symptoms with reduced fever and malaise and less efficient viral clearance
Delayed decline in inflammatory cytokines induced by an infectious stimulation	Longer period during which inflammatory cytokines produce a prothrombotic state (e.g., risk for thromboembolic stroke, myocardial infarction)
Reduced T-cell help	Reduced protection from vaccine, and reduced longevity of protection from vaccine
Increased memory T-cell count with imbalance of Th1 and Th2 responses	Reduced response to vaccine and new infection
Decreased T-cell response to IL-2	Reduced T-cell help in orchestrating adaptive immune response and reduced vaccine response
Decreased B-cell responses to new antigens and increased autoantibodies	Reduced response to vaccine and increased autoimmunity
Decreased NK-cell cytotoxicity	Reduced innate immunity
Reduced nutrition	Reduced physiologic reserve, impaired immune response, and more difficult rehabilitation
Brain aging	Greater likelihood of delirium, sleep and appetite disturbance with cytokine release associated with infection and stress

FEV1, forced expiratory volume in one second.

burden of *S. pneumoniae* in adults is related to pneumonia; however, it has the capacity of causing a wide range of diseases, similar to that in other ages.[39] Manifestations can be roughly grouped into two categories: (1) invasive pneumococcal disease (IPD) and noninvasive pneumococcal disease (NIPD). McLaughlin et al. estimated that the annual cost for pneumococcal disease in the US in 2013 was $5.1 billion for adults aged 50 years and older, including $3.8 billion for those aged 65 years and older.[3]

IPD may be defined as an infectious episode where *S. pneumoniae* is isolated from a normally sterile site, usually blood or cerebrospinal fluid, regardless of clinical syndrome. In the elderly, these episodes are mainly represented by bloodstream infection with or without pneumonia and/or meningitis. Other less common manifestations include endocarditis, purulent pericarditis, osteomyelitis, septic arthritis, chest empyema,

spontaneous bacterial peritonitis, pyelonephritis, endophthalmitis, and purulent thyroiditis.[40]

NIPD includes a wide range of manifestations, from upper respiratory tract infections (e.g., acute otitis media, sinusitis, and epiglottitis) to gastrointestinal infections (e.g., cholecystitis and cholangitis), skin and soft-tissue infections (e.g., erysipelas, cellulitis), and nonbacteremic pneumonia. *S. pneumoniae* is the most common bacterial cause for community-acquired pneumonia (CAP). Importantly, more than 75% of pneumococcal pneumonia (PP) cases are thought to be nonbacteremic, based on epidemiologic studies, and, therefore, classified as NIPD. Nonbacteremic PP remains an important cause of mortality in the US, where an estimated 25,000 related deaths occur annually in adults over the age of 50 years.[41]

S. pneumoniae is responsible for most deaths related to bacterial respiratory infections worldwide in all age groups, including the elderly. The CDC estimates that about 25%–30% of all patients with PP experience bacteremia, and overall there are approximately 400,000 PP-related hospitalizations annually in the US.[42] The incidence and severity of pneumococcal disease starts to increase with age beginning in the sixth decade of life. Data from the CDC Active Bacterial Core surveillance report indicate that a US resident over the age of 65 years has a 40-fold increased risk of dying compared with that of a young adult of the age group 18–34 years.[43]

The clinical manifestation of pneumococcal disease varies greatly with age. Bacteremic pneumonia constitutes the majority of IPD in the adult population, including the elderly, up to 80% in some studies. On the other hand, meningitis is much more common at the other extreme of age; in one study, 5%–7% of adults with IPD had meningitis compared with >30% of infants younger than 2 years.[40]

In the US the case fatality rate (CFR) for PP is estimated at 5%–7% for the general population, 20% for individuals aged 65 years or older and more than 50% in older nursing home residents.[44] Estimates suggest that there are an additional 12,000 cases of pneumococcal bacteremia annually, with a general CFR of 20%, but up to 60% in the elderly. In addition, pneumococci are responsible for an estimated 3000–6000 cases of meningitis yearly, with a CFR of 22% among adults.[44] One study reported that the 30-day mortality rate of patients with IPD before the pneumococcal conjugate vaccine introduction in Denmark was 15.4 per 100,000 for individuals aged 65 years or older compared with 3.8 per 100,000 for those of age range 50–64 years and less than 0.6 per 100,000 for adults aged 18–49 years over the period of 2000–07.[45]

The increased susceptibility to *S. pneumoniae* is attributed to the senescence of the innate and adaptive immune system (refer the previous section), as well as to comorbidity stacking. Older patients with pneumonia frequently have multiple morbidities, and the interaction between aging and these additional morbidities likely further exacerbate the severity in this group. However, data are conflicting on the relative importance of these factors and on the contribution of comorbidities on outcomes in different age groups. Some studies suggest that age has an exacerbating effect on the outcome of CAP that is independent of the presence of comorbidities.[46] In a study looking at a subgroup of healthy and well-functioning adults hospitalized for bacteremic pneumonia, older patients had higher mortality than younger patients with a similar comorbidity profile, serotype, severity of presentation, and provided with similar care.[47] Another study that explored an international database of older individuals hospitalized with CAP suggested that age alone is not a factor for poor outcomes except among the oldest, i.e., those patients with little or no comorbidities aged 80 years and older.[48] Some data suggest that the commonly used Pneumonia Severity Index (PSI) and CURB-65 score may underestimate the severity of pneumonia in the elderly. Cilloniz et al., for example, demonstrated that the impact of comorbidities on mortality is more pronounced at an older age, suggesting an interaction between these factors, as opposed to risk stacking.[49–51]

Pneumonia is associated with impaired mobility and delirium in the elderly. It remains a major cause of hospitalization and, subsequently, contributes to declining physical function and could be considered vaccine-preventable disability.[52] This may lead to loss of independence and the need for full-time care. Early rehabilitation may not be enough to prevent this decline in many at-risk individuals.[53] This is true for community-acquired pneumonia, as well as nursing home and hospital-acquired pneumonia (i.e., healthcare-associated pneumonia [HCAP]).

Studies have shown a link between CAP and CV adverse events and complications.[54] Cangemi et al. found that 18% of individuals hospitalized with CAP had a CV event, including myocardial infarction or new episode of atrial fibrillation.[55] Violi et al. prospectively followed up 1182 CAP admissions for 30 days and found that 32% had a CV event within 30 days with a 3-fold greater mortality than those with CAP that did not have a CV event.[56] The proportion with cardiac complications increased with age and PSI-determined pneumonia severity.[57]

AGE AND PRESENTATION OF HZ

It is estimated that >95% of American adults have a latent varicella zoster virus (VZV) infection; among those, 1 million develop HZ each year, with a lifetime incidence of 20%–30% in the general population.[58] About half of all adults who live until the age of 85 years will develop HZ. Multiple studies show an increased incidence of HZ in recent years in the US, similar to other countries. In a longitudinal cohort in Minnesota, for example, incidence increased by 40% between 1991 and 2010 among the Medicare-insured population aged 65 years or older (Fig. 3.3). The overall incidence increases with age, from less than four per

HZ Incidence Increases with Age and over Time

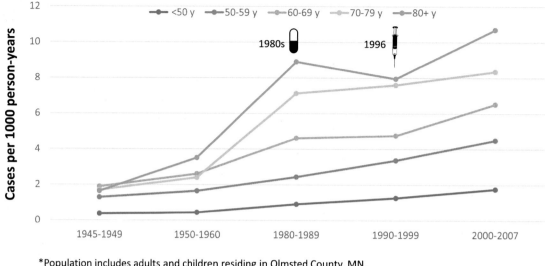

*Population includes adults and children residing in Olmsted County, MN.

Introduction of antivirals (i.e., oral acyclovir) into treatment of acute HZ	Introduction of universal varicella vaccination in U.S.

FIG. 3.3 HZ incidence increases with age and over time.[59]

1000 person-years for persons younger than 60 years to more than 10 per 1000 person-years after the age of 80 years.[60–62]

The estimated cost of HZ in adults aged 65 years old and older was $3 billion in 2013.[3] Varghese et al. suggest that, as the US population ages, the number of yearly HZ cases among those aged 65 years or older is likely to increase 2.5- to 4.5-fold between 2015 and 2030.[63]

Acute HZ has a substantial functional impact on older individuals. Katz et al. observed that acute zoster pain has a significant impact of health-related quality of life (HRQL).[64] Schmader et al. found that the pain from HZ interfered with all ADL, but the greatest effect was on enjoyment of life, sleep, general activity, leisure activities, getting out of the house, and shopping.[65] Others have used the 36-Item Short Form Survey (SF-36) to assess function and quality of life and found that postherpetic neuralgia (PHN) impairs sleep and energy, adversely affects cognitive and functional status, and diminishes quality of life. PHN is also associated with insomnia, chronic fatigue, anorexia,

weight loss, depression, social withdrawal, difficulty in decision-making, and loss of autonomy. Although some of these effects may be in part attributed to neurotropic medications used in the management of this complication, chronic pain itself is a known stressor and can affect attention, memory, and mood.[66,67]

Accumulating evidence suggests that HZ is associated with CV and cerebrovascular events. A recent systematic review and meta-analysis that included 12 studies examining 7.9 million patients up to 28 years found that there is an increase in CV and cerebrovascular events associated with HZ and HZ ophthalmicus, with a specific increased risk for stroke near 33% (95% CI, 1.22–1.46) for the first 3 months after HZ and 22% (95% CI, 1.15–1.29) up to a year.[68] Others have similar findings.[69–71] Although the exact mechanism is obscure, HZ may induce systemic inflammation, autoimmune responses, or hemodynamic changes that result in thrombotic events.[70,72,73] Individuals who develop HZ have elevated inflammatory markers including C-reactive protein (CRP) that are similar to markers that identify cardiac risk.

AGE AND VACCINE IMPACT ON OUTCOMES

Age and Protective Efficacy of Influenza Vaccine

Influenza vaccine effectiveness is thwarted by age-related declines in vaccine response[74,75] (Fig. 3.4). The search for improved effectiveness was not answered with a double-dose influenza vaccine or adding a second booster dose.[76] Rather, the vaccines introduced into the US market with improved immunogenicity and efficacy needed to do more. These include two higher dose vaccines (an inactivated vaccine with four times the usual 15 μg of antigen, and a recombinant vaccine with three times the antigen) and a vaccine adjuvanted with MF59. In older adults, the evidence is strongest for the highest dose vaccine, with two major randomized controlled trials (RCTs) over different influenza seasons, indicating a 12.7% reduction in respiratory hospitalization of nursing home residents compared with regular-dosed influenza vaccines and a 24% relative reduction in laboratory-confirmed influenza compared with community-dwelling elderly who received regular dose vaccine with higher relative efficacy for vaccine-type infection.[77,78] Two other metadata-type studies report concordant findings.[79,80] The adjuvanted vaccine has several nonrandomized controlled studies suggesting a similar effect compared with the regular-dose influenza vaccine.[81-83] A single RCT indicated that recombinant vaccine compared with regular-dose vaccine resulted in a 30% reduction in ILI.[84]

Age and Protective Efficacy of Pneumococcal Vaccine

The currently recommended vaccine regimen for individuals over the age of 65 years involves two vaccines. One is the 23-valent pneumococcal polysaccharide vaccine (PPV23), and the other is the 13-valent pneumococcal conjugate vaccine (PCV13). PPV23 is less immunogenic but covers 10 more strains than the PCV13, whereas PCV13 is more immunogenic and produces better immunologic memory to its antigens than PPV23. A large double-blind RCT in individuals aged 65 years and older reported a 45% efficacy of PCV13 in preventing strain-matched CAP.[85] Falkenhorst et al. performed a systematic literature review and meta-analysis of the vaccine efficacy/effectiveness of PPV23 against IPD and PP in adults aged 60 years and older living in industrialized countries; separate pooled analyses of RCTs, case-control, and cohort studies found a significant vaccine efficacy against IPD and PP by any

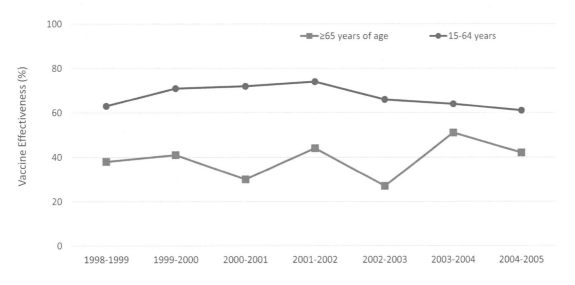

FIG. 3.4 Age and protective efficacy of influenza vaccine.[75]

serotype in the elderly.[86] Because the PCV13 and PPV23 together offer potentially additive advantages, the recommended schedule includes using both the vaccines.[87]

Declines in IPD were observed in the adult population, including older adults, as early as 2001, shortly after the introduction of the 7-valent pneumococcal conjugate vaccine (PCV7) for children in 2000, and more than a decade before the introduction of PCV13 in the adult population. This is attributed to herd immunity, achieved with reduced colonization and spread by those receiving the conjugated vaccine because it reduced incidence of vaccine strain serotype-related disease in both vaccinated and unvaccinated populations in the Unites States. Overall, IPD in older adults decreased from 59 per 100,000 to 23 per 100,000 between 1998 and 2015; the incidence of IPD attributed to serotypes covered by PCV13 decreased from 44 per 100,000 to 5 per 100,000 over the same period. In addition, the incidence of IPD attributed to serotypes covered by PPV23 (licensed in 1983) declined during the same period (from 51 per 100,000 to 13 per 100,000), but this is attributed to declines in IPD caused by serotypes common with PCV13.[42]

Age and Protective Efficacy of Zoster Vaccine

There are two FDA-approved vaccines for shingles prevention. One is an attenuated live vaccine (ZVL) that was FDA approved in 2005, and the other is an adjuvanted recombinant subunit vaccine (RZV), approved in October 2017. In a large RCT, ZVL had an efficacy of 51% in protecting against HZ and reduced PHN by 66.5% when all age groups over 60 years were included together.[60] The primary reduction in PHN was the result of persons not getting shingles in the first place. Examining the efficacy by decades of life, ZVL was 70% effective in 50- to 59-year-old group, 64% in 60- to 69-year-old group, 41% in 70- to 79-year-old group, and only 18% effective in persons over the age of 80 years.[88] Because of both the declining efficacy with age and room for improvement in all age groups, there was impetus to find a more effective vaccine, leading to the development of the adjuvanted zoster vaccine.

There are several differences in RZV compared to ZVL. RZV requires two doses for full effectiveness compared with a single dose for ZVL. RZV is a subunit vaccine adjuvanted with Adjuvant System (AS01), a novel adjuvant, and is stored at normal refrigeration (2–8°C), rather than in a freezer (−50°C to −15°C), as required for ZVL. Two large RCTs focused on subjects aged 50 years and over and then specifically on those

aged 70 years and older.[89,90] The results demonstrated an overall efficacy of >96% and efficacy of 89% in subjects over the age of 80 years. Too few cases of zoster occurred in the vaccine group to determine whether the vaccine confers an added benefit to prevent PHN beyond that of the primary prevention of shingles.

The large difference in the prevention of shingles after RZV compared to that reported previously with ZVL convinced the Advisory Committee on Immunization Practices (ACIP) to preferentially recommend RZV over ZVL.[91] They recommended RZV for persons starting at the age of 50 years and older even if they received prior ZVL. Expert opinion, however, suggests that RZV should not be administered to an individual within 2 months of receiving ZVL. Because of the new preferential vaccination status of RZV, including revaccination with RZV for individuals previously vaccinated, it may reset the progress toward national goals for HZ vaccination coverage, such as by the CDC for Healthy People 2020.[92] Currently there are no data about the safety of RZV in the context of functionally impaired elderly. Clinically important, though transient, arm soreness related to the RZV could affect the use of a walker or assistive device and potentially impact acute independence.

There are no data yet to inform us about the safety of RZV in the context of functionally impaired elderly, whereas the not infrequent transient adverse event of arm soreness may impact the use of a walker or assistive device, potentially acutely affecting independence.

Vaccine Impact on Thrombotic and CV Disease

As discussed previously, there are emerging data that inflammation induced by VPD leads to a prothrombotic effect. The potential for vaccines to prevent these thrombotic complications is apparent in an evolving body of literature. Most of the data on the connection of a vaccine and protection from thrombotic events are with influenza vaccine. A meta-analysis of Udell et al.'s on 5 clinical trials of over 6000 patients with varying degrees of CV risk which evaluated the link between influenza vaccine and CV outcomes found that influenza vaccine was associated with 36% lower incidence of major CV events within a year of vaccination.[93] In patients with recent acute coronary syndrome, influenza vaccine was associated with a 55% lower risk of major adverse CV events (MACEs). In an unblinded prospective RCT with a blinded endpoint, Phromminti-kul et al. evaluated the impact of influenza vaccine on MACE.[94] MACE outcomes included a broad definition including death, hospitalization from acute coronary syndrome, heart failure, and/or stroke. These outcomes occurred less frequently in the vaccine group than in the control group (9.5% vs. 19.3%; adjusted hazard ratio [HR], 0.67 [0.51−0.86]; P = .005). There was no specific mortality difference, however. The beneficial effects associated with the influenza vaccine persisted even after adjustment for variables affecting MACE and in every patient subgroup.

A Cochrane analysis included eight influenza vaccination trials comparing a population that received either placebo or no vaccination with 12,029 subjects that received at least one vaccination to evaluate vaccine-related reduction in CV mortality and combined CV events.[28,95] They concluded that influenza vaccination was associated with a reduction in CV disease and MACE but noted a risk of bias in some studies making for inconsistent results and a need for additional higher quality evidence to confirm the relationship. In patients with known coronary disease, the reduction in acute myocardial infarction associated with influenza vaccination was estimated to be in the range of reductions associated with well-established coronary prevention measures such as smoking cessation, statin therapy, or antihypertensive therapy (17%−43%).[26,93,96]

There is an ongoing clinical trial of high-dose versus standard-dose influenza vaccine in adults with known recent myocardial infarction or heart failure to assess if the high-dose vaccine has a differential benefit even including those under the age of 65 years (NCT02787044). As of early 2018, this trial was continuing to recruit, with an anticipated completion by early 2021, and may settle any uncertainty about the likely benefits of influenza vaccine in the reduction of CV outcomes for this high-risk population.

The first study of the potential preventive effect of influenza vaccination on venous thromboembolism was carried out by Zhu et al., who reported that influenza vaccination reduces the risk of venous thromboembolism by 26%.[97]

There are data on the relationship of pneumococcal or shingles vaccines to vascular consequences of their respective infections. A large population-based cohort study that assessed the clinical effectiveness of the 23-valent polysaccharide pneumococcal vaccine (PPV23) against acute myocardial infarction and ischemic stroke in older adults found a significant benefit against ischemic stroke, but not myocardial infarction.[98] In a meta-analysis of observational studies by Ren et al., the use of PPV was found to be associated with a significant decrease of acute CV events in elderly patients, but not of stroke; none of the outcomes was decreased in the general study population or the younger subgroup.[99] Vlachopoulos et al. conducted a metadata analysis that showed that PPV is associated with a significant decrease of CV events and death; the protective effect of vaccination tends to increase at older age and in subjects with high−CV-risk factors.[100] In contrast, Minassian et al. conducted a case series analysis in vaccinated and unvaccinated older residents in the US and reported that stroke and myocardial infarction rates were transiently increased after exposure to HZ but that there was no evidence for a role of live attenuated zoster vaccination in these associations.[70] This study was limited, however, by its small sample size. Data will likely emerge in the coming years to better assess any thromboprotective benefit or risk from the new more efficacious recombinant adjuvanted zoster vaccine, RZV.

IMMUNOSENESCENCE AND FACTORS THAT AFFECT IT

Immunosenescence is defined as the gradual decline in immune function as a consequence of the normal aging process. This is determined by genetic disposition and influenced by external factors that affect immunosenescence severity. Some of these factors may overlap with those that are associated with the general aging process. There are nonmodifiable factors such as sex, oxidative stress, chronic viral infections (e.g., cytomegalovirus [CMV] and possibly Epstein−Barr virus), and potentially modifiable risks related to sociodemographic factors, comorbidities, medications, health behaviors, nutritional status, stress, and exercise.[101−103]

Immunosenescence can be described as an outcome of the sum of multiple age-associated defects that result in immune dysregulation. Collectively these changes result in more than just poor vaccine responses in late life but also allow infections to run longer unchecked, as symptoms from the underlying disease driven by cytokines alter the clinical presentation where potentially even lethal infection appears initially to be clinically more benign. Some of the known clinical implications of cytokine changes associated with aging are indicated in Table 3.2.

The clinical relevance of this change means that older adults who are infected present differently, and their infection may be delayed or go entirely unrecognized. For example, patients with influenza who are hospitalized often go undiagnosed, and the contribution of influenza as the cause of the hospitalization event gets missed. In a recent RCT we described a difference in hospitalization rates of nursing home residents who lived in facilities that were randomized at the facility level to either standard dose or a four-fold higher dose influenza vaccine; the outcomes were determined from the Medicare claims and the Minimal Dataset discharge records. There were nearly 300 fewer hospitalizations of residents in the facilities that offered high-dose vaccine than those that gave standard-dose vaccine; 27 individuals had a Medicare claim of influenza, with only 6 from facilities receiving the more immunogenic high-dose vaccine. Two-third of the hospitalization difference of nearly 300 in this influenza vaccine RCT could be accounted for by hospitalizations for nonrespiratory primary diagnoses involving the CV system. In other words the clinicians had either not listed the influenza diagnosis as part of their insurance claim or influenza presented in an unrecognized form, related to immunosenescence consequences of altered presentation and immune dysregulation and a pro-thrombotic state resulting in a CV rather than respiratory presentation for hospitalization.[77,104]

There are multiple specific defects in the aging immune system which culminate in immunosenescence and likely are additive in their effects. The defects described in older individuals encompass all the immune cells that are critical for optimal vaccine–induced responses. Defects that are relevant to vaccine response are found in antigen-presenting cells, T cells, and B cells. There is evidence in older individuals of a reduced phagocytic capacity and cell migration in dendritic cells and macrophages that are critically involved in the initial vaccine uptake and presentation.[105,106] T follicular helper cells (Tfh) are required for optimal antibody titers in most vaccines that are T dependent. Tfh have been found to be reduced in number and in their helper function with aging.[107,108] B cells produce the antibodies that are the critical effector molecules in protection induced by vaccine. B cells in older persons have multiple defects including a reduced number of naive B cells in the periphery and lymph nodes with aging, whereas the number of memory B cells increases with age.[109] There is also a defect in isotype switching and somatic hypermutation with aging that leads to a decline in high-affinity IgG antibodies.[110] Finally, there is reduced B cell diversity, fewer antigen-specific antibodies, and increased amounts of nonspecific antibodies produced in older individuals.[111,112]

With aging, there develops a chronic low-level inflammatory state. This has been termed "inflammaging." The chronic inflammation of aging is likely a very important process as most age-related diseases have inflammation as one of the drivers of their pathogenesis.[2] The chronic inflammation could be the result of one of many causes including the accumulation of damaged macromolecules and cells, harmful products from gut microbiota, senescent cells secreting proinflammatory cytokines, chronic viral infections such as CMV, and Epstein–Barr virus (EBV) to name a few. This chronic inflammation is demonstrated by elevated inflammatory cytokines such IL-6 and TNF-alpha and inflammatory markers such as CRP and erythrocyte sedimentation rate (ESR).

STRATEGIES TO OVERCOME THE EFFECTS OF IMMUNOSENESCENCE

There have been a number of efforts to develop vaccines specifically designed to help overcome the reduced vaccine response related to immunosenescence in older persons. Two primary strategies have resulted in FDA-approved products focused on older population so far. One strategy is to increase the dose of the immunogen in the vaccine. There are currently three licensed products that have used this strategy. There is the high-dose influenza vaccine that is the identical vaccine composition to the standard-dose influenza vaccine, except this vaccine has 4-fold higher antigen doses. This high-dose influenza vaccine has been shown to have increased immunogenicity with higher antibody titers elicited and, more importantly, had a 24% reduced rate of protocol-defined clinical and laboratory-confirmed influenza than standard-dose vaccine.[113–115] The second product is the recombinant influenza vaccine, which uses three times the antigen of the regular vaccine. It has similar immunogenicity by traditional measures to the standard-dose vaccine but improved clinical protection in elderly individuals.[84,116] The third product is the live attenuated zoster vaccine. It has a 14-fold higher dose than the chickenpox vaccine, although it is the same live attenuated virus strain.

The second strategy for vaccine enhancement is the use of an adjuvant. By enhancing the inflammatory responses at the injection site to the antigen, adjuvants contribute to the initiation of the innate immune response, with mostly localized and short-lived effects.[117] An adjuvanted influenza vaccine has been available in Europe since the late 1990's, but the first licensed adjuvanted influenza product in the US became available in late 2015. The adjuvanted influenza vaccine improves immunogenicity and heterologous immunity to drifted influenza strains compared with the standard-dose vaccine.[118,119] The added immunogenicity offers the potential for improved protection in seasons where the predominant clinical strain does not closely match the strain in the vaccine. In October

2017 a new vaccine was licensed to prevent shingles that includes AS01 adjuvant. This vaccine, in contrast to the live shingles vaccine, appears to largely maintain its high clinical efficacy even in older individuals.[60,89,90]

There are other adjuvants that have not been specifically targeted for products in older populations, but they may hold promise because they are potent immune stimulants. CpG 1018, a novel Toll-Like Receptor (TLR)-based adjuvant in the new HEPLISAV-B Hepatitis B vaccine, Monophosphoryl lipid A adjuvant used in one human papillomavirus (HPV) vaccines, and AS03 adjuvant used in a licensed pandemic influenza vaccine are three emerging options. Other approaches that focus on delivery of the antigen as a mechanism of enhancement including use of a virus-like particles (VLPs) or viral vector–based vaccines show promise in general but, like the newer adjuvants, need to be tested specifically to determine if they enhance vaccine efficacy in older populations.[120]

There are several indirect strategies that can be used to help overcome infection risks derived from immunosenescence. Such strategies do not involve the older person's immune system. Some are within the control of the individual, and some are societal measures. For example, an individual could avoid getting infected during the height of the influenza season by avoiding social situations using social distancing. Group or societal interventions can have broader benefits. Because influenza spreads from person to person, older adults often contract the disease after contact with children or other younger adults, including healthcare providers. These contacts are typically in younger age groups where influenza vaccine is most effective. There are several reports correlating influenza vaccination uptake in healthcare workers with a reduced risk of influenza outbreaks.[121–123] There are data in the community setting showing that when influenza vaccination of children and younger adults decline, more influenza cases occur in older adults, thus supporting the concept of herd immunity.[124,125]

BARRIERS TO VACCINATION

There are many barriers to vaccination. Vaccine access and acceptance is determined by multiple factors, such as language, transportation availability, social support, and legal status. Access is one of the hardest to modify. As people age and disease burden increases, they may become functionally impaired. Older adults who no longer drive or have access to affordable transportation require dependence on friends, family, or public transportation systems.[126,127]

Elderly individuals are more likely to receive a vaccine if it is readily available to them, such as in convenient community locations, whether their local pharmacy, shopping center, senior center, or faith-based community center. A report on the 2014 Behavioral Risk Factor Surveillance System, a state-based observational survey of US adults, found that, compared to younger adults, individuals aged 65 years and older were more likely to choose a pharmacy to a doctor's office for influenza immunization. In 2018, all 50 states allow pharmacist vaccination in some capacity.[128] Some adults may avoid contact with the healthcare system altogether, including direct contact with pharmacies or vaccination clinics, due to a fear for legal repercussions related to signing forms that require their names and addresses.

In the US, the cost of influenza and pneumococcal vaccination for older adults is covered by Medicare for US citizens, limiting cost as a barrier for most. The shingles vaccine is currently covered but requires varying copays depending on insurance type.

VACCINE USE IN LTC

The LTC resident population is frail and at a particularly high risk for increased morbidity and mortality from all the VPD. This population, however, is substantially understudied for many reasons, including the administrative effort required to enroll subjects, because many potential subjects are unable to consent for themselves and require approval from legally authorized representatives. They are, however, a population that requires expensive care, particularly if their illness leads to hospitalization. There are a small number of LTC-focused studies that evaluate vaccine immunogenicity and clinical effectiveness. Nace et al. reported immunogenicity data that high-dose influenza vaccine that produced superior antibody responses works better in LTC residents than standard-dose vaccine.[115] Two cluster randomized trials in LTC followed the effort of Nace et al. The first, a small-scale pilot in 39 NHs with a predominant H3N2 season, reported a 32% relative reduction in hospitalization compared with standard-dose vaccine.[129] The second, a large-scale trial of 823 NHs with a predominant H1N1 season, demonstrated a nearly 13% relative reduction in hospitalization for respiratory illness in those residents who received high-dose influenza vaccine compared with standard-dose.[77] Maruyama et al. also studied an LTC population and found that PPV23 prevented PP and reduced mortality.[130]

Contrary to evidence for vaccine efficacy in nursing home residents, the vaccination rates in this population remain suboptimal. Black et al. reported that influenza vaccination coverage increased 3.3% (71.4%–75.7%) between the 2005–06 and 2014–15 influenza seasons and pneumococcal vaccination coverage increased 11% (67.4%–78.4%) between 2006 and 2014, despite Healthy People 2010 and 2020 targets of 90% for both the groups.[131]

There is evidence of racial inequality in influenza and pneumococcal vaccine uptake. In a study of vaccination rates in Michigan nursing homes, African-Americans disproportionately lived in nursing homes where vaccination rates were the lowest. In this study the low rates were attributed to facility-level differences in offering vaccination.[14,132] This concern may now be addressed to some degree, in which changes in nursing home regulations in more recent years require that all NH residents be offered influenza and pneumococcal vaccine.

The presence of several immunization strategies in nursing homes, including standing orders for influenza vaccinations, verbal consent allowed for vaccinations, and routine review of facility-wide vaccination rates, is associated with higher vaccination coverage in nursing home residents.[14] Other factors in nursing homes associated with more vaccine coverage include written protocols for immunizations and refusal documentation, provider reminders, and documenting vaccination status in a consistent place in medical records.[133,134]

The importance of maximizing healthcare worker compliance with vaccination is discussed elsewhere in this review. MMWR reported recently on the 2016–17 influenza vaccination rates and found that vaccination coverage continued to be higher among hospital healthcare workers than LTC healthcare workers, at 92.3% versus 68.0%, respectively. High staff turnover in NHs also contributes to staff vaccination coverage at the facility level and needs to be considered in an overall strategy.[135,136] The authors suggest implementing workplace strategies, including mandatory vaccination requirements and active promotion of on-site vaccinations at no cost to help maximize vaccine coverage in healthcare workers.[137]

Influenza outbreaks occur in NHs despite high vaccine coverage or good match to the circulating vaccine strain, which may indicate insufficient vaccine effectiveness to contain the spread of the influenza virus.[138,139] This underscores the importance of maintaining high vaccination rates among residents, caregivers, and staff. It is also important for the nursing home staff to remain vigilant to recognize clinical illness that accompanies an influenza outbreak and take appropriate infection control measures that can include facility, resident, and staff-wide antiviral therapy or chemoprophylaxis. Pneumococcus, although not considered as much of a communicable infectious disease, has still led to outbreaks in LTC facilities with low vaccine coverage and presumably high rates of nasopharyngeal carriage of *S. pneumoniae* in their residents.[140,141]

WHAT WE NEED IN THE FUTURE

Investigators and manufacturers need to advance vaccine research that specifically addresses the characteristics that make older adults more vulnerable to VPD, such as immunosenescence and high disease burden, and to develop vaccine formulations targeting them. Older populations are often understudied and systematically excluded from clinical trials due to the complexity of their inclusion. This is short-sighted given that they have the greatest need medically and will be the greatest proportion of the population worldwide in the next 35 years.[142]

Preliminary evidence from clinical trials in the frailest populations suggest that the older immune system, even in the face of immunosenescence, still has sufficient functional reserve available for enhanced protection when using higher dose or adjuvant vaccine strategies.

Currently, we still lack specific knowledge about waning protection from shingles and *S. pneumoniae* vaccines and how to boost vaccine response. The combination of characteristics that produce a more durable response and is universal, creating response against many strains of influenza, would have tremendous value for the vaccine armamentarium. There remains a debate as to whether to give certain vaccines at younger ages, when eliciting a response is more preserved, as an approach to generate more durable responses. These are essential questions, with much work to do in the field of vaccines for older adults.

SUMMARY

There are many challenges around vaccination and the older population, a group with great need. Immunosenescence has proven to be a significant challenge in optimal vaccine design and is a key feature relating to increased infectious disease morbidity and mortality with age and vaccine failure. One lesser appreciated aspect of immunosenescence is its relationship to "inflammaging" and the increasingly prothrombotic state that expands during the window of risk after infection. Emerging data with influenza and pneumococcal vaccines suggest the promise of vaccine-preventable outcomes that are beyond just the infection and also the potential for preventing vascular thrombotic events in older adults. Vaccines' effect on preventing functional decline is particularly relevant in the older, multimorbid population, where loss of function from an acute illness often leads to lasting decline.

The field has come a long way in the last several decades, adding several substantially improved vaccines and vaccine design approaches, from higher dose offerings to adjuvants and conjugation, all resulting in greater protection from clinical disease in older individuals. Increasingly, even though there is ample room for further improvement, our challenge is expanding beyond just "better vaccines" to developing and implementing strategies to increasing vaccine uptake as no vaccine can be effective when left on the shelf.

REFERENCES

1. Yoshikawa TT, Norman DC. Geriatric infectious diseases: current concepts on diagnosis and management. *J Am Geriatr Soc*. 2017;65:631–641.
2. Franceschi C, Campisi J. Chronic inflammation (inflammaging) and its potential contribution to age-associated diseases. *J Gerontol A Biol Sci Med Sci*. 2014; 69(suppl 1):S4–S9.
3. McLaughlin JM, McGinnis JJ, Tan L, Mercatante A, Fortuna J. Estimated human and economic burden of four major adult vaccine-preventable diseases in the United States, 2013. *J Prim Prev*. 2015;36:259–273.
4. Palache A, Abelin A, Hollingsworth R, et al. Survey of distribution of seasonal influenza vaccine doses in 201 countries (2004-2015): the 2003 World Health Assembly resolution on seasonal influenza vaccination coverage and the 2009 influenza pandemic have had very little impact on improving influenza control and pandemic preparedness. *Vaccine*. 2017;35:4681–4686.
5. Williams WW, Lu PJ, O'Halloran A, et al. Surveillance of vaccination coverage among adult populations—United States, 2015. *MMWR Surveill Summ*. 2017;66:1–28.
6. Nagata JM, Hernandez-Ramos I, Kurup AS, Albrecht D, Vivas-Torrealba C, Franco-Paredes C. Social determinants of health and seasonal influenza vaccination in adults ≥65 years: a systematic review of qualitative and quantitative data. *BMC Public Health*. 2013;13:388.
7. Schmid P, Rauber D, Betsch C, Lidolt G, Denker ML. Barriers of influenza vaccination Intention and behavior - a systematic review of influenza vaccine hesitancy, 2005-2016. *PLoS One*. 2017;12:e0170550.
8. Kamis A, Zhang Y, Kamis T. A multiyear model of influenza vaccination in the United States. *Int J Environ Res Public Health*. 2017;14.
9. Wheelock A, Parand A, Rigole B, et al. Sociopsychological factors driving adult vaccination: a qualitative study. *PLoS One*. 2014;9:e113503.
10. Wu LA, Kanitz E, Crumly J, D'Ancona F, Strikas RA. Adult immunization policies in advanced economies: vaccination recommendations, financing, and vaccination coverage. *Int J Public Health*. 2013;58:865–874.
11. Fabiani M, Riccardo F, Di Napoli A, Gargiulo L, Declich S, Petrelli A. Differences in influenza vaccination coverage between adult Immigrants and Italian citizens at risk for influenza-related complications: a cross-sectional study. *PLoS One*. 2016;11.
12. Lu P, Rodriguez-Lainz A, O'Halloran A, Greby S, Williams WW. Adult vaccination disparities among foreign born populations in the United States, 2012. *Am J Prev Med*. 2014;47:722–733.
13. Bardenheier BH, Shefer AM, Lu PJ, Remsburg RE, Marsteller JA. Are standing order programs associated with influenza vaccination?—NNHS, 2004. *J Am Med Dir Assoc*. 2010;11:654–661.
14. Bardenheier B, Wortley P, Ahmed F, Gravenstein S, Hogue CJ. Racial inequities in receipt of influenza vaccination among long-term care residents within and between facilities in Michigan. *Med Care*. 2011;49: 371–377.
15. Cox NJ. Prevention and control of influenza. *Lancet (London, Engl)*. 1999;354(suppl:SIV30).
16. Cox NJ, Fukuda K. Influenza. *Infect Dis Clin North Am*. 1998;12:27–38.
17. Gravenstein S, Pop-Vicas A, Ambrozaitis A. The 2009 A/H1N1 pandemic influenza and the nursing home. *Med Health R*. 2010;93:382–384.
18. Falsey AR, Baran A, Walsh EE. Should clinical case definitions of influenza in hospitalized older adults include fever? *Influenza Other Respir Viruses*. 2015;9(suppl 1): 23–29.
19. Falsey AR, Formica MA, Hennessey PA, Criddle MM, Sullender WM, Walsh EE. Detection of respiratory syncytial virus in adults with chronic obstructive pulmonary disease. *Am J Respir Crit Care Med*. 2006;173: 639–643.
20. Drinka PJ, Gravenstein S, Krause P, et al. Non-influenza respiratory viruses may overlap and obscure influenza activity. *J Am Geriatr Soc*. 1999;47:1087–1093.
21. Gozalo PL, Pop-Vicas A, Feng Z, Gravenstein S, Mor V. Effect of influenza on functional decline. *J Am Geriatr Soc*. 2012;60:1260–1267.
22. Barker WH, Borisute H, Cox C. A study of the impact of influenza on the functional status of frail older people. *Arch Intern Med*. 1998;158:645–650.
23. Falsey AR, Walsh EE. Respiratory syncytial virus infection in elderly adults. *Drugs Aging*. 2005;22:577–587.
24. McElhaney JE, Andrew MK, McNeil SA. Estimating influenza vaccine effectiveness: evolution of methods to better understand effects of confounding in older adults. *Vaccine*. 2017;35:6269–6274.
25. Andrew MK, Shinde V, Ye L, et al. The importance of frailty in the assessment of influenza vaccine effectiveness against influenza-related hospitalization in elderly people. *J Infect Dis*. 2017;216:405–414.

26. Barnes M, Heywood AE, Mahimbo A, Rahman B, Newall AT, Macintyre CR. Acute myocardial infarction and influenza: a meta-analysis of case-control studies. *Heart.* 2015;101:1738−1747.

27. Naghavi M, Barlas Z, Siadaty S, Naguib S, Madjid M, Casscells W. Association of influenza vaccination and reduced risk of recurrent myocardial infarction. *Circulation.* 2000;102:3039−3045.

28. LeBras MH, Barry AR. Influenza vaccination for secondary prevention of cardiovascular events: a systematic review. *Can J Hosp Pharm.* 2017;70:27−34.

29. Kwong JC, Schwartz KL, Campitelli MA, et al. Acute myocardial infarction after laboratory-confirmed influenza infection. *N Engl J Med.* 2018;378:345−353.

30. Smeeth L, Thomas SL, Hall AJ, Hubbard R, Farrington P, Vallance P. Risk of myocardial infarction and stroke after acute infection or vaccination. *N Engl J Med.* 2004;351: 2611−2618.

31. Walters KA, D'Agnillo F, Sheng ZM, et al. 1918 pandemic influenza virus and Streptococcus pneumoniae co-infection results in activation of coagulation and widespread pulmonary thrombosis in mice and humans. *J Pathol.* 2016;238:85−97.

32. Falsey AR, Hennessey PA, Formica MA, Cox C, Walsh EE. Respiratory syncytial virus infection in elderly and high-risk adults. *N Engl J Med.* 2005;352:1749−1759.

33. Nagler RM, Hershkovich O. Age-related changes in unstimulated salivary function and composition and its relations to medications and oral sensorial complaints. *Aging Clin Exp Res.* 2005;17:358−366.

34. Miranda-Rius J, Brunet-Llobet L, Lahor-Soler E, Farré M. Salivary secretory disorders, inducing drugs, and clinical management. *Int J Med Sci.* 2015;12(10):811−824.

35. Richalet JP, Lhuissier FJ. Aging, Tolerance to high Altitude, and Cardiorespiratory response to hypoxia. *High Alt Med Biol.* 2015;16:117−124.

36. Black S, Nicolay U, Del Giudice G, Rappuoli R. Influence of statins on influenza vaccine response in elderly individuals. *J Infect Dis.* 2016;213:1224−1228.

37. Chinen J, Shearer WT. Advances in basic and clinical immunology in 2007. *J Allergy Clin Immunol.* 2008;122: 36−41.

38. Fomin I, Caspi D, Levy V, et al. Vaccination against influenza in rheumatoid arthritis: the effect of disease modifying drugs, including TNFα blockers. *Ann Rheum Dis.* 2006;65:191−194.

39. Rueda AM, Serpa JA, Matloobi M, Mushtaq M, Musher DM. The spectrum of invasive pneumococcal disease at an adult tertiary care hospital in the early 21st century. *Med Baltim.* 2010;89:331−336.

40. Backhaus E, Berg S, Andersson R, et al. Epidemiology of invasive pneumococcal infections: manifestations, incidence and case fatality rate correlated to age, gender and risk factors. *BMC Infect Dis.* 2016;16:367.

41. Weycker D, Strutton D, Edelsberg J, Sato R, Jackson LA. Clinical and economic burden of pneumococcal disease in older US adults. *Vaccine.* 2010;28:4955−4960.

42. Centers for Disease Control, Prevention. Epidemiology of vaccine-preventable diseases: pneumococcal disease. In: Hamborsky J, Kroger A, Wolfe S, eds. *The Pink Book.* 13 ed. Washington, DC: Public Health Foundation; 2015.

43. Active Bacterial Core Surveillance (ABCs) Report. *Emerging Infections Program Network, Streptococcus Pneumoniae, 2013.* 2013. https://www.cdc.gov/abcs/reports-findings/survreports/spneu13.pdf.

44. Pneumococcal Disease. *Surveillance and Reporting.* 2015. https://www.cdc.gov/pneumococcal/surveillance.html.

45. Harboe ZB, Dalby T, Weinberger DM, et al. Impact of 13-valent pneumococcal conjugate vaccination in invasive pneumococcal disease incidence and mortality. *Clin Infect Dis.* 2014;59:1066−1073.

46. Yende S, Angus DC, Ali IS, et al. Influence of comorbid conditions on long-term mortality after pneumonia in older people. *J Am Geriatr Soc.* 2007;55:518−525.

47. Ruiz LA, Espana PP, Gomez A, et al. Age-related differences in management and outcomes in hospitalized healthy and well-functioning bacteremic pneumococcal pneumonia patients: a cohort study. *BMC Geriatr.* 2017; 17:130.

48. Luna CM, Palma I, Niederman MS, et al. The impact of age and comorbidities on the mortality of patients of different age groups admitted with community-acquired pneumonia. *Ann Am Thorac Soc.* 2016;13: 1519−1526.

49. Cilloniz C, Polverino E, Ewig S, et al. Impact of age and comorbidity on cause and outcome in community-acquired pneumonia. *Chest.* 2013;144:999−1007.

50. Pelton SI, Shea KM, Weycker D, Farkouh RA, Strutton DR, Edelsberg J. Rethinking risk for pneumococcal disease in adults: the role of risk stacking. *Open Forum Infect Dis.* 2015;2:ofv020.

51. Curcio D, Cane A, Isturiz R. Redefining risk categories for pneumococcal disease in adults: critical analysis of the evidence. *Int J Infect Dis.* 2015;37:30−35.

52. Ferrucci L, Guralnik JM, Pahor M, Corti MC, Havlik RJ. Hospital diagnoses, medicare charges, and nursing home admissions in the year when older persons become severely disabled. *JAMA.* 1997;277:728−734.

53. Kato T, Miyashita N, Kawai Y, et al. Changes in physical function after hospitalization in patients with nursing and healthcare-associated pneumonia. *J Infect Chemother.* 2016;22:662−666.

54. Rae N, Finch S, Chalmers JD. Cardiovascular disease as a complication of community-acquired pneumonia. *Curr Opin Pulm Med.* 2016;22:212−218.

55. Cangemi R, Calvieri C, Falcone M, et al. Relation of cardiac complications in the early phase of community-acquired pneumonia to long-term mortality and cardiovascular events. *Am J Cardiol.* 2015;116:647−651.

56. Violi F, Cangemi R, Falcone M, et al. Cardiovascular complications and short-term mortality risk in community-acquired pneumonia. *Clin Infect Dis.* 2017;64: 1486−1493.

57. Feldman C, Anderson R. Prevalence, pathogenesis, therapy, and prevention of cardiovascular events in patients with community-acquired pneumonia. *Pneumonia (Nathan Qld)*. 2016;8:11.

58. Shingles (Herpes Zoster). *Shingles Surveillance*. 2017. https://www.cdc.gov/shingles/surveillance.html.

59. Kawai K, Yawn BP, Wollan P, Harpaz R. Increasing incidence of herpes zoster over a 60-year period from a population-based study. *Clin Infect Dis*. 2016;63: 221–226.

60. Oxman MN, Levin MJ, Johnson GR, et al. A vaccine to prevent herpes zoster and postherpetic neuralgia in older adults. *N Engl J Med*. 2005;352:2271–2284.

61. Yawn BP, Saddier P, Wollan PC, St Sauver JL, Kurland MJ, Sy LS. A population-based study of the incidence and complication rates of herpes zoster before zoster vaccine introduction. *Mayo Clin Proc*. 2007;82:1341–1349.

62. Schmader K. Herpes zoster. *Clin Geriatr Med*. 2016;32: 539–553.

63. Varghese L, Standaert B, Olivieri A, Curran D. The temporal impact of aging on the burden of herpes zoster. *BMC Geriatr*. 2017;17:30.

64. Katz J, Cooper EM, Walther RR, Sweeney EW, Dworkin RH. Acute pain in herpes zoster and its impact on health-related quality of life. *Clin Infect Dis*. 2004; 39:342–348.

65. Schmader KE, Sloane R, Pieper C, et al. The impact of acute herpes zoster pain and discomfort on functional status and quality of life in older adults. *Clin J Pain*. 2007;23:490–496.

66. Pickering G, Pereira B, Clere F, et al. Cognitive function in older patients with postherpetic neuralgia. *Pain Pract*. 2014;14:E1–E7.

67. Pickering G, Leplege A. Herpes zoster pain, postherpetic neuralgia, and quality of life in the elderly. *Pain Pract*. 2011;11:397–402.

68. Erskine N, Tran H, Levin L, et al. A systematic review and meta-analysis on herpes zoster and the risk of cardiac and cerebrovascular events. *PLoS One*. 2017;12:e0181565.

69. Yawn BP, Wollan PC, Nagel MA, Gilden D. Risk of stroke and myocardial infarction after herpes zoster in older adults in a us community population. *Mayo Clin Proc*. 2016;91:33–44.

70. Minassian C, Thomas SL, Smeeth L, Douglas I, Brauer R, Langan SM. Acute cardiovascular events after herpes zoster: a Self-controlled case series analysis in vaccinated and unvaccinated older residents of the United States. *PLoS Med*. 2015;12:e1001919.

71. Kim MC, Yun SC, Lee HB, et al. Herpes zoster increases the risk of stroke and myocardial infarction. *J Am Coll Cardiol*. 2017;70:295–296.

72. Breuer J, Pacou M, Gautier A, Brown MM. Herpes zoster as a risk factor for stroke and TIA: a retrospective cohort study in the UK. *Neurology*. 2014;83:e27–e33.

73. Josephson C, Nuss R, Jacobson L, et al. The varicella-autoantibody syndrome. *Pediatr Res*. 2001;50:345–352.

74. Monto AS, Ansaldi F, Aspinall R, et al. Influenza control in the 21st century: optimizing protection of older adults. *Vaccine*. 2009;27:5043–5053.

75. Legrand J, Vergu E, Flahault A. Real-time monitoring of the influenza vaccine field effectiveness. *Vaccine*. 2006; 24:6.

76. Roos-Van Eijndhoven DG, Cools HJ, Westendorp RG, Ten Cate-Hoek AJ, Knook DL, Remarque EJ. Randomized controlled trial of seroresponses to double dose and booster influenza vaccination in frail elderly subjects. *J Med Virol*. 2001;63:293–298.

77. Gravenstein S, Davidson HE, Taljaard M, et al. Comparative effectiveness of high-dose versus standard-dose influenza vaccination on numbers of US nursing home residents admitted to hospital: a cluster-randomised trial. *Lancet Respir Med*. 2017;5:738–746.

78. DiazGranados CA, Dunning AJ, Robertson CA, Talbot HK, Landolfi V, Greenberg DP. Effect of previous-year vaccination on the efficacy, immunogenicity, and safety of high-dose inactivated influenza vaccine in older adults. *Clin Infect Dis*. 2016;62: 1092–1099.

79. Izurieta HS, Thadani N, Shay DK, et al. Comparative effectiveness of high-dose versus standard-dose influenza vaccines in US residents aged 65 years and older from 2012 to 2013 using Medicare data: a retrospective cohort analysis. *Lancet Infect Dis*. 2015;15:293–300.

80. Shay DK, Chillarige Y, Kelman J, et al. Comparative effectiveness of high-dose versus standard-dose influenza vaccines among us medicare beneficiaries in preventing postinfluenza deaths during 2012-2013 and 2013-2014. *J Infect Dis*. 2017;215:510–517.

81. Mannino S, Villa M, Apolone G, et al. Effectiveness of adjuvanted influenza vaccination in elderly subjects in northern Italy. *Am J Epidemiol*. 2012;176:527–533.

82. Iob A, Brianti G, Zamparo E, Gallo T. Evidence of increased clinical protection of an MF59-adjuvant influenza vaccine compared to a non-adjuvant vaccine among elderly residents of long-term care facilities in Italy. *Epidemiol Infect*. 2005;133:687–693.

83. Van Buynder PG, Konrad S, Van Buynder JL, et al. The comparative effectiveness of adjuvanted and unadjuvanted trivalent inactivated influenza vaccine (TIV) in the elderly. *Vaccine*. 2013;31:6122–6128.

84. Dunkle LM, Izikson R, Patriarca P, et al. Efficacy of recombinant influenza vaccine in adults 50 years of age or older. *N Engl J Med*. 2017;376:2427–2436.

85. Bonten MJ, Huijts SM, Bolkenbaas M, et al. Polysaccharide conjugate vaccine against pneumococcal pneumonia in adults. *N Engl J Med*. 2015;372:1114–1125.

86. Falkenhorst G, Remschmidt C, Harder T, Hummers-Pradier E, Wichmann O, Bogdan C. Effectiveness of the 23-valent pneumococcal polysaccharide vaccine (PPV23) against pneumococcal disease in the elderly: systematic review and meta-analysis. *PLoS One*. 2017;12: e0169368.

87. Tomczyk S, Bennett NM, Stoecker C, et al. Use of 13-valent pneumococcal conjugate vaccine and 23-valent pneumococcal polysaccharide vaccine among adults aged ≥65 years: recommendations of the Advisory Committee on Immunization Practices (ACIP). *MMWR Morb Mortal Wkly Rep.* 2014;63:822–825.

88. Schmader KE, Levin MJ, Gnann Jr JW, et al. Efficacy, safety, and tolerability of herpes zoster vaccine in persons aged 50-59 years. *Clin Infect Dis.* 2012;54:922–928.

89. Cunningham AL, Lal H, Kovac M, et al. Efficacy of the herpes zoster subunit vaccine in adults 70 years of age or older. *N Engl J Med.* 2016;375:1019–1032.

90. Lal H, Cunningham AL, Godeaux O, et al. Efficacy of an adjuvanted herpes zoster subunit vaccine in older adults. *N Engl J Med.* 2015;372:2087–2096.

91. Dooling KLGA, Patel M, Lee GM, Moore K, Belongia EA, Harpaz R. Recommendations of the Advisory Committee on immunization practices for use of herpes zoster vaccines. *MMWR Morb Mortal Wkly Rep.* 2018;67:6.

92. 2014. 2017. (Accessed December 15, 2017, at https://www.healthypeople.gov/2020/topics-objectives/topic/immunization-and-infectious-diseases/objectives.)

93. Udell JA, Zawi R, Bhatt DL, et al. Association between influenza vaccination and cardiovascular outcomes in high-risk patients: a meta-analysis. *JAMA.* 2013;310:1711–1720.

94. Phrommintikul A, Kuanprasert S, Wongcharoen W, Kanjanavanit R, Chaiwarith R, Sukonthasarn A. Influenza vaccination reduces cardiovascular events in patients with acute coronary syndrome. *Eur Heart J.* 2011;32:1730–1735.

95. Clar C, Oseni Z, Flowers N, Keshtkar-Jahromi M, Rees K. Influenza vaccines for preventing cardiovascular disease. *Cochrane Database Syst Rev.* 2015;5(5):Cd005050.

96. MacIntyre CR, Mahimbo A, Moa AM, Barnes M. Influenza vaccine as a coronary intervention for prevention of myocardial infarction. *Heart.* 2016;102:1953–1956.

97. Zhu T, Carcaillon L, Martinez I, et al. Association of influenza vaccination with reduced risk of venous thromboembolism. *Thromb Haemost.* 2009;102:1259–1264.

98. Vila-Corcoles A, Ochoa-Gondar O, Rodriguez-Blanco T, et al. Clinical effectiveness of pneumococcal vaccination against acute myocardial infarction and stroke in people over 60 years: the CAPAMIS study, one-year follow-up. *BMC Public Health.* 2012;12:222.

99. Ren S, Newby D, Li SC, et al. Effect of the adult pneumococcal polysaccharide vaccine on cardiovascular disease: a systematic review and meta-analysis. *Open Heart.* 2015;2:e000247.

100. Vlachopoulos CV, Terentes-Printzios DG, Aznaouridis KA, Pietri PG, Stefanadis CI. Association between pneumococcal vaccination and cardiovascular outcomes: a systematic review and meta-analysis of cohort studies. *Eur J Prev Cardiol.* 2015;22:1185–1199.

101. Ongradi J, Kovesdi V. Factors that may impact on immunosenescence: an appraisal. *Immun Ageing.* 2010;7:7.

102. Koch S, Larbi A, Ozcelik D, et al. Cytomegalovirus infection: a driving force in human T cell immunosenescence. *Ann N Y Acad Sci.* 2007;1114:23–35.

103. Bauer ME, Muller GC, Correa BL, Vianna P, Turner JE, Bosch JA. Psychoneuroendocrine interventions aimed at attenuating immunosenescence: a review. *Biogerontology.* 2013;14:9–20.

104. Gravenstein SDH, Taljaard M, Ogarek JA, Han LF, Gozalo PL, Mor V. *Impact on Cardiorespiratory Outcomes of High Versus Standard Dose Influenza Vaccine in US Nursing Homes Results of a Cluster-randomized Controlled Trial.* San Francisco: GSA; 2017.

105. Agrawal A, Agrawal S, Cao JN, Su H, Osann K, Gupta S. Altered innate immune functioning of dendritic cells in elderly humans: a role of phosphoinositide 3-kinase-signaling pathway. *J Immunol.* 2007;178:6912–6922.

106. Ashcroft GS, Horan MA, Ferguson MW. Aging alters the inflammatory and endothelial cell adhesion molecule profiles during human cutaneous wound healing. *Lab Invest.* 1998;78:47–58.

107. Herati RS, Reuter MA, Dolfi DV, et al. Circulating CXCR5+PD-1+ response predicts influenza vaccine antibody responses in young adults but not elderly adults. *J Immunol.* 2014;193:3528–3537.

108. Linterman MA. How T follicular helper cells and the germinal centre response change with age. *Immunol Cell Biol.* 2014;92:72–79.

109. Lazuardi L, Jenewein B, Wolf AM, Pfister G, Tzankov A, Grubeck-Loebenstein B. Age-related loss of naive T cells and dysregulation of T-cell/B-cell interactions in human lymph nodes. *Immunology.* 2005;114:37–43.

110. Frasca D, Riley RL, Blomberg BB. Humoral immune response and B-cell functions including immunoglobulin class switch are downregulated in aged mice and humans. *Semin Immunol.* 2005;17:378–384.

111. Gibson KL, Wu YC, Barnett Y, et al. B-cell diversity decreases in old age and is correlated with poor health status. *Aging Cell.* 2009;8:18–25.

112. Howard WA, Gibson KL, Dunn-Walters DK. Antibody quality in old age. *Rejuvenation Res.* 2006;9:117–125.

113. DiazGranados CA, Dunning AJ, Kimmel M, et al. Efficacy of high-dose versus standard-dose influenza vaccine in older adults. *N Engl J Med.* 2014;371:635–645.

114. Falsey AR, Treanor JJ, Tornieporth N, Capellan J, Gorse GJ. Randomized, double-blind controlled phase 3 trial comparing the immunogenicity of high-dose and standard-dose influenza vaccine in adults 65 years of age and older. *J Infect Dis.* 2009;200:172–180.

115. Nace DA, Lin CJ, Ross TM, Saracco S, Churilla RM, Zimmerman RK. Randomized, controlled trial of high-dose influenza vaccine among frail residents of long-term care facilities. *J Infect Dis.* 2015;211:1915–1924.

116. Dunkle LM, Izikson R, Patriarca PA, Goldenthal KL, Muse D, Cox MMJ. Randomized Comparison of immunogenicity and safety of Quadrivalent recombinant versus inactivated influenza vaccine in healthy adults 18-49 years of age. *J Infect Dis.* 2017;216:1219–1226.

117. Di Pasquale A, Preiss S, Tavares Da SF, Garcon N. Vaccine adjuvants: from 1920 to 2015 and beyond. *Vaccines.* 2015;3:320−343.

118. Frey SE, Reyes MR, Reynales H, et al. Comparison of the safety and immunogenicity of an MF59(R)-adjuvanted with a non-adjuvanted seasonal influenza vaccine in elderly subjects. *Vaccine.* 2014;32:5027−5034.

119. Ansaldi F, Bacilieri S, Durando P, et al. Cross-protection by MF59-adjuvanted influenza vaccine: neutralizing and haemagglutination-inhibiting antibody activity against A(H3N2) drifted influenza viruses. *Vaccine.* 2008;26:1525−1529.

120. Fuenmayor J, Godia F, Cervera L. Production of virus-like particles for vaccines. *N Biotechnol.* 2017;39:174−180.

121. Potter J, Stott DJ, Roberts MA, et al. Influenza vaccination of health care workers in long-term-care hospitals reduces the mortality of elderly patients. *J Infect Dis.* 1997;175:1−6.

122. Hayward AC, Harling R, Wetten S, et al. Effectiveness of an influenza vaccine programme for care home staff to prevent death, morbidity, and health service use among residents: cluster randomised controlled trial. *BMJ.* 2006;333:1241.

123. Lemaitre M, Meret T, Rothan-Tondeur M, et al. Effect of influenza vaccination of nursing home staff on mortality of residents: a cluster-randomized trial. *J Am Geriatr Soc.* 2009;57:1580−1586.

124. Taksler GB, Rothberg MB, Cutler DM. Association of influenza vaccination coverage in younger adults with influenza-related illness in the elderly. *Clin Infect Dis.* 2015;61:1495−1503.

125. Reichert TA, Sugaya N, Fedson DS, Glezen WP, Simonsen L, Tashiro M. The Japanese experience with vaccinating schoolchildren against influenza. *N Engl J Med.* 2001;344:889−896.

126. Heier Stamm JL, Serban N, Swann J, Wortley P. Quantifying and explaining accessibility with application to the 2009 H1N1 vaccination campaign. *Health Care Manag Sci.* 2017;20:76−93.

127. Eilers R, Krabbe PF, de Melker HE. Factors affecting the uptake of vaccination by the elderly in Western society. *Prev Med.* 2014;69:224−234.

128. Inguva S, Sautter JM, Chun GJ, Patterson BJ, McGhan WF. Population characteristics associated with pharmacy-based influenza vaccination in United States survey data. *J Am Pharm Assoc.* 2003;2017(57):654−660.

129. Gravenstein S, Davidson HE, Han LF, et al. Feasibility of a cluster-randomized influenza vaccination trial in U.S. nursing homes: lessons learned. *Hum Vaccin Immunother.* 2017;14:736−743.

130. Maruyama T, Taguchi O, Niederman MS, et al. Efficacy of 23-valent pneumococcal vaccine in preventing pneumonia and improving survival in nursing home residents: double blind, randomised and placebo controlled trial. *BMJ.* 2010;340:c1004.

131. Black CL, Williams WW, Arbeloa I, et al. Trends in influenza and pneumococcal vaccination among us nursing home residents, 2006-2014. *J Am Med Dir Assoc.* 2017;18:735.e1−e14.

132. Li Y, Mukamel DB. Racial disparities in receipt of influenza and pneumococcus vaccinations among US nursing-home residents. *Am J Public Health.* 2010;100(suppl 1):S256−S262.

133. Bardenheier BH, Shefer A, McKibben L, Roberts H, Rhew D, Bratzler D. Factors predictive of increased influenza and pneumococcal vaccination coverage in long-term care facilities: the CMS-CDC standing orders program Project. *J Am Med Dir Assoc.* 2005;6:291−299.

134. Black CL, Williams WW, Warnock R, Pilishvili T, Kim D, Kelman JA. Pneumococcal vaccination among Medicare Beneficiaries occurring after the Advisory Committee on immunization practices Recommendation for routine Use of 13-valent pneumococcal conjugate vaccine and 23-valent pneumococcal polysaccharide vaccine for adults aged ≥65 Years. *MMWR Morb Mortal Wkly Rep.* 2017;66:728−733.

135. Nace DA, Perera S, Handler SM, Muder R, Hoffman EL. Increasing influenza and pneumococcal immunization rates in a nursing home Network. *J Am Med Dir Assoc.* 2011;12:678−684.

136. Ofstead CL, Amelang MR, Wetzler HP, Tan L. Moving the needle on nursing staff influenza vaccination in long-term care: results of an evidence-based intervention. *Vaccine.* 2017;35:2390−2395.

137. Black CL, Yue X, Mps, et al. Influenza vaccination coverage among health care Personnel - United States, 2016-17 influenza season. *MMWR Morb Mortal Wkly Rep.* 2017;66:1009−1015.

138. Castilla J, Cia F, Zubicoa J, Reina G, Martínez-Artola V, Ezpeleta C. Influenza outbreaks in nursing homes with high vaccination coverage in Navarre, Spain, 2011/12. *Euro Surveill.* 2012;17.

139. Ansaldi F, Zancolli M, Durando P, et al. Antibody response against heterogeneous circulating influenza virus strains elicited by MF59- and non-adjuvanted vaccines during seasons with good or partial matching between vaccine strain and clinical isolates. *Vaccine.* 2010;28:4123−4129.

140. Tan CG, Ostrawski S, Bresnitz EA. A preventable outbreak of pneumococcal pneumonia among unvaccinated nursing home residents in New Jersey during 2001. *Infect Control Hosp Epidemiol.* 2003;24:848−852.

141. Nuorti JP, Butler JC, Crutcher JM, et al. An outbreak of multidrug-resistant pneumococcal pneumonia and bacteremia among unvaccinated nursing home residents. *N Engl J Med.* 1998;338:1861−1868.

142. He WGD, Kowal P. An aging World: 2015. In: *U.S Census Bureau IPR.* Washington, D.C: U.S. Government Publishing Office; 2016.

CHAPTER 4

Herpes Zoster Vaccines: What's New?

ANTHONY L. CUNNINGHAM, MBBS, MD • MYRON J. LEVIN, MD •
THOMAS C. HEINEMAN, MD, PHD

HERPES ZOSTER

Clinical

Herpes zoster (HZ) is a neurocutaneous disease characterized by a pathognomonic dermatomal (area of skin innervated by a single sensory ganglion) papulo-vesicular rash evolving through pustular and crusting stages (Fig. 4.1).[1] The rash is usually accompanied by pain in the area of the rash. Pain may start before the rash appears (prodromal pain) and can persist for weeks to months even after the resolution of the rash (designated postherpetic neuralgia [PHN]). The most widely accepted definition of PHN is pain of at least moderate severity persisting for more than 90 days after the rash onset. The incidence of HZ correlates strongly with the immune competence of an individual, such that the incidence is very high in patients with immune-compromising illnesses (e.g., HIV) or those receiving chemotherapy, high-dose steroids, biological modifiers, or hematopoietic stem cell and organ transplantation.[2,3] In the USA, such patients account for 10% of HZ.[3]

Severity of HZ is also related to the degree of immune compromise.[3] The most frequent cause of immune decline is that it accompanies aging (called immune senescence), such that 60% of HZ cases occur in people aged at least 50 years (Fig. 4.2).[2,3] This pattern is the same worldwide. Complications of HZ include eye involvement, including blindness, neurologic damage, superinfection of the rash, and most importantly, prolonged and severe pain (PHN).[2–4] Not only does the incidence of HZ increase with age but also the incidence, duration, and severity of pain and the likelihood of complications[4] (Fig. 4.3). Prolonged pain and complications of HZ have a profound effect on the quality of life of many elderly individuals.[5]

Pathophysiology

Latency

The potential to develop HZ begins with the initial (primary) infection with the varicella-zoster virus (VZV), which is clinically apparent as varicella (chickenpox). During varicella the cervical and peripheral sensory ganglia become latently infected with VZV, either because of the retrograde spread of VZV from skin lesions and/or because the VZV viremia that occurs during varicella facilitates VZV access to sensory ganglia.

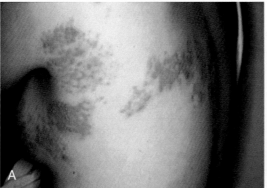
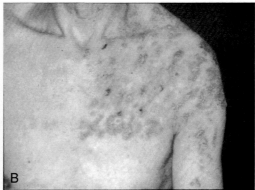

FIG. 4.1 The dermatomal rash of herpes zoster. **(A)** Thoracic dermatome, early papulo-vesicular stage. **(B)** Cervical (C3-4) dermatome, later pustular stage. (Courtesy of Dr Ken Schmader.)

Vaccinations. https://doi.org/10.1016/B978-0-323-55435-0.00004-5

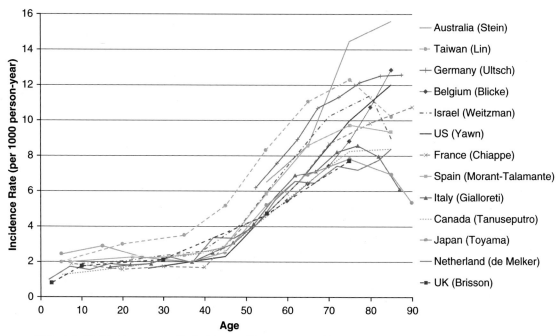

FIG. 4.2 Worldwide age-specific incidence of herpes zoster. (Reproduced from Kawai K et al. Systematic review of incidence and complications of herpes zoster: towards a global perspective. *BMJ Open* 2014;4: https://doi.org/10.1136/bmjopen-2-14-004833.)

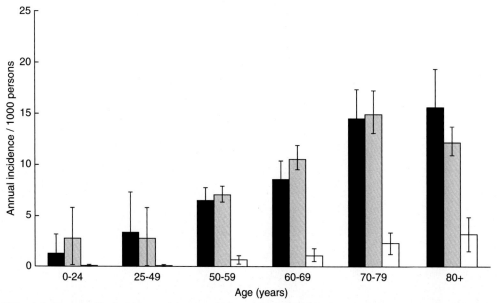

FIG. 4.3 Age-specific incidence of herpes zoster and of postherpetic neuralgia in Australia. This was estimated using general practice data from Bettering the Evaluation and Care of Health (BEACH) (April 2000 to September 2006) extrapolated to the Australian population (black bars) and based on number of prescriptions for direct-acting antiviral drugs available on the Pharmaceutical Benefits Scheme (1998–2005) (gray bars). Age-specific incidence of PHN was estimated using BEACH data, extrapolated to the Australian population (white bars). (Reproduced from Stein A et al. *Vaccine* 2009;27:520.)

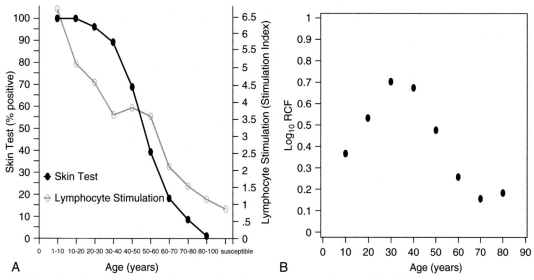

FIG. 4.4 Cell-mediated immunity to varicella-zoster virus declines with age. **(A)** Lymphocyte proliferation/skin test. **(B)** Responder cell frequency (RCF). (**(A)** Adapted from Berger R et al. *Infect Immun* 1981;32:24; Burke BL et al. *Arch Int Med* 1982;142;291. **(B)** Adapted from Weinberg et al. *J Infect Dis* 2010;201:1024.)

VZV remains latent in sensory ganglia for life.[6] At postmortem, about one in 20 sensory neurons contains VZV DNA.[7] Latency of VZV is associated with limited transcription of viral genes, but new infectious viral particles are not produced. Because 95% of adults in the developed world have had varicella by the age of 30 years, almost everyone in the world is at risk to develop HZ.

VZV-specific immunity and latency

There is evidence that VZV sporadically reactivates asymptomatically, but the frequency of this is not known.[8,9] Importantly, reactivation events rarely lead to HZ. This is because the VZV-specific humoral and VZV-specific cell-mediated immune (VZV-CMI) responses that develop during varicella persist into adulthood. Memory immune responses are sufficient not only to prevent second cases of varicella but also to prevent HZ after sporadic VZV reactivation. The evidence for the importance of CMI is largely clinical: (1) An increased incidence of HZ does not occur in patients with B-cell malignancies associated with antibody synthesis until chemotherapy is administered and CMI is suppressed; (2) Inborn genetic errors associated with γ-globulin defects are not associated with severe varicella or severe HZ[10]; (3) Efficacy of an investigational nonlive HZ vaccine (described in the following) correlated with VZV-CMI and not specific antibody[11,12]; (4) In several chemotherapy and transplant settings,

HZ incidence correlated with deficits in VZV-CMI, while specific antibody was present; and (5) HZ is greatly increased in hematopoietic stem cell transplants, even though intravenous γ-globulin containing high titers of VZV-specific antibody is administered as posttransplantation care.

These observations indicate that VZV-CMI is necessary and sufficient to prevent HZ. This is consistent with the observations that VZV-CMI declines with age, with an accelerated decline in the 4th decade of life and further decline for each decade thereafter[13–15] (Fig. 4.4). This age-related decline in VZV-CMI correlates with an increase in HZ risk and appears to be universal across populations (see Fig. 4.2), strongly suggesting that VZV-CMI is required to maintain VZV latency.

Clinical correlates when VZV-CMI fails to limit a reactivation event

Sporadic reactivation of latent VZV occurs, but HZ is uncommon because of the presence of sufficient VZV-CMI. However, when reactivation occurs and VZV-CMI is inadequate, replication of VZV continues, resulting in ganglionitis that is characterized by destruction and/or inflammation of sensory neurons[16] (Fig. 4.5). This explains the prodromal neuropathic pain characteristic of HZ. Meanwhile, when VZV continues to replicate in the single ganglion (or adjacent ganglia) at the site of

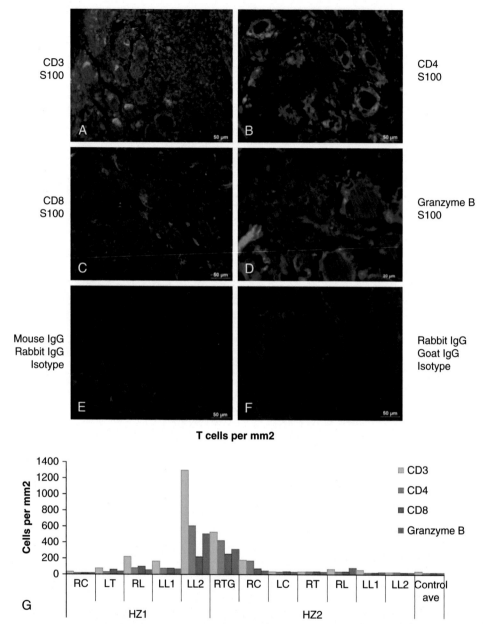

FIG. 4.5 Immunohistology of herpes zoster in dorsal root ganglion immediately postmortem, showing predominance of infiltrating CD4 and CD8 T cells around VZV-infected neurons T cell subsets in ganglia during herpes zoster. **(A to D)** Immunofluorescent staining was performed with CD3, CD4, CD8, granzyme B, and S100 B. **(E and F)** There was no specific staining with isotype control antibodies. **(G)** The number of positive cells per mm^2 was determined from two independent stains and averaged. (Reproduced from Staein et al. *J Virol* 2014;88:2704.)

reactivation, anterograde movement to the skin results in the dermatomal rash. The duration of the prodrome reflects the time from the onset of the early ganglionitis and the time required for VZV to reach and replicate in the skin to produce the vesicular rash.[17,18] Skin damage from the rash contributes to the pain through pain receptors in the skin (nociceptive pain). Damaged neurons in the affected ganglion may heal slowly, with scarring, and this also results in aberrant higher order spinal and cerebral connections and signaling. The exact pathogenesis of the persistence of this pain long after the skin heals (PHN) is only partially understood. Steroids have no significant effect and antivirals a minimal effect on prolonged pain.[4] Because VZV-specific immune memory declines with age, the severity and duration of all these events, including the incidence of complications, increase with age, reflecting delay in resolution of the VZV burden.[18]

HERPES ZOSTER VACCINE—LIVE

Pivotal Trial—If the root cause of HZ is inadequate VZV-CMI, whether from age or medically related causes, it follows that immunizing with a virus similar to that which stimulates immune memory should provide a level of protection characteristic of younger (or more immune competent) people and thereby prevent or delay the occurrence of HZ. Even if HZ is not prevented by vaccination, the episode of HZ should be shorter and less severe because recovery starting from a higher level of specific immune memory would lead to a more rapid response to the infection, even if this was not sufficient to completely prevent the reactivation.

Preparations to test this hypothesis were undertaken from 1984 to 1999. A series of phase I and II trials that used formulations of the Oka/Merck strain of VZV (being developed for the varicella vaccine and licensed in 1995) were directed toward dose finding, defining immune assays needed to evaluate an HZ vaccine, and determining the immunogenicity and safety of the candidate vaccine for people ≥60 years of age (YOA).[19]

Based on these clinical experiments, a double-blind, placebo-controlled efficacy trial of 38,500 people ≥60 YOA was undertaken with a vaccine containing ∼24,500 pfu of VZV, 14-fold more than the varicella vaccine.[20] This study included 17,800 subjects ≥70 YOA and ∼2500 ≥ 80 YOA. HZ cases were diagnosed by PCR for 90% of cases and by an expert adjudication committee for suspected cases that lacked evaluable lesion samples. Pain and effects on the quality of life in subjects who developed HZ were measured with validated methods.

The candidate HZ vaccine licensed in 2005 (ZVL, Zostavax) was an important advance. Overall, 51% of vaccine recipients ≥60 YOA were protected against HZ over a median period of 3.1 years. Age-specific efficacy was 64% for those 60−69 YOA at the time of vaccination, fell to 41% for those 70−79 YOA, and was even lower for older vaccinees (Table 4.1).[20] ZVL prevented PHN in 67% of vaccinees through ages 70−79 years, with some protection against PHN even into the 8th decade of life, demonstrating an attenuating effect when HZ was not prevented (Table 4.1). The vaccine also largely preserved the quality of life of the older vaccinees, as measured by standardized measures of life activities.[21]

The age effect on response to the vaccine somewhat reduces the overall value of the vaccine. Moreover, the pivotal trial followed up subjects for a mean of 3.1 years. Subsequent longer term follow-up studies for 10 years indicated waning of protection to clinically insignificant levels by 7−8 years after vaccination.[22,23]

Immunogenicity substudy of the pivotal trial—A prespecified cohort of 1200 subjects (divided equally between vaccine and placebo recipients) provided serum and peripheral blood mononuclear cells at entry, 3 months, and annually for 3 years.[24] VZV-specific antibody (gpELISA) and VZV-CMI responses (by responder cell frequency [RCF] and ELISPOT) were determined (See Fig. 4.5 legend). Baseline levels of antibody did not

TABLE 4.1
Efficacy of the Live Zoster Vaccine (ZVL)

CLINICAL ENDPOINT	EFFICACY (%)				
Age	50−59	60−80+	60−69	70−79	≥80
HZ	70	51	64	41	18
PHN	—	66.5	65.7	66.8	—
Preserving the quality of life	—	66	70	61	59

M Oxman et al. *N Engl J Med* 2005;352:2271; Schmader et al. *Clin Infect Dis* 2012;54:922−928, Merck Package insert, 2006: Schmader et al. *J Am Geriatr Soc* 2010;58:1634.

vary with age, whereas VZV-CMI correlated negatively with increasing age, confirming the selective effect of age on VZV-CMI. A roughly 1.7- to 2.0-fold increase in all immune responses occurred at 3 months after vaccination, but the VZV-CMI responses were increasingly lower with each 5-year increase in age (Fig. 4.6). This also correlated well with, and presumably explains, the clinical outcome. In addition, all immune responses decreased over the 3-year follow-up, again consistent with clinical observations, although substantial immunity was retained at the latest time point evaluated. Because this cohort was also observed for HZ, it was possible to determine on a population basis that higher antibody or VZV-CMI levels correlated with protection from HZ, but it was not possible to define a specific level of response with any measure that defined protection on an individual basis (surrogate of protection).

Efficacy trial in subjects 50−59 YOA—An additional large efficacy trial was undertaken in 22, 500 subjects 50−59 YOA. This 2-year trial, with a design similar to the pivotal trial for older subjects, demonstrated a 69.8% efficacy against HZ. Higher efficacy would have been expected among younger vaccinees who retained a greater proportion of their varicella-induced immunity.[25] Sera were obtained at baseline and at 6 weeks after vaccination. Higher antibody level correlated overall with protection against HZ, but a specific level that strongly predicted protection was not apparent. This was considered to be a nonmechanistic correlate of protection.[26] A post hoc analysis determined that a fourfold increase in antibody after vaccination strongly predicted protection; the strength of this relationship increased as the magnitude of the rise in antibody increased.[27]

Effectiveness studies—Many of the findings of the pivotal trial were confirmed by an effectiveness study of 303,000 members of a managed care organization, followed for up to 3 years. This showed efficacy against HZ of 55% and also determined that hospitalization for HZ was reduced by 67%.[28] Waning of protection was confirmed in another large effectiveness study (704,000 participants) but provided encouraging results of a different nature, namely, that protection was 45%−50% well into the 8th decade of life and that efficacy was not diminished by comorbidities such as diabetes and kidney, heart, and liver disease.[29] A subsequent effectiveness study (~5 million people) confirmed that 5-year protection (~50%) was little affected by the age of the vaccinee and that protection against PHN remained high regardless of age for at least 6 years after vaccination.[23] Another important finding of the effectiveness study was that vaccinated people

who subsequently developed malignancy and received treatment were significantly protected from HZ after they were immune suppressed with chemotherapy.[30]

Attempts to improve these clinical outcomes—Studies were undertaken to improve the immune response to ZVL, with the underlying hypothesis that improving the immune response would translate into improved efficacy. The limitation of these studies was the absence of a specific immune surrogate for protection to guide potential interventions. Given this obstacle, increasing the dose of vaccine did not appreciably enhance immune responses, although there is some evidence that duration of immunity was increased with larger doses (Merck Research Laboratories, unpublished; Levin MJ. unpublished). Two doses separated by 6−12 weeks did not improve the sustained immune responses.[31,32] Intradermal administration induced higher responses than the subcutaneous route (as licensed), and there was an indication that VZV-CMI central memory responses were enhanced.[33] No additional studies with this approach have been undertaken.

Attempts to reverse the decline in immune protection—A study was conducted comparing VZV-CMI (ELISPOT) in two age-matched cohorts, one receiving the live vaccine for the first time and the comparator receiving a second dose a decade after receiving the previous dose. Vaccinees >70 YOA receiving a booster dose had baseline VZV-CMI responses greater than first-time recipients (i.e., retained some immunity from their past immunization), and responses in the boosted cohort were significantly higher at 1 year.[34] This effect declined by 3 years after reimmunization, but T cell memory and effector memory responses remained above preimmunization levels.[35] This experiment indicated that decline in waning immunity could be restored. The implications for efficacy are unknown.

HERPES ZOSTER VACCINE—INACTIVATED

Heat-inactivated or γ-irradiated zoster vaccine—Since the live vaccine was licensed as unsuitable for immune-compromised patients, there has been much research over the past 12 years to develop an inactivated (either by heat or irradiation) vaccine based on the Oka/Merck strain. The initial study was in hematopoietic cell transplant recipients, in which the administration schedule was one dose before immune-suppressive therapy and three additional monthly doses. Attenuation or prevention of HZ was demonstrated, and protection was correlated with induction of VZV-CMI, but not antibody.[11,12] Subsequent studies demonstrated immunogenicity and safety in patients with

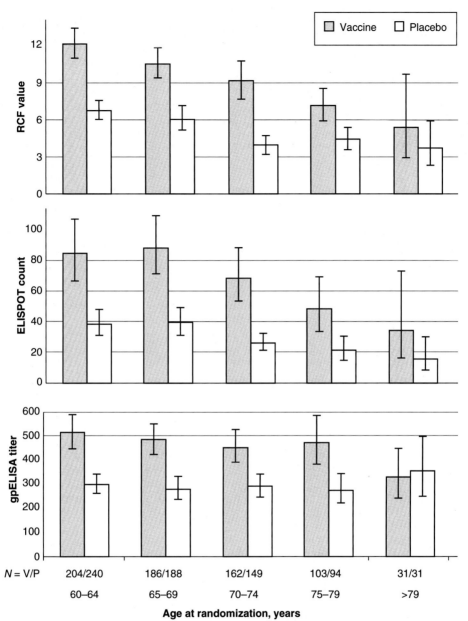

FIG. 4.6 Immunogenicity of live attenuated zoster vaccine (ZVL). Varicella-zoster virus–specific immune responses at 6 weeks after vaccination, according to age group. Responder cell frequency (RCF) value, no. of responding cells per 10^5 peripheral blood mononuclear cells (PBMCs); ELISPOT counts, no. of spot-forming cells per million PBMCs; and glycoprotein ELISA (gpELISA) titer, gpELISA units/mL. *Error bars*, 95% confidence intervals for geometric mean. *N*, no. of subjects who had blood samples obtained within the time interval; *V*, no. of subjects in the vaccine group for each age range; *P*, no. of subjects in the placebo group for each age range. Among vaccinees there was a significant linear age effect (age slope) as measured by RCF and ELISPOT ($P < 0.001$). There was a lesser association between age and gpELISA response ($P = 0.034$). (Reproduced from Levin M et al. *J Infect Dis* 2008;197:825.)

the following conditions: patients with solid and hematologic tumors receiving chemotherapy, patients with autoimmune diseases receiving immune-modifying therapies, and patients with HIV (CD4 counts <200/μL). The inactivated vaccine was not immunogenic in allogeneic stem cell transplant recipients.[36,37] A phase III trial in autologous stem cell transplant recipients using the four-dose schedule and γ-irradiated VZV demonstrated an efficacy against HZ of 64%, against complications of HZ of 74%, and against PHN of 84%.[38] No long-term protection data are available. It is unclear how this vaccine will be used given the requirement for four doses and the alternative nonlive subunit vaccine discussed in the following. However, it is well tolerated and has no adjuvant. It might have value as a vaccine administered before the current live vaccine or as a booster after either of the licensed vaccines.

HERPES ZOSTER VACCINE—SUBUNIT
Rationale and Composition
The introduction of ZVL represented an important advance in reducing the burden of HZ in older adults; nonetheless, opportunities to improve HZ prevention remained. Most notably, the declining efficacy of ZVL with age left a substantial unmet medical need in people 70 YOA, a large and expanding demographic. In addition, ZVL is contraindicated in significantly immune-compromised individuals in whom HZ is common and often severe. To address these needs, an adjuvanted subunit vaccine against HZ, HZ/su (for "herpes zoster/subunit"), was developed. Although the ability of a subunit vaccine to elicit immune responses capable of preventing HZ remained to be proven, this approach was attractive for several reasons. First, the development of new adjuvant systems offered the promise of eliciting strong cellular and humoral responses to a peptide antigen. Second, a nonlive vaccine would avoid potential safety concerns associated with administering a replicating virus to immunocompromised people. Finally, the manufacturing simplicity and stability of a subunit vaccine would be advantageous in supplying a large and expanding market.

HZ/su consists of 50 μg of VZV glycoprotein E (gE) and the AS01$_B$ adjuvant system.[39] gE is the most abundant glycoprotein expressed by VZV-infected cells and in the envelope of VZV virions and is essential for viral replication.[40,41] It was selected as the HZ/su vaccine antigen primarily because of its prominence as a target of humoral and cellular immune responses during VZV infection.[42–45] The recombinant gE used in HZ/su lacks its transmembrane domain, a modification that facilitates its purification by permitting cellular secretion. It is expressed in Chinese hamster ovary cells and thus retains native mammalian posttranslational modifications including glycosylation.[46]

Typical of purified protein antigens, gE is only modestly immunogenic.[46] To enhance and broaden the immune responses to gE, HZ/su also contains the AS01$_B$ adjuvant system. AS01$_B$ consists of liposomes containing 50 μg each of two immunostimulants, 3-O-desacyl-4-monophosphoryl lipid A (MPL) and *Quillaja saponaria* Molina, fraction 21 (QS21, Antigenics).[47] Preclinical studies in mice demonstrated that gE combined with AS01$_B$ stimulates robust cellular and humoral immune responses.[46]

HZ/su Efficacy Against HZ
Early phase clinical trials established the ability of HZ/su to elicit strong gE-specific humoral and cellular immune responses in adults ≥50 YOA and older, including those ≥70 YOA[39,48,49] (Fig. 4.7). Moreover, these studies demonstrated that while a single dose of HZ/su was clearly immunogenic, addition of a second dose substantially enhanced vaccine-induced immune responses.[48]

Based on these results, as well as acceptable safety and tolerability profiles from several phase 1 and 2 studies,[39,48–50] HZ/su efficacy and safety were evaluated in two large phase 3 studies, ZOE-50 and ZOE-70.[51,52] The ZOE-50 study was designed to assess the efficacy of HZ/su in preventing HZ in a representative population of immunocompetent adults ≥50 YOA. The ZOE-70 study was conducted to provide additional efficacy and safety data in adults ≥70 YOA, a population at high risk for HZ and in which the efficacy of the live attenuated zoster vaccine is diminished. The enrollment of a large number of subjects ≥70 YOA was also necessary to assess HZ/su efficacy for the prevention of PHN as the incidence of PHN is highest in that age group.

ZOE-50 and ZOE-70 were blinded, randomized, placebo-controlled studies and were conducted in parallel at the same study sites in 18 countries. In both the studies HZ/su or placebo (saline) was administered intramuscularly 2 months apart, and subjects were followed up for the development of HZ and PHN.[51,52]

In ZOE-50 a total of 15,411 evaluable subjects were randomized to receive HZ/su or placebo. Subjects were stratified into three age cohorts, 50–59, 60–69, and ≥ 70 YOA, and were followed up for a mean of 3.2 years. The mean age of the participants was 62.3 years. During the follow-up period, HZ occurred

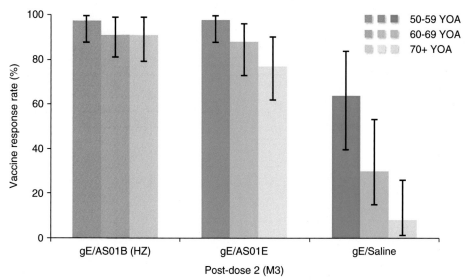

FIG. 4.7 Specific T cell response rates to HZ/su (gE/AS01B) but not gE without the adjuvant were well preserved with subject age. (Data from *J Infect Dis* 2013;208(12):1953—1961 and also reproduced with permission from Cunningham AL *Expert Rev Biol Ther* 2016;16(2):265—271.)

in six HZ/su recipients (0.3 cases/1000 person-years) and 210 placebo recipients (9.1 cases/1000 person-years) for a vaccine efficacy of 97.2% (95% confidence interval [CI], 93.7—99.0; $P < .001$). Vaccine efficacy was similar (96.4%—97.9%) and statistically significant ($P < .001$) in each of the study age cohorts[51] (Fig. 4.8).

In ZOE-70 13,900 evaluable subjects were randomized to receive HZ/su or placebo and stratified into two age cohorts, 70—79 and ≥ 80 YOA (mean age, 75.6 years) (Table 4.2). During a mean follow-up period of 3.7 years, HZ occurred in 23 HZ/su recipients (0.9/1000 person-years) and 223 placebo recipients (9.2/1000 person-years) for a vaccine efficacy against HZ of 89.8% (95% CI, 84.2—93.7; $P < .001$). The parallel design of the ZOE-50 and ZOE-70 studies allowed data from participants ≥ 70 YOA from both the studies (16,596 participants) to be pooled for analysis. This provided a more robust assessment of vaccine efficacy and demonstrated that HZ/su prevented HZ in persons ≥ 70 YOA with an efficacy of 91.3% (95% CI, 86.8—94.5; $P < .001$).[52] The pooled analysis also confirmed that HZ/su efficacy against HZ was similar (91.3%—91.4%) and statistically significant ($P < .001$) in both the 70—79 and ≥ 80 YOA cohorts.[52] Analysis of the ZOE-50 and ZOE-70 data for adults ≥ 70 YOA also provides insight into the durability of HZ/su protection (Fig. 4.9). During 1—4 years after vaccination HZ/su efficacy was insignificantly different at 97.6%, 92.0%, 84.7%, and 87.9%, respectively ($P < .001$ HZ/su

compared to placebo for each year after vaccination for each yearly efficacy assessment) (Table 4.2).

The data from the ZOE-50 and ZOE-70 studies demonstrate that HZ/su has very high efficacy against HZ in adults ≥ 50 YOA. Remarkably HZ/su efficacy is largely unaffected by age at the time of vaccination, remaining above 90% in people ≥ 80 YOA.[52] This contrasts with the HZ efficacy of ZVL, which markedly declines as the age of the vaccine recipient increases.[20,53] In addition, the efficacy of HZ/su shows little evidence of waning during the early years after vaccination, remaining >87% in year 4. Long-term evaluation of HZ/su recipients is ongoing to assess the persistence of its efficacy beyond 4 years.

HZ/su efficacy against PHN

The ZOE-50 and ZOE-70 studies also evaluated the efficacy of HZ/su against PHN, the most common complication of HZ and the greatest source of HZ-associated morbidity. While no uniform definition of PHN exists, in the ZOE-50 and ZOE-70 studies, it was defined as significant HZ-associated pain that persists or develops more than 90 days after the onset of HZ rash, a definition that had been used in the pivotal trial of ZVL.[20,51,52]

In the ZOE-50 and ZOE-70 studies combined, four cases of PHN occurred in HZ/su recipients (0.1 case/1000 person-years) and 46 cases occurred in placebo recipients (0.9 cases/1000 person-years) for a vaccine efficacy of 91.2% in adults ≥ 50 YOA (95% CI,

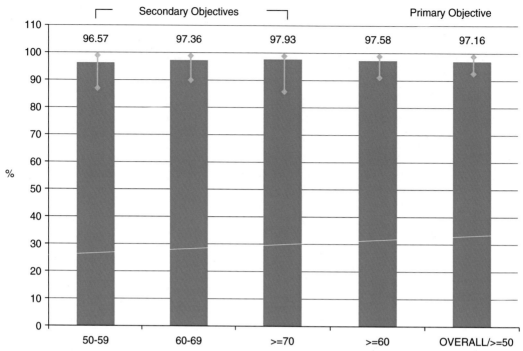

FIG. 4.8 HZ/su vaccine efficacy against first/only episode of herpes zoster stratified by age group. (Data from *N Engl J Med* 2015;372(22):2087–2096 and also reproduced with permission from Cunningham AL *Expert Rev Biol Ther* 2016.)

75.9–97.7; $P < .001$). In subjects $\geq$70 YOA HZ/su efficacy against PHN was 88.8% (95% CI, 68.7–97.1; $P < .001$). No cases of PHN occurred in HZ/su recipients younger than 70 YOA compared to 10 cases in age-matched placebo recipients[52] (Fig. 4.9).

ZVL efficacy against PHN is substantially and significantly higher than its efficacy against HZ, especially in people $\geq$70 YOA (66.8% vs. 37.6%)[20] (Table 4.1), indicating that ZVL provides some protection against PHN in vaccinated people who develop breakthrough HZ.[29] In the ZOE-50 and ZOE-70 studies the efficacy of HZ/su against HZ and PHN was similar. This indicates that HZ/su efficacy against PHN is driven primarily by its ability to prevent HZ, and these studies provide no evidence that HZ/su offers additional efficacy against PHN in vaccine recipients with breakthrough HZ.[52] However, the high efficacy of HZ/su in the ZOE-50 and ZOE-70 studies resulted in very few breakthrough cases HZ, thereby limiting the ability to assess HZ/su efficacy in reducing the incidence of PHN in vaccinated people who develop HZ (Table 4.3).

Despite the paucity of HZ cases in the ZOE-50 and ZOE-70 groups, the impact of vaccination on the course of breakthrough HZ was assessed by comparing

HZ-associated pain in vaccine and placebo recipients. In subjects $\geq$70 YOA with confirmed HZ the average maximum daily pain scores were 4.5/10 compared to 5.6/10 for HZ/su and placebo recipients, respectively ($P = .04$). Similarly, HZ/su recipients with breakthrough HZ also reported lower overall maximum pain scores during their HZ episodes (5.7/10 vs. 7.0/10; $P = .03$).[54] Therefore HZ/su appears to not only reduce the risk of HZ but also the severity of pain associated with HZ in vaccine recipients with breakthrough disease.[55]

The ZOE-50 and ZOE-70 studies also assessed the effect of vaccination on non-PHN complications (HZ-associated vasculitis, stroke, and disseminated, ophthalmic, neurologic, and visceral diseases). The most commonly reported complications were ophthalmic disease and disseminated HZ. Among ZOE-50 and ZOE-70 participants combined, 1 HZ/su recipient and 16 placebo recipients developed an HZ complication other than PHN (vaccine efficacy 93.7%; 95% CI, 59.5%–99.9%).[56] Therefore in addition to providing high efficacy in preventing HZ, HZ/su provides equally strong protection against the complications of HZ, most notably PHN. HZ/su prevents HZ

TABLE 4.2
Vaccination against Herpes zoster and Post Herpetic Neuralgia in the modified vaccinated cohort

CONDITION AND COHORT	HZ/SU GROUP				PLACEBO GROUP				VACCINE EFFICACY[†]
	Participants (number)	Cases	Cumulative Follow-up Period[‡] (person-years)	Incidence Rate (Cases/1000 person-years)	Participants (number)	Cases	Cumulative Follow-up Period[‡] (person-years)	Incidence Rate (Cases/1000 person-years)	% (95% CI)
POOLED ZOE-70 AND ZOE-50									
Age Group									
Overall	8250	25	30,725.5	0.8	8346	284	30,414.7	9.3	91.3 (86.8–94.5)
70–79 years	6468	19	24,410.9	0.8	6554	216	24,262.8	8.9	91.3 (86.0–94.9)
≥80 years	1782	6	6314.6	1.0	1792	68	6151.9	11.1	91.4 (80.2–97.0)
Year									
1	8250	2	8156.2	0.2	8346	83	8206.2	10.1	97.6 (90.9–99.8)
2	8039	7	7916.9	0.9	8024	87	7860.5	11.1	92.0 (82.8–96.9)
3	7736	9	7612.2	1.2	7661	58	7488.4	7.7	84.7 (69.0–93.4)
4	7426	7	7040.3	1.0	7267	56	6859.6	8.2	87.9 (73.3–95.4)
Postherpetic Neuralgia									
POOLED ZOE-70 AND ZOE-50									
≥70 years	8250	4	30,760.3	0.1	8346	36	30,942.0	1.2	88.8 (68.7–97.1)
≥50 years	13,881	4	53,171.5	0.1	14,035	46	53,545.0	0.9	91.2 (75.9–97.7)
Age Group									
50–59 years	3491	0	13,789.7	0.0	3523	8	13,928.7	0.6	100.0 (40.8–100.0)
60–69 years	2140	0	8621.4	0.0	2166	2	8674.4	0.2	100.0 (−442.9 to 100.0)
70–79 years	6468	2	24,438.8	0.1	6554	29	24,660.4	1.2	93.0 (72.4–99.2)
≥80 years	1782	2	6321.5	0.3	1792	7	6281.6	1.1	71.2 (−51.6 to 97.1)

The modified vaccinated cohort excluded participants who did not receive the second dose of the herpes zoster subunit vaccine (HZ/su) or placebo or who had a confirmed episode of herpes zoster within 30 days after the second dose.
[†]Vaccine efficacy was calculated by means of the Poisson method. Vaccine efficacy in each age group was adjusted for region, and overall vaccine efficacy was adjusted for age group and region. $P < .001$ for all comparisons of the efficacy against herpes zoster of the vaccine versus placebo. For the comparison of efficacy against postherpetic neuralgia of the vaccine versus placebo, $P = .008$ in the 50—59-years age group and $P = .001$ in the ≥50-years, ≥70-years, and 70—79-years age groups. $P = .008$ in the 50—59-years age group; the numbers of cases in the placebo group were not sufficient to obtain a significant result in the 60—69 years (P– 0.51) and ≥80 years (P–0.18) age groups.
Adapted from Cunningham AL et al. *N Engl J Med* 2016 15:375.

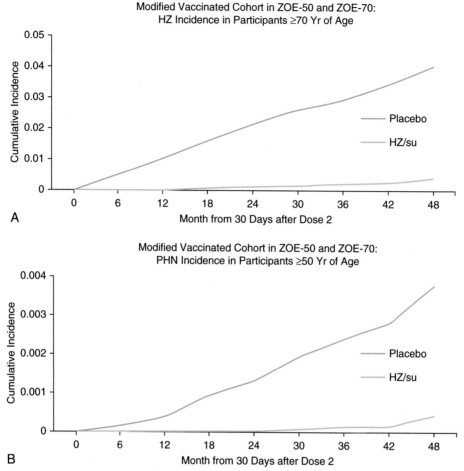

FIG. 4.9 Risk of development of herpes zoster or postherpetic neuralgia after vaccination. **(A)** Cumulative incidence of herpes zoster in adults aged 70 years and above as Kaplan-Meier estimates from 30 days after receiving the second dose of HZ/su to the end of follow-up (4 years) in all cases pooled from ZOE-50 and ZOE-70 (cf Cunningham AL et al.). **(B)** Cumulative incidence of postherpetic neuralgia in adults aged 50 years and above as Kaplan-Meier estimates from 30 days after receiving the second dose of HZ/su to the end of follow-up (4 years) in all cases pooled from ZOE-50 and ZOE-70. (From Cunningham AL et al. Efficacy of the herpes zoster subunit vaccine in adults 70 years of age or older. *N Engl J Med* 2016;375:1019–1032 © 2016 Massachusetts Medical Society. Reprinted with permission from Massachusetts Medical Society.)

complications primarily by preventing HZ itself rather than through preventing complications in people with breakthrough disease. Nonetheless, HZ/su does appear to ameliorate of the course of HZ beyond simple prevention.[54]

HZ/su safety and tolerability

Most HZ/su safety data come from the large ZOE-50 and ZOE-70 studies. In those studies 14,548 adults ≥50 YOA received HZ/su, and 14,663 received the saline placebo. All serious adverse events (SAEs)

TABLE 4.3
Strengths and Weaknesses of the Two Vaccines ZVL and HZ/SU

Consideration	ZVL	HZ/SU
Antigen	Live, attenuated virus	Virus component (gE)
Prior experience	~38 million doses	17,800
Adjuvant	None	AS01B (new in the USA)
Efficacy	51% overall	~91% overall
Age effect	Yes	No
Reactogenic	Like other vaccines	Significantly greater
Persistence	~5 years	4 years to date; immunity ↑ at 6–9 years
Doses	One	Two (0–2 to 6 months)
Protection with one dose	Yes	Some, but limited

Briefing document for the FDA hearing Sept 13, 2017; AL Cunningham. *Exp Opin Biol Ther* 2016;16:265.

were collected for 1 year after vaccination, and fatalities were collected for the duration of the study (4.1 years). Because HZ/su contains the previously unlicensed adjuvant, AS01$_B$, potential immune-mediated diseases (PIMDs) were also collected for the duration of the study to assess any excess risk of these events associated with vaccine-induced immune stimulation.

During the year after vaccination, SAEs were reported in similar proportions of HZ/su and placebo recipients (10.1% and 10.4%, respectively). Likewise, and over the duration of the study, fatalities (4.3% and 4.6%, respectively) and PIMDs (1.2% and 1.4%, respectively) occurred with comparable frequencies in the vaccine and placebo groups.[57] No temporal relationship between HZ/su administration and any of these events was observed. A small number of SAEs, fatalities, and PIMDs were considered related to vaccine by investigators; however, these events were evenly distributed between the vaccine and placebo groups. Together, these data suggest that HZ/su has an acceptable safety profile in older adults, which may allay concerns about the potential of AS01$_B$ adjuvant to increase the risk of autoimmune disease. Postlicensure studies are planned to further monitor HZ/su safety.

The most comprehensive data describing HZ/su-associated reactions come from the ZOE-50 study. In that study solicited local reactions (injection site pain, redness, and swelling) and systemic symptoms (fatigue, myalgia, headache, gastrointestinal symptoms, fever, and shivering) were collected in 4460 HZ/su and 4466 placebo recipients during the 7 days after vaccine or placebo administration.[51] Solicited injection-site reactions were substantially more frequent in HZ/su recipients than in placebo recipients (81.5% vs. 11.9%). The most common local reaction was pain, reported by 79.1% of HZ/su recipients. Similarly, solicited systemic reactions were more frequent after HZ/su, occurring in 66.1% of vaccine recipients compared to 29.5% of placebo recipients, with the most common symptoms being myalgia and fatigue. Grade 3 local and systemic reactions, defined as preventing normal daily activity, occurred in 9.5% and 11.4% of HZ/su recipients and in 0.4% and 2.4% of placebo recipients, respectively. Vaccine-associated reactions were transient, with overall median durations of 1–3 days (1–2 days for grade 3 reactions). Despite the reactogenicity of HZ/su, second-dose compliance was high, approximately 95%, in both the ZOE-50 and ZOE-70 studies, which was comparable to that in the placebo groups, suggesting that the vaccine was generally well tolerated.

HZ/su in immunocompromised populations

One advantage of nonreplicating vaccines is that they circumvent safety concerns associated with the use of live vaccines in highly immunocompromised individuals, such as the possibility of vaccine-related disseminated disease [Zostavax USPI]. Indeed, recent postmarketing surveillance over 10 years showed two cases of disseminated HZ in severely immunocompromised patients proven to be caused by the vaccine strain, one in hematologic malignancy and the other on immunosuppressive medication.[58] Accordingly, an adjuvanted subunit vaccine, HZ/su, was developed so that it could be safely used in populations at high risk for HZ due to immunodeficiency.

The safety and reactogenicity of HZ/su has been evaluated in several immunocompromised populations including autologous stem cell transplant recipients, HIV-infected adults, renal transplant recipients and people with hematologic or solid organ malignancies.[55,59–61] No safety concerns arose in any immunocompromised group, including no association with transplant rejection in renal transplant recipients. In all cases the HZ/su reactogenicity profile was similar to that observed in older adults in the ZOE-50 and ZOE-70 trials and did not affect the underlying disease.

In terms of HZ/su dosing it was initially hypothesized that three doses of HZ/su may be needed to elicit strong immune responses in immunocompromised individuals rather than the two doses used in older adults. Therefore, studies of HZ/su in HIV-infected adults and autologous transplant recipients compared two- and three-dose schedules. In HIV-infected adults (mean $CD4^+$ T-cell count of 594 cells/mL at baseline) two doses of HZ/su elicited gE-specific cellular and humoral responses comparable to those observed in older adults, and a third dose offered little additional benefit.[59] In autologous stem cell transplant patients two doses of HZ/su (at months 2 and 3 after transplant) stimulated strong cellular and humoral immune responses.[60] Addition of a third dose only modestly boosted immune responses. Notably, cellular immune responses after two doses of HZ/su were at least as high as those observed in older adults. It should be noted that humoral responses to HZ/su were lower in stem cell transplant patients with non-Hodgkin B-cell lymphoma, presumably due to B-cell depletion induced by the anti-CD20 monoclonal antibody rituximab, which is often given to these patients before transplant. Based on these results, a large randomized, controlled study to evaluate the efficacy of two doses of HZ/su in preventing HZ in autologous stem cell transplant recipients was initiated.

Two doses of HZ/su also induced strong humoral and cellular immune responses in adults with hematologic malignancies. The proportion of subjects achieving a cellular immune response to HZ/su (based on predetermined criteria) was 84%, and the median magnitude of cellular responses was similar to that observed in older adults.[61] In a small study of patients with solid organ malignancies, HZ/su also induced substantial cellular and humoral immune responses, although the overall cellular response rate and magnitude of response were lower than in patients with hematologic malignancies.[55]

In renal transplant recipients, the final immunocompromised population in which HZ/su has been evaluated to date, the vaccine again proved highly immunogenic when administered as two doses after transplantation.[55] Humoral and cellular immune response rates were approximately 80% and 70%, respectively, and the median cellular responses to HZ/su were only slightly lower than those observed in immunocompetent older adults.

HZ/su in previous ZVL recipients or prior HZ
Thirty-eight million older adults in the US and elsewhere have been vaccinated with ZVL.[62] Because of the waning efficacy of ZVL over time,[22] they are at significant risk for HZ and may benefit from HZ/su revaccination. To assess the potential of HZ/su to be used in this population, the safety and immunogenicity of HZ/su were compared between ZVL-naïve adults ≥50 YOA and those who had received ZVL at least 5 years prior.[63] Previous vaccination with ZVL had no effect on either cellular or humoral immune responses to HZ/su or the reactogenicity profile. Therefore HZ/su may be used to revaccinate prior ZVL recipients (as now recommended by the US Advisory Committee on Immunization Practices).

Coadministration with other vaccines in the aging
Coadministration of HZ/su with a quadrivalent seasonal inactivated influenza vaccine in a phase 3, open-label, randomized clinical trial in adults aged ≥50 years was safe and showed no interference in the immune responses to either vaccine[64] Studies in older adults have also been conducted to evaluate HZ/su when coadministered with a tetanus, diphtheria, and acellular pertussis vaccine (Boostrix, GSK) and with a pneumococcal vaccine (Pneumovax 23, Merck). Results from these studies have not yet been published.

MECHANISM OF ACTION AND IMMUNOGENICITY OF HZ/SU
VZV-Specific Immunity and Response to Reactivation
The results obtained with HZ/su may also provide insight into the immunologic mechanism(s) responsible for preventing HZ. Current theories suggest that latent infection, which is present only in sensory neurons, is maintained by (1) VZV-specific T cells that interact with latently infected neurons to provide signals required to maintain latency and/or (2) sporadic reactivation of latent VZV, for which there is growing evidence, that is aborted by systemic VZV-CMI before replication proceeds to clinical disease (i.e., subclinical reactivation). Since the HZ/su stimulates only gE-specific CMI and since latently infected neurons make a limited number of VZV transcripts and proteins, and gE is not among them (when measured less than 9 hours after death),[65] this suggests that latency is maintained by surveillance for, and rapid resolution of, sporadic VZV reactivation by the gE-specific CMI induced by HZ/su (Shingrix).[65] This is yet to be proven.

Although a decline in VZV-specific T-cell immunity is known to precede HZ, the exact type or level of immunological correlate of HZ protection has not been identified. However, both $CD4^+$ and $CD8^+$ T cells appear to be important in preventing VZV reactivation. In contrast, the role of humoral immunity in reducing the risk of HZ is less clear.[16,66–68] Nonetheless, a correlate of protection analysis performed in subjects vaccinated with ZVL indicated that a fourfold rise in VZV-specific antibody titers, as measured by a glycoprotein-based enzyme-linked immunosorbent assay, was a good nonmechanistic correlate of protection.[67]

Immune responses to HZ/su in the two subcohorts of the ZOE-50 and ZOE-70 trials were measured in antibody (n = 3293) and cell-mediated (n = 466) immune assays. Serum anti-gE antibodies and CD4 T cells expressing ≥ 2 activation markers (CD4^{2+}) after stimulation with gE peptides were measured in each cohort: 97.8% of HZ/su and 2.0% of placebo recipients showed a humoral response to vaccination, defined as a $\geq$ fourfold increase in anti-gE antibody concentrations; geometric mean concentrations increased 39.4-fold (M1) and 8.8-fold (M36) over baseline in HZ/su recipients. Humoral responses were similar between participants 70–79 and $\geq$ 80 YOA throughout the 36 months of observation. 93.3% of HZ/su and 0% of placebo recipients showed a gE-specific CD4^{2+} T-cell response. Median CD4^{2+} T-cell frequencies increased 24.6-fold (M1) and 7.9-fold (M36) over baseline in HZ/su recipients. CD4^{2+} T-cell frequencies remained >5.6-fold above baseline in all age groups for 3 years after immunization. Although after vaccination, increases in CD4^{2+} T-cell frequencies were higher in HZ/su recipients $\geq$70 YOA than in those <70 YOA, median frequencies were still greatly elevated over baseline at all time points. They initially declined over the first year but then plateaued. The proportion of CD4 T cells expressing all four activation markers increased over time in all age groups for up to 4 years.[69]

CD8 T cell responses to the vaccine have been detected by sensitive assays (Weinberg et al., Clin Invest (In Press) 2018). The few HZ cases in HZ/su recipients in ZOE-50 and ZOE-70 and the modest number of subjects contributing to CD4 T cell data from these studies due to practical limitations make it impossible to define an exact quantitative immunological correlate of protection. Nevertheless, future analyses of HZ/su immunogenicity in these individual cases will be of great scientific interest because it may help explain how a strong but highly focused immune response, targeting a single VZV antigen, can induce strong age-independent protection against HZ.[70]

The most important finding of the HZ/su phase I/II and III trials is that a single viral protein combined with an adjuvant can provide strong protection against HZ. VZV gE appears to be an excellent immunogen that can elicit both neutralizing antibody and CD4 T cells

responses. gE-specific immune responses to HZ/su in both older and immunocompromised populations were greatly boosted by the AS01$_B$ adjuvant system.[46,71,72] In the phase I–II studies, gE combined with AS01$_B$ stimulated higher gE-specific CD4$^+$ T cell and humoral immune responses than gE without AS01 or with lower amounts of the MPL and QS21 immunostimulants.[46,49,72]

MPL, present in both AS01$_B$ and AS04 adjuvants, stimulates TLR4 on antigen-presenting cells. The mechanism of QS21, present in AS01$_B$ but not AS04, is not fully elucidated in humans. In mice, QS21 stimulates the inflammasomes in innate immune cells, probably first in injected muscle but definitely later when it contacts peripheral macrophages in draining lymph nodes. This has a downstream stimulatory effect on blood monocyte-derived dendritic cells and resident lymph node dendritic cells that present the gE to T cells via release of interferon gamma (IFN-γ).[71,73] Furthermore, in humans and animal models, AS01$_B$ stimulated the release of IFN-γ from CD8 T and natural killer (NK) cells.[74] This cytokine is an essential antiviral component of the immune response to viral infections, in general. Therefore it is likely that QS21 contributes to the excellent efficacy of single viral protein/adjuvant combinations against HZ, whereas the efficacy of a similar vaccine for primary genital herpes adjuvanted with AS04, which lacks QS21, had limited efficacy. Both are herpesvirus diseases with similar pathogenesis. Nevertheless, HZ is a reactivation disease and easier to prevent than initial genital herpes, which requires induction of naïve immune responses.

HZ/su also appears to overcome immunosenescence as shown by the maintenance of excellent vaccine efficacy even in those older than 80 YOA in ZOE-50 and ZOE-70, together with a minimal decrease in immunogenicity with increasing age in phase I/II trial data.[49,75,76]

COST-EFFECTIVENESS OF ZVL AND HZ/SU

Cost-effectiveness of the two vaccines was calculated by teams constituted by each of the manufacturers, GlaxoSmithKline and Merck, by the CDC, and by independent investigators.[77] These analyses were reviewed at the US Advisory Committee on Immunization Practices on October 25, 2017 (https://www.cdc.gov/vaccines/acip/meetings/slides-2017-10.html).

Both manufacturers used cost-effectiveness ratios (CERs) defined as

Costs of vaccination–Costs of no vaccination/Outcomes with vaccination–Outcomes without vaccination = changes in costs/change in outcomes = $/quality-adjusted life-year (QALY). These were calculated for the following comparisons: HZ/su versus no vaccine; ZVL versus no vaccine; and HZ/su versus ZVL.

For HZ/su versus no vaccine, the base case cost per QALY gained was $12,000 (GSK) and $107,000 (Merck). For ZVL versus no vaccine, the base case CERs were $120,000 (GSK) and $83,000 (Merck) per QALY gained. The CDC model showed $19,000 and $80,000 per QALY for HZ/su and Zostavax, respectively, whereas Le et al. reported $30,000 and $67,000 per QALY for HZ/su and Zostavax, respectively. For HZ/su versus ZVL, both the latter models showed HZ/su to be dominant versus ZVL (base case).

The results varied by age at immunization and were sensitive to estimates of the duration of vaccine efficacy, incidence of HZ, PHN, and their cost per episode. The differences between the models reflected different assumptions for these variables in addition to two-dose uptake and vaccine costs. These all may differ from country to country.

HZ/su was licensed in the USA, Canada, Europe, and Japan for individuals aged 50 years and above in 2017.

SIGNIFICANCE OF THE EFFICACY OF HZ/SU IN AGING SUBJECTS

The high efficacy of HZ/su suggests that using one or a few target antigens combined with relevant adjuvants could be extended to prophylactic or therapeutic vaccines for diseases such as genital herpes that is caused by a related pathogen and also for improving the limited efficacy of other vaccines, such as influenza or pneumococcus in aging subjects.

Future Topics

1. Comparative studies between the live and recombinant vaccines will be limited to immunogenicity and reactogenicity. A relevant trial is now being analyzed.
2. How long will the protection from HZ/su last given that the immunogenicity studies on phase I/II trials show persistence of VZV gE-specific CD4$^+$ T cell immunity for 9 years?[29,78]
3. Will effectiveness studies validate the results of controlled trials?
4. What is the likely compliance with a two-dose HZ/su regimen in the "real world"?
5. Will HZ/su be efficacious in severely immunocompromised patients for whom the live vaccine is contraindicated? Data from the phase III trial addressing this will soon be available.

6. What is the efficacy of HZ/su with a single dose? Is there any setting in which the second dose should be omitted?
7. Can exact immunologic correlates of protection be established, extending data soon to be published from the ZOE-50 trial?

REFERENCES

1. Cohen JI. Clinical practice: herpes zoster. *N Engl J Med.* 2013;369:255−263.
2. Kawai K, Yawn BP, Wollan P, Harpaz R. Increasing incidence of herpes zoster over a 60-year period from a population-based study. *Clin Infect Dis.* 2016;63: 221−226.
3. Yawn BP, Saddier P, Wollan PC, St Sauver JL, Kurland MJ, Sy LS. A population-based study of the incidence and complication rates of herpes zoster before zoster vaccine introduction. *Mayo Clin Proc.* 2007;82:1341−1349.
4. Johnson RW, Rice AS. Clinical practice. Postherpetic neuralgia. *N Engl J Med.* 2014;371:1526−1533.
5. Johnson RW, Bouhassira D, Kassianos G, Leplege A, Schmader KE, Weinke T. The impact of herpes zoster and post-herpetic neuralgia on quality-of-life. *BMC Med.* 2010;8:37.
6. Mitchell BM, Bloom DC, Cohrs RJ, Gilden DH, Kennedy PG. Herpes simplex virus-1 and varicella-zoster virus latency in ganglia. *J Neurovirol.* 2003;9:194−204.
7. Levin MJ, Cai GY, Manchak MD, Pizer LI. Varicella-zoster virus DNA in cells isolated from human trigeminal ganglia. *J Virol.* 2003;77:6979−6987.
8. Ljungman P, Lonnqvist B, Gahrton G, Ringden O, Sundqvist VA, Wahren B. Clinical and subclinical reactivations of varicella-zoster virus in immunocompromised patients. *J Infect Dis.* 1986;153:840−847.
9. Wilson A, Sharp M, Koropchak CM, Ting SF, Arvin AM. Subclinical varicella-zoster virus viremia, herpes zoster, and T lymphocyte immunity to varicella-zoster viral antigens after bone marrow transplantation. *J Infect Dis.* 1992;165:119−126.
10. Good RA, Zak SJ. Disturbances in gamma globulin synthesis as experiments of nature. *Pediatrics.* 1956;18:109−149.
11. Hata A, Asanuma H, Rinki M, et al. Use of an inactivated varicella vaccine in recipients of hematopoietic-cell transplants. *N Engl J Med.* 2002;347:26−34.
12. Redman RL, Nader S, Zerboni L, et al. Early reconstitution of immunity and decreased severity of herpes zoster in bone marrow transplant recipients immunized with inactivated varicella vaccine. *J Infect Dis.* 1997;176:578−585.
13. Burke BL, Steele RW, Beard OW, Wood JS, Cain TD, Marmer DJ. Immune responses to varicella-zoster in the aged. *Arch Inter Med.* 1982;142:291−293.
14. Miller AE. Selective decline in cellular immune response to varicella-zoster in the elderly. *Neurology.* 1980;30: 582−587.

15. Weinberg A, Lazar AA, Zerbe GO, et al. Influence of age and nature of primary infection on varicella-zoster virus-specific cell-mediated immune responses. *J Infect Dis.* 2010;201:1024−1030.

16. Steain M, Sutherland JP, Rodriguez M, Cunningham AL, Slobedman B, Abendroth A. Analysis of T Cell responses during active varicella zoster virus reactivation in human ganglia. *J Virol.* 2013.

17. Ku CC, Besser J, Abendroth A, Grose C, Arvin AM. Varicella-Zoster virus pathogenesis and immunobiology: new concepts emerging from investigations with the SCIDhu mouse model. *J Virol.* 2005;79:2651−2658.

18. Gershon AA, Gershon MD. Pathogenesis and current approaches to control of varicella-zoster virus infections. *Clin Microbiol Rev.* 2013;26:728−743.

19. Levin MJ. Use of varicella vaccines to prevent herpes zoster in older individuals. *Arch Virol Suppl.* 2001:151−160.

20. Oxman MN, Levin MJ, Johnson GR, et al. A vaccine to prevent herpes zoster and postherpetic neuralgia in older adults. *N Engl J Med.* 2005;352:2271−2284.

21. Schmader KE, Johnson GR, Saddier P, et al. Effect of a zoster vaccine on herpes zoster-related interference with functional status and health-related quality of life measures in older adults. *J Am Geriatr Soc.* 2010;58:1634−1641.

22. Morrison VA, Johnson GR, Schmader KE, et al. Long-term persistence of zoster vaccine efficacy. *Clin Infect Dis.* 2015; 60:900−909.

23. Baxter R, Bartlett J, Fireman B, et al. Long-term effectiveness of the live zoster vaccine in preventing shingles: a cohort study. *Am J Epidemiol.* 2018;187:161−169.

24. Levin MJ, Oxman MN, Zhang JH, et al. Varicella-zoster virus-specific immune responses in elderly recipients of a herpes zoster vaccine. *J Infect Dis.* 2008;197:825−835.

25. Schmader KE, Levin MJ, Gnann Jr JW, et al. Efficacy, safety, and tolerability of herpes zoster vaccine in persons aged 50−59 years. *Clin Infect Dis.* 2012;54:922−928.

26. Levin MJ, Schmader KE, Gnann JW, et al. Varicella-zoster virus-specific antibody responses in 50-59-year-old recipients of zoster vaccine. *J Infect Dis.* 2013;208: 1386−1390.

27. Gilbert PB, Gabriel EE, Miao X, et al. fold rise in antibody titers by measured by glycoprotein-based enzyme-linked immunosorbent assay is an excellent correlate of protection for a herpes zoster vaccine, demonstrated via the vaccine efficacy curve. *J Infect Dis.* 2014.

28. Tseng HF, Smith N, Harpaz R, Bialek SR, Sy LS, Jacobsen SJ. Herpes zoster vaccine in older adults and the risk of subsequent herpes zoster disease. *Jama.* 2011;305:160−166.

29. Tseng HF, Harpaz R, Luo Y, et al. Declining effectiveness of herpes zoster vaccine in adults aged >/=60 years. *J Infect Dis.* 2016;213:1872−1875.

30. Tseng HF, Tartof S, Harpaz R, et al. Vaccination against zoster remains effective in older adults who later undergo chemotherapy. *Clin Infect Dis.* 2014;59:913−919.

31. Diaz C, Dentico P, Gonzalez R, et al. Safety, tolerability, and immunogenicity of a two-dose regimen of high-titer varicella vaccine in subjects > or =13 years of age. *Vaccine.* 2006;24:6875−6885.

32. Vermeulen JN, Lange JM, Tyring SK, et al. Safety, tolerability, and immunogenicity after 1 and 2 doses of zoster vaccine in healthy adults >/=60 years of age. *Vaccine.* 2012;30:904−910.

33. Beals CR, Railkar RA, Schaeffer AK, et al. Immune response and reactogenicity of intradermal administration versus subcutaneous administration of varicella-zoster virus vaccine: an exploratory, randomised, partly blinded trial. *Lancet Infect Dis.* 2016;16:915−922.

34. Levin MJ, Schmader KE, Pang L, et al. Cellular and humoral responses to a second dose of herpes zoster vaccine administered 10 years after the first dose among older adults. *J Infect Dis.* 2016;213:14−22.

35. Weinberg A, Levin M, Schmader K, et al. *Varicella Zoster Virus (VZV) Cell-mediated Immunity 3 Years after the Administration of Zoster Vaccine to Septuagenarians Immunized 10 Years Previously. Poster #1715. Session: ID Week, New Orleans, LA; 10/27/2016.* 2016.

36. Eberhardson M, Hall S, Papp KA, et al. Safety and immunogenicity of inactivated varicella-zoster virus vaccine in adults with autoimmune disease: a phase 2, randomized, double-blind, placebo-controlled clinical trial. *Clin Infect Dis.* 2017;65:1174−1182.

37. Mullane KM, Winston DJ, Wertheim MS, et al. Safety and immunogenicity of heat-treated zoster vaccine (ZVHT) in immunocompromised adults. *J Infect Dis.* 2013;208: 1375−1385.

38. Winston DJ, Mullane KM, Boeckh MJ, et al. A Phase III, Double-Blind, Randomized, Placebo-Controlled, Multicenter Clinical Trial to Study the Safety, Tolerability, Efficacy, and Immunogenicity of Inactivated Vzv Vaccine (ZVIN) in Recipients of Autologous Hematopoietic Cell Transplants (Auto-HCTs). Abstract #6. In: BMT Tandem Meetings. (Orlando, FL).

39. Leroux-Roels I, Leroux-Roels G, Clement F, et al. A phase 1/2 clinical trial evaluating safety and immunogenicity of a varicella zoster glycoprotein e subunit vaccine candidate in young and older adults. *J Infect Dis.* 2012;206: 1280−1290.

40. Grose C. Glycoproteins encoded by varicella-zoster virus: biosynthesis, phosphorylation, and intracellular trafficking. *Annu Rev Microbiol.* 1990;44:59−80.

41. Mallory S, Sommer M, Arvin AM. Mutational analysis of the role of glycoprotein I in varicella-zoster virus replication and its effects on glycoprotein E conformation and trafficking. *J Virol.* 1997;71:8279−8288.

42. Bergen RE, Sharp M, Sanchez A, Judd AK, Arvin AM. Human T cells recognize multiple epitopes of an immediate early/tegument protein (IE62) and glycoprotein I of varicella zoster virus. *Viral Immunol.* 1991;4:151−166.

43. Brunell PA, Novelli VM, Keller PM, Ellis RW. Antibodies to the three major glycoproteins of varicella-zoster virus: search for the relevant host immune response. *J Infect Dis.* 1987;156:430−435.

44. Fowler WJ, Garcia-Valcarcel M, Hill-Perkins MS, et al. Identification of immunodominant regions and linear B cell epitopes of the gE envelope protein of varicella-zoster virus. *Virology.* 1995;214:531−540.

45. Malavige GN, Jones L, Black AP, Ogg GS. Varicella zoster virus glycoprotein E-specific CD4+ T cells show evidence of recent activation and effector differentiation, consistent with frequent exposure to replicative cycle antigens in healthy immune donors. *Clin Exp Immunol.* 2008;152: 522–531.

46. Dendouga N, Fochesato M, Lockman L, Mossman S, Giannini SL. Cell-mediated immune responses to a varicella-zoster virus glycoprotein E vaccine using both a TLR agonist and QS21 in mice. *Vaccine.* 2012;30: 3126–3135.

47. Garcon N, Van Mechelen M. Recent clinical experience with vaccines using MPL- and QS-21-containing adjuvant systems. *Exp Rev Vaccines.* 2011;10:471–486.

48. Chlibek R, Bayas JM, Collins H, et al. Safety and immunogenicity of an AS01-adjuvanted varicella-zoster virus subunit candidate vaccine against herpes zoster in adults >=50 years of age. *J Infect Dis.* 2013;208:1953–1961.

49. Chlibek R, Smetana J, Pauksens K, et al. Safety and immunogenicity of three different formulations of an adjuvanted varicella-zoster virus subunit candidate vaccine in older adults: a phase II, randomized, controlled study. *Vaccine.* 2014;32:1745–1753.

50. Lal H, Zahaf T, Heineman TC. Safety and immunogenicity of an AS01-adjuvanted varicella zoster virus subunit candidate vaccine (HZ/su): a phase-I, open-label study in Japanese adults. *Hum Vaccin Immunother.* 2013;9:1425–1429.

51. Lal H, Cunningham AL, Godeaux O, et al. Efficacy of an adjuvanted herpes zoster subunit vaccine in older adults. *N Engl J Med.* 2015;372:2087–2096.

52. Cunningham AL, Lal H, Kovac M, et al. Efficacy of the herpes zoster subunit vaccine in adults 70 years of age or older. *N Engl J Med.* 2016;375:1019–1032.

53. Schmader KE, Oxman MN, Levin MJ, et al. Persistence of the efficacy of zoster vaccine in the shingles prevention study and the short-term persistence substudy. *Clin Infect Dis.* 2012;55:1320–1328.

54. Dea C. *Quality-of-Life Impact of an Investigational Subunit-adjuvanted Herpes Zoster Vaccine in Adults ≥50 Years of Age.* 2016.

55. Vink P. Immunogenicity and safety of a candidate subunit adjuvanted herpes zoster vaccine (HZ/su) in adults post renal transplant: a phase III randomized clinical trial. *Open Forum Infect Dis.* 2017;4:S417-S.

56. Kovac M, Lal H, Cunningham AL, et al. Complications of herpes zoster in immunocompetent older adults: incidence in vaccine and placebo groups in two large phase 3 trials. *Vaccine.* 2018. In press.

57. López-Fauqued ea M. *Results of a Safety Pooled Analysis of an Adjuvanted Herpes Zoster Subunit Vaccine in More than 14,500 Participants Aged 50 Years or Older.* 2017.

58. Willis ED, Woodward M, Brown E, et al. Herpes zoster vaccine live: a 10 year review of post-marketing safety experience. *Vaccine.* 2017;35:7231–7239.

59. Berkowitz EM, Moyle G, Stellbrink HJ, et al. Safety and immunogenicity of an adjuvanted herpes zoster subunit candidate vaccine in HIV-infected adults: a phase 1/2a randomized, placebo-controlled study. *J Infect Dis.* 2015;211: 1279–1287.

60. Stadtmauer EA, Sullivan KM, Marty FM, et al. A phase 1/2 study of an adjuvanted varicella-zoster virus subunit vaccine in autologous hematopoietic cell transplant recipients. *Blood.* 2014;124:2921–2929.

61. Oostvogels L. *Immunogenicity and Safety of an Adjuvanted Herpes Zoster Subunit Candidate Vaccine in Adults with Hematologic Malignancies: A Phase III, Randomized Clinical Trial.* 2017 (Poster Abstract Session: Herpes Zoster Vaccine.).

62. Zhang D, Johnson K, Newransky C, Acosta CJ. Herpes zoster vaccine coverage in older adults in the U.S, 2007–2013. *Am J Prevent Med.* 2017;52:e17–e23.

63. Grupping K, Campora L, Douha M, et al. Immunogenicity and safety of the HZ/su adjuvanted herpes zoster subunit vaccine in adults previously vaccinated with a live-attenuated herpes zoster vaccine. *J Infect Dis.* 2017.

64. Schwarz TF, Aggarwal N, Moeckesch B, et al. Immunogenicity and safety of an adjuvanted herpes zoster subunit vaccine co-administered with seasonal influenza vaccine in adults aged 50 years and older. *J Infect Dis.* 2017.

65. Kennedy PG, Rovnak J, Badani H, Cohrs RJ. A comparison of herpes simplex virus type 1 and varicella-zoster virus latency and reactivation. *J General Virol.* 2015;96: 1581–1602.

66. Arvin AM. Humoral and cellular immunity to varicella-zoster virus: an overview. *J Infect Dis.* 2008;197(suppl 2): S58–S60.

67. Gilbert PB, Gabriel EE, Miao X, et al. Fold rise in antibody titers by measured by glycoprotein-based enzyme-linked immunosorbent assay is an excellent correlate of protection for a herpes zoster vaccine, demonstrated via the vaccine efficacy curve. *J Infect Dis.* 2014;210: 1573–1581.

68. Gowrishankar K, Steain M, Cunningham AL, et al. Characterization of the host immune response in human Ganglia after herpes zoster. *J Virol.* 2010;84:8861–8870.

69. Cunningham AL, Heineman TC, Lal H, et al. Immune responses to a recombinant glycoprotein E herpes zoster vaccine in adults aged >/=50 years. *J Infect Dis.* 2018.

70. Leroux-Roels G, Marchant A, Levy J, et al. Impact of adjuvants on CD4(+) T cell and B cell responses to a protein antigen vaccine: results from a phase II, randomized, multicenter trial. *Clin Immunol.* 2016;169: 16–27.

71. Didierlaurent AM, Collignon C, Bourguignon P, et al. Enhancement of adaptive immunity by the human vaccine adjuvant AS01 depends on activated dendritic cells. *J Immunol.* 2014;193:1920–1930.

72. Vandepapeliere P, Horsmans Y, Moris P, et al. Vaccine adjuvant systems containing monophosphoryl lipid A and QS21 induce strong and persistent humoral and T cell responses against hepatitis B surface antigen in healthy adult volunteers. *Vaccine.* 2008;26:1375—1386.

73. Didierlaurent AM, Laupeze B, Di Pasquale A, Hergli N, Collignon C, Garcon N. Adjuvant system AS01: helping to overcome the challenges of modern vaccines. *Exp Rev Vaccine.* 2017;16:55—63.

74. Coccia M, Collignon C, Hervé C, et al. Cell d molecular synergy in AS01-adjuvanted vaccines results in an early IFNγ response promoting vaccine immunogenicity. *NPJ Vaccine.* 2017;2.

75. Dorrington MG, Bowdish DM. Immunosenescence and novel vaccination strategies for the elderly. *Front Immunol.* 2013;4:171.

76. Linton PJ, Dorshkind K. Age-related changes in lymphocyte development and function. *Nat Immunol.* 2004;5: 133—139.

77. Le P, Rothberg MB. Cost-effectiveness of the adjuvanted herpes zoster subunit vaccine in older adults. *JAMA Intern Med.* 2018;178:248—258.

78. Baxter R, Bartlett J, Fireman B, et al. *Effectiveness of Live Zoster Vaccine in Preventing Postherpetic Neuralgia. Abstract #128. In: IDWeek.* 2016 (New Orleans).

CHAPTER 5

Zika Vaccines: Current State

RICHARD B. KENNEDY, PHD • INNA G. OVSYANNIKOVA, PHD •
PRITISH K. TOSH, MD, FIDSA, FACP •
GREGORY A. POLAND, MD, FIDSA, MACP, FRCP (LONDON)

HISTORY AND EPIDEMIOLOGY OF ZIKA

Initially identified in 1947, Zika virus (ZIKV) infection was declared a public health emergency of international concern early in 2016.[1] Spread primarily through the bite of infected *Aedes aegypti* or *Aedes albopictus* mosquitoes, ZIKV infection leads to complications such as birth defects and neurologic diseases. With the global distribution of endemic infections continuing to expand, a safe and effective vaccine to protect against Zika infection is needed.

ZIKV was first identified in 1947 in a rhesus monkey in the Zika Forest of Uganda as part of a yellow fever surveillance program.[2] Blood from the febrile monkey was injected into Swiss albino mice that subsequently became ill; harvesting of the brains yielded a novel filterable and transmissible agent. The virus was subsequently isolated from mosquitoes trapped in the same area and given the name Zika virus. For the next several decades, Zika was largely an obscure flavivirus without any clear or obvious impact on humans.

In 2007, an outbreak of fever and rash on Yap Island in the South Pacific led to 49 confirmed and 59 probable cases of ZIKV, and a household survey found that nearly three quarters of those tested had antibodies consistent with prior Zika infection.[3] In 2013, a larger outbreak in French Polynesia resulted in nearly 300 confirmed cases and over 19,000 suspected cases. For the first time, an increase in cases of Guillain-Barré syndrome (GBS) was observed.[4,5] Sporadic outbreaks continued in 2015, as cases were identified in Brazil, where, for the first time, instances of microcephaly were identified in children born to women infected with ZIKV while pregnant.[6] By Spring 2016, Zika became endemic in Brazil and elsewhere in South and Central America. By 2017, 48 countries in the Western Hemisphere had evidence of human ZIKV transmission, and ZIKV was found to be endemic throughout large parts of the Americas, central Africa, Southeast Asia, and the South Pacific.[7-10] In addition, small and nonsustained outbreaks occurred in parts of Florida and Texas, although no ongoing transmission has been documented.

ZIKA DISEASE

ZIKV is maintained in its natural reservoir of nonhuman primates through the sylvatic cycle, where the virus is spread from primate to primate through a mosquito vector.[11] Urban cycles of human transmission occur after a person is infected from the bite of a mosquito from the zoonotic reservoir; transmission is primarily sustained within human populations through the bite of infected female *Aedes aegypti* or, to a lesser degree, other mosquitoes such as *Aedes albopictus*.[12] Less commonly, Zika can be transmitted in utero from a woman infected while pregnant as well as sexually through blood transfusion or other bodily secretions, including semen and vaginal secretions.[13,14] Although the duration of Zika viremia is usually less than a week, the virus can persist in semen for well over a month even in asymptomatic patients, leading to an ongoing risk of Zika transmission long after individuals leave an area where the virus is endemic.[15,16]

The incubation period is 3–10 days, with 80% of infections resulting in asymptomatic disease.[3,12] For those with symptoms, 97% develop a maculopapular rash; other common symptoms include arthralgia, myalgia, headache, and conjunctivitis. For those with symptomatic disease, the disease is usually self-limited and symptoms usually resolve within 1 week; however, Zika infection has become a major public health concern because it has been shown to cause microcephaly and other birth defects in children born to mothers infected during pregnancy and because of long-term persistence in semen. Although this association was suspected in early outbreaks, pathologic and epidemiologic evidence has emerged making clear such causality.[17-21] US data

Vaccinations. https://doi.org/10.1016/B978-0-323-55435-0.00005-7

75

on pregnant women with laboratory-proven ZIKV infection have found a 5% overall risk of congenital Zika syndrome—the highest risk (15%) occurring when infection happens during the first trimester.[22] In addition to congenital Zika syndrome, surveillance data from seven countries in Central and South America have found a 2- to 10-fold increase in the rate of GBS following the start of the Zika outbreak compared to baseline levels.[23] Other neurologic complications of Zika infection have been described, including encephalitis, transverse myelitis, and chronic inflammatory demyelinating polyneuropathy.[24]

PUBLIC HEALTH MEASURES

There are ongoing public health efforts to prevent Zika infection and its complications.[25] Pregnant women are encouraged not to travel to areas with endemic Zika transmission and to abstain from sex with partners who have traveled to Zika-endemic areas or to use barrier protection. It is also recommended that women wait 8 weeks and men wait 6 months after returning from a Zika-endemic area before attempting to conceive. For those living in Zika-endemic areas or who must travel to Zika-endemic areas, it is advised to wear long sleeves and pants and apply insect repellent to exposed skin and to reduce mosquito breeding grounds by eliminating areas of standing water near homes. Efforts are also underway to limit the spread of Zika-infected mosquitoes through various mosquito-control efforts. Finally, individuals returning from Zika-endemic areas should continue to use insect repellent for an additional 3 weeks.[25,26]

Symptomatic travelers returning from Zika-endemic areas should be tested for ZIKV with nucleic acid testing (NAT) if the exposure was within 2 weeks or IgM serology if the exposure was after 2 weeks.[27] At each clinic visit, pregnant women should be asked about their travel or the travel of their sex partners to Zika-endemic regions.[27] Those with potential ZIKV exposure due to travel in at-risk areas within 8 weeks or the travel of their male sex partners within 6 months should be tested for ZIKV by NAT or serology regardless of their symptoms and have an anatomic ultrasound performed looking for microcephaly in the developing fetus.[27] Amniocentesis with testing for ZIKV should be offered for those with a positive NAT/serologic test or an abnormal ultrasound result.[27]

Although these recommendations will likely reduce the risk of Zika infection and therefore the risks associated with Zika infection among those living in areas where Zika is not endemic, the geographic distribution of mosquitoes capable of carrying Zika is large and

growing; more is needed to provide protection for those living in Zika-endemic areas.[28] Mosquito-control programs may not be successful as a stand-alone effort in preventing the spread of Zika and may have many unintended consequences.[29,30] The asymptomatic nature of most Zika infections further complicates targeted interventions and makes development of antivirals impractical as a stand-alone strategy to reduce complications. As such, the most compelling global solution to the ongoing Zika outbreak is for the rapid development of safe and effective vaccines before Zika becomes endemic globally.[29] Natural infection with Zika generally confers immunity, but also carries risk (e.g., GBS). This gives promise to the development of a protective vaccine—but also caution including the potential for vaccine-induced GBS—as different vaccine strategies are explored.[31]

IMMUNOLOGY OF ZIKA INFECTION

Our present understanding of ZIKV biology and immunological responses to Zika infection in humans is incomplete and inadequately understood. ZIKV is a single-stranded RNA virus with a genome encoding a polyprotein that is cleaved by viral and host proteases into three structural (C, prM/M, and Env) and seven nonstructural (NS) proteins.[32] Aedes mosquitoes deposit virus in the epidermis and dermis of the bitten host's skin. Several entry receptors and adhesion factors, including DC-SIGN/CD209, TAM (AXL), and TIM family members, are involved in ZIKV infection.[33,34] AXL and its ligand GAS6 (a cellular protein involved in cell growth and survival) play a major role in ZIKV entry and modulation of innate immune responses in human glial cells.[34] Specifically, ZIKV-GAS6 complexes activate a signaling molecule AXL that mediates ZIKV entry by the clathrin-mediated endocytosis pathway and dampens innate immunity. When ZIKV enters epidermal keratinocytes, dermal fibroblasts, and immature dendritic cells, the virus induces the expression of pathogen recognition receptors and innate genes (such as TLR3, RIG-I, and MDA-5) that then trigger the expression of type I and type II IFNs, interferon inducible genes (including OAS2, MX-1, and ISG-15), and inflammatory cytokine genes. In this regard, the antiviral effects of both type I and type II IFNs in protection against ZIKV infection have been described. Specifically, a significant role of type I interferon (IFN) responses that are characterized by increased IFN-β gene expression in regulating/controlling ZIKV infection in mice has been demonstrated.[35] Likewise, it has been demonstrated that ZIKV NS5 protein binds and inhibits human STAT2, suppressing type I IFN signaling and promoting virus propagation.[36]

Although antibody (Ab) is an immune correlate of protection (e.g., Ab response titer) for ZIKV, a defined protective titer has not yet been established. Recent vaccine challenge studies in rhesus macaques have suggested a putative correlate of protection (as 1:10 PRNT50 neutralizing Ab titer).[37,38] ZIKV infection induces robust humoral (IgG and IgM neutralizing antibodies) and polyfunctional T cell (CD4+ and CD8+) adaptive immune responses that are essential for resolving virus infection. Humoral immunity has been shown to play a critical role in ZIKV protection in both rhesus monkey and mouse models.[39-43] Studies of individuals with ZIKV disease reveal the presence of IgG and IgM neutralizing antibodies; however, these antibodies provided only partial protection in mice against lethal ZIKV and were cross-reactive with antibodies against other flaviviruses, specifically dengue virus (DENV) and yellow fever virus (YFV).[3] Prior infection with, or immunization against, other flaviviruses may also influence the severity of ZIKV illness or vice versa, although scant data currently exist.

Promising results using both mouse and nonhuman primate models to develop ZIKV vaccines that elicit protective immune responses have been published.[39,42,44,45] In a mouse study, a plasmid prM-Env DNA vaccine induced ZIKV-specific antibodies and protected against infection and/or disease after a single immunization.[42] This study demonstrated that envelope (Env)-specific Ab titers to ZIKV following a plasmid prM-Env DNA vaccine can be considered an immunologic correlate of protection. Since Env glycoprotein is crucial for ZIKV attachment, entry, and replication, it may be useful as a potential vaccine target.[46] Notably, anti-Env neutralizing antibodies have been recognized as correlates of protection for vaccines against other flaviviruses, including YFV, Japanese encephalitis, and tick-borne encephalitis viruses. Further, data suggest that immunity induced by a ZIKV protein (MR766) may offer cross-protective immune responses against various ZIKV strains in a rhesus macaque model.[37]

To date, relatively little is known regarding B cell and T cell responses to ZIKV. B cell ZIKV epitopes have been mapped to several viral proteins, including the Env, precursor membrane (prM), and NS proteins.[41,47,48] Among the NS proteins, NS1 glycoprotein (~48 kDa) is a conserved membrane-associated multifunctional virulence factor that has been proposed to play a role in viral replication, immune evasion, and Ab recognition.[49] Sequence similarity between NS1 proteins of ZIKV and closely related flavivirus DENV have been

shown to be about 55%.[41] The sero cross-reactivity of ZIKV and DENV antibodies makes it difficult to serologically diagnose ZIKV infection. However, preexisting DENV- or YFV-specific antibodies do not cross-protect against ZIKV disease and are unable to neutralize ZIKV. It has also been reported that DENV-specific antibodies in individuals with previous DENV infections may cause enhanced ZIKV replication and infection via an antibody-dependent enhancement (ADE) mechanism that can cause a fatal shock syndrome.[50,51] A lipid nanoparticle (LNP)-derived modified prM-E RNA ZIKV vaccine introduced mutations in the conserved fusion-loop epitope in the Env protein, which reduced the production of dengue-enhancing antibodies in both cell culture and mice compared to the unmutated fusion-loop.[52] A better understanding of the interaction between DENV and ZIKV infections is important for vaccine design, as well as for the development of strategies to combat these infections—particularly in areas where both diseases commonly occur.

While the importance of Ab responses in protection against ZIKV infection has been established in animal models,[41,42,53] protective effects conferred by T cells have also been clearly demonstrated.[54] T cell activity contributes to protection and viral clearance in other flavivirus models, such as WNV and DENV.[55,56] A recent study by Ngono et al. has found that adoptive transfer of ZIKV-specific CD8+ T cells reduced viral burdens, while CD8+ KO (H-2^b) mice exhibited higher mortality—confirming the importance of T cell activity in controlling ZIKV replication.[54] The authors demonstrated that ZIKV infection induced strong CD8+ T cell responses that target viral prM, Env, and NS5 proteins in mice and identified CD8+ T cell-reactive peptides (26 peptides for ZIKV African lineage strain and 15 peptides for ZIKV Asian lineage strain).[54] An immunodominant CD8+ T cell epitope has also been recently mapped to ZIKV Env protein (Env294-302), which is 99% conserved across all available full-length ZIKV polyprotein sequences.[57]

Analysis of T cell responses to ZIKV revealed the presence of the following responses: a Th1-polarized CD4+ T cell response, which is characterized by production of interferon gamma (IFN-γ), tumor necrosis factor alpha (TNF-α), and interleukin-2; and a robust effector CD8+ T cell response, which is characterized by production of effector cytokines and cytolytic molecules in immunocompetent mice.[57] While CD4+ T cells support antiviral proinflammatory responses and assist in the development and maturation of Ab responses,[58] CD8+ T cell responses can prevent ADE of DENV disease.[59] It has been demonstrated that pregnancy suppresses adaptive CD8+ and CD4+ T cell responses (such as T cell activation and proliferation) to ZIKV infection in mice.[35]

CURRENT VACCINE DEVELOPMENT ACTIVITIES

In relatively short order, Zika went from an obscure viral illness to an international public health concern. The rapid geographic spread of Zika, as well as its links to neurologic sequelae in adults and the potentially devastating effects on developing fetuses, has resulted in a significant effort to develop effective preventive measures.[58,60,61] Vaccines play center stage in those efforts as they have the potential to provide long-term protection to individuals, induce herd immunity in susceptible populations, and reduce disease transmission. A large variety of vaccine types exist, and researchers are developing Zika vaccines that cover the entire gamut of potential formulations.[62]

At the current time, there are no licensed vaccines to prevent ZIKV infection and disease. A number of vaccines (such as DNA, mRNA, inactivated whole-virion, or live attenuated) are currently either close to or in early Phase 1 and/or Phase 2 clinical trials.[63,64] These clinical trials may offer immune markers of protection and/or provide a surrogate endpoint that may forecast the clinical benefit of ZIKV vaccines (e.g., prevention of ZIKV disease or infection).[65]

Given the unique nature of Zika, successful vaccine products must address multiple issues: safety in target populations that include pregnant women, infants and young children, and immunocompromised and immunosenescent individuals; the need for rapid development of immunity (i.e., a preference for single-dose vaccines); the effect of previous flavivirus exposure; potential effects of Zika vaccine-induced immunity on subsequent flavivirus infection; cold chain needs; cost considerations; and availability and ease of deployment/use in regions affected by Zika.[66] The World Health Organization (WHO) has published a target product profile (TPP) outlining the idea attributes of a vaccine.[67] Here, we describe recent work in this area, with a focus on the vaccines that are furthest along in their development.

Live viral vaccines are among the most immunogenic of all vaccine types and typically provide robust and long-lasting, if not life-long, immunity. In most cases, the virus used is attenuated in some manner; however, due to the presence of live virus and/or the possibility that the virus may revert to a more pathogenic form, there are safety concerns associated with this type of vaccine. Live viral vaccines are typically contraindicated in the immunocompromised, very young infants, and pregnant women. These safety concerns are likely to be enhanced given our current, albeit incomplete, understanding of Zika pathogenesis and the documented link to developmental defects.

A live-attenuated ZIKV vaccine has been developed by introducing a 10-nucleotide deletion in a noncoding region of the viral region.[68] This vaccine elicited high-titer neutralizing Ab and robust T cell responses. Vaccinated animals (both immunocompetent CD-1 and immunocompromised A129 strains) developed sterilizing immunity that fully protected against subsequent high-dose viral challenge. Mosquitoes fed a blood meal containing the attenuated vaccine virus were not infected. The deletion has been shown to decrease viral RNA synthesis and increase viral sensitivity to IFN-β.

Additional attenuated vaccines have been created by introducing segments of the ZIKV genome into viral vectors. These chimeric and recombinant vector vaccines typically contain the E and prM proteins from ZIKV.[69–71] The E protein is the main target of neutralizing Abs, and inclusion of the prM protein allows for the production of subviral particles from infected cells, thereby increasing the in vivo antigen dose. One such live virus vaccine candidate has been created by replacing the prM-E genes in DENV with the ZIKV homolog.[72] The chimeric ZIKV vaccine on the DENV-2 backbone elicited high-titer neutralizing Ab and protected A129 mice against an intraperitoneal challenge with 10^4 PFU ZIKV. Vector-based vaccines incorporate specific Zika-derived sequences (e.g., the prM or E proteins) into an existing viral vector with proven immunogenicity. Adenoviruses, poxviruses, and lentiviruses are among the most commonly used vectors, as they facilitate long-term expression of the proteins of interest and are highly immunogenic. Preexisting immunity to the vector is a major disadvantage of these types of vaccines, although the use of rare strains or and/or prime-boost regimens with different formulations can be used to overcome this limitation.

An adenovirus-based ZIKV vaccine containing the E protein (BeH815744 strain) fused to the T4 fibritin foldon trimerization domain was created and administered subcutaneously (s.c.) to C57BL/6 mice in two doses (10^{11} PFU/dose).[73] Robust Ab responses, including high-titer neutralizing Ab, were detectable 2 weeks after administration of a booster dose. Maternal Ab elicited by this vaccine also provided complete protection to the 7-day-old pups challenged intraperitoneally (i.p.) with 10^5 PFU ZIKV DAKAR41542. Another group developed a rhesus adenovirus serotype

52-based ZIKV vaccine that expresses prM and E proteins.[42] A single dose of 10^{11} viral particles induced strong neutralizing Ab and IFN-γ producing T cell responses 2 weeks after vaccination. Furthermore, vaccinated rhesus macaques were completely protected (no detectable virus in serum) upon subsequent s.c. challenge with 10^3 PFU of Brazil/ZKV2015 strain. This protection was provided by a single dose administered intramuscularly (i.m.). The use of the rhesus adenovirus serotype avoids the problems with preexisting immunity that are typically observed with human adenovirus-based vaccines. Another vector-based ZIKV vaccine used recombinant vesicular stomatitis virus backbone and found that a prime-boost regimen of two intravenous (i.v.) doses induced strong humoral and cellular immune responses in BL/6 and Balb/c mice.[74] Ab titers were higher in the constructs that included prM and E proteins compared to E protein alone (both constructs used sequences from the ZikaSPH2015 strain). Additional vectors, such as measles virus, have also been utilized in the creation of ZIKV vaccines.[61]

Inactivated vaccines rely on chemical or physical processes to "kill" the virus. The resulting vaccine delivers a full complement of viral proteins, but the viral particles are unable to cause infection. Similarly, protein and peptide-based vaccines also lack infectious viral particles and are formulated to contain immunogenic proteins or epitopes. Vaccines containing synthetic peptides representing B and T cell epitopes with appropriate adjuvants that induce protective humoral and cellular immune responses may offer potential advantages over conventional whole-virion inactivated immunization. Peptide-based vaccines against viral pathogens (including Zika) are advantageous because of the lack of genetic material; they permit the immune response to focus only on immunodominant epitopes, allow for a relative ease of production, and they can be administered to pregnant women and persons with immunosuppressive disorders. Moreover, synthetic peptides are thermostable, biologically safe, and inexpensive to manufacture; they can be combined with adjuvants and are easily administered.[75,76] However, by themselves, peptides are not very immunogenic and therefore must be formulated with an adjuvant or other mechanism to enhance immunogenicity.

Viral-like particle (VLP) vaccines are typically composed of an empty viral shell. This shell is composed of the viral proteins usually targeted by humoral immune responses, but it lacks the viral genome and is therefore unable to replicate. These VLP vaccines retain the three-dimensional structure of the intact virus and contain both linear and conformational B cell epitopes. A purified formalin-inactivated ZIKV vaccine formulated with Alhydrogel given in a prime-boost regimen (with doses 21 days apart) was strongly immunogenic in both Balb/c and AG129 mice, eliciting high-titer neutralizing Ab.[77] Vaccinated AG129 mice were protected against an i.v. challenge with 10^5 PFU ZIKV MR766. Vaccinated animals also developed a strong anamnestic response upon virus challenge. Passive immunization using antisera from immunized rabbits prevented viremia in Balb/c mice challenged 6 hours postimmunization. This vaccine also protected against heterotypic virus challenge of AG129 mice using the FS 13025 strain of ZIKV.

Another purified alum-adjuvanted, formalin-inactivated ZIKV vaccine based on the PRVABC59 strain provided complete protection against viral challenge in both Balb/c mice and rhesus macaques.[39,42] In this study, both i.m. and s.c. immunization was studied, with s.c. vaccination generating lower Ab titers. Low-level viremia was also detected in two of the five mice vaccinated by the s.c. route, demonstrating that the route of vaccine administration can affect vaccine efficacy. A protein subunit vaccine consisting of the ZIKV E protein (BeH815744 strain) has been developed and tested after transcutaneous administration using a microneedle array.[73] Two doses of this vaccine, given 14 days apart, generated Ab responses 1 month after the booster vaccination. Immunized females were bred with nonimmunized males 3 weeks after vaccination, and pups were challenged i.p. with a lethal dose (10^5 PFU) of ZIKV DAKAR4152. The microneedle protein vaccine resulted in reduced weight loss, but only increased survival rates from 12.5% (pups from unimmunized mothers) to 50%. This study indicated that maternal immunization can provide passive protection to neonates, a promising result for future use of a ZIKV vaccine in pregnant women. A VLP-based ZIKV vaccine has also been developed and tested.[78] Cells expressing the capsid, premembrane, and Env structural proteins, together with the nonstructural NS2B/NS3B protease, produced high-titer VLPs based on the ZIKV H/PF/2013 genome. The resulting VLPs are recognized by monoclonal antibodies targeting conformational epitopes as well as by sera from Zika-infected patients. A single dose of vaccine (containing 1 or 4 µg of protein with or without Addavax—a squalene oil-in-water emulsion) elicited high-titer serum IgG and neutralizing Ab. Both the presence of adjuvant and higher antigen dose enhanced the humoral response. Ab responses to this vaccine did not enhance DENV-2 infection in vitro—an important finding that enhances confidence that this type of vaccine could be safely used in DENV-endemic areas.

Nucleic acid-based vaccines rely on the injection of DNA or RNA encoding viral proteins. Upon uptake by host cells, the viral proteins are produced, providing a sustained source of antigen and resulting in the development of Ab and antigen-specific T cells. A plasmid DNA vaccine encoding the prM and E proteins of Zika has been tested in Balb/c mice. Animals vaccinated with a single 50 μg dose of plasmid had detectable Ab responses 3 weeks after vaccination.[42] As with other vaccines described above, the formulation containing the full-length prM + E elicited higher Env-specific Ab titers than the formulation containing the E protein alone. This vaccine also induced both antigen-specific CD4+ and CD8+ T cell responses. A single dose of this vaccine also protected against an intranasal challenge with either ZIKV Brazil/ZKV2015 or PRVABC59, as immunized animals had no detectable viremia following challenge with either virus. Depletion of CD4+ and/or CD8+ T cells after vaccination and before viral challenge had no effect on protection, suggesting that humoral immunity is sufficient for protection. Note, however, that this experiment did not address the need for T cell help during the development of that humoral response. This same vaccine has been tested in nonhuman primates using a 5 mg dose administered i.m.[39] A single dose elicited minimal Ab titers, while a prime-boost regimen resulted in the development of fairly robust humoral immunity 2 weeks after the priming dose. As with the mouse studies, vaccinated macaques were fully protected and had no detectable viremia following subcutaneous challenge with 10^3 PFU of ZIKV Brazil/ZKV2015.

Dowd et al. developed two DNA plasmid vaccines containing the prM-E sequence from the French Polynesian ZIKV isolate H/PF/2013.[44] The first variant (VRC5283) replaced the ZIKV prM signal sequence with the JEV sequence; the second variant (VRC5288) replaced both the prM signal sequence and the stem/transmembrane E protein sequences with the corresponding JEV region. Both variants elicited high-titer virus binding and virus neutralizing Ab responses after electroporation of 50ug DNA into the quadriceps muscle of Balb/c and BL/6 mice. Immunogenicity in rhesus macaques was also evaluated; animals received a single 1 mg dose, a prime-boost regimen with 1 mg per dose, or a prime-boost regimen with 4 mg per dose. All groups developed neutralizing Ab responses, although titers were significantly lower in the single-dose group. Differences in immunogenicity between the two vaccine constructs were minimal. Protection was evaluated in

these same vaccination groups by evaluating serum viral load following an s.c. challenge with 10^3 PFU of the PRVABC59 strain of ZIKV. Virus was undetectable in all animals vaccinated twice with VR5283 (JEV signal peptide and full-length ZIKV prM-E), regardless of dose. A single animal vaccinated twice with 1 mg of VR5288 (ZIVK prM-E with JEV signal peptide/transmembrane/stem regions) had transient, low-level viral load on Day 3 and Day 7. In contrast, mice vaccinated once with 1 mg of VRC5288 all experienced moderate to high-level viremia, indicating that this vaccine dose elicited subprotective Ab titers. Inovio Pharmaceuticals and GeneOne Life Science were among the first to develop a Zika vaccine. This product, a DNA vaccine based on a ZIKV prM-E consensus sequence, has been found to elicit ZIKV-specific T cells capable of producing TNF-α and IFN-γ in both C5BL/6 and IFNAR KO mice.[79] The vaccine was administered 3× at 2-week intervals through intramuscular electroporation. The same vaccine regimen induced robust binding and neutralizing Ab titers in both strains of mice. The consensus sequence vaccine was found to elicit stronger humoral and cellular immune responses than versions containing either the Brazilian or Puerto Rican sequences. Protective efficacy in IFNAR KO mice was also evaluated following infection with 1 or 2×10^6 PFU of ZIKV-PR209. Vaccinated mice exhibited 100% survival compared to 30% (1×10^6 PFU) or 10% (2×10^6 PFU) survival in control animals. Vaccinated animals had no evidence of weight loss or clinical signs of illness. Adoptive transfer of immune sera from vaccinated animals into IFNAR KO mice reduced weight loss and protected 80% of passively immunized animals. Experiments using intradermal immunization of rhesus macaques (two doses: 2 mg each, 2 weeks apart) confirmed the immunogenicity of the vaccine formulation, as both humoral and cellular immune responses were readily detectable 6 weeks after vaccination. This DNA vaccine has also shown promise in clinical trials.[80]

Several RNA vaccines have also been developed and have shown promise in animal studies. Pardi et al. have developed a nucleoside-modified mRNA encoding the prM-E proteins of ZIKV H/PF/2013.[46] The modification avoids innate immune responses and enhances mRNA translation. The mRNA is also encapsulated in lipid nanoparticles to further enhance protein expression. A single intradermal injection induces E protein-specific Th1 responses and high-titer neutralizing antibodies in both C57BL/6 and Balb/c mice. Single-dose vaccination prevents viremia in Balb/c mice challenged 2 or 20 weeks after vaccination with 200 PFU of ZIKV PRVABC59. The vaccine was also tested at 600, 200, and 50 μg doses in rhesus macaques. Five weeks later, vaccination was followed by s.c. injection of 10^4 tissue culture infectious dose 50% ($TCID_{50}$) of ZIKV PRVABC59. One vaccinated animal (recipient of 600 μg of vaccine) experienced a transient low-level viremia of 100 viral RNA copies per ml on Day 3, whereas all control animals exhibited 1000−10,000 copies per ml. Another nucleoside-modified RNA vaccine was constructed encoding the ZIKV prM-E sequence with optimized 5′ and 3′ untranslated regions (UTRs) and a signal sequence from human IgE.[52] A variant of this construct lacking the cross-reactive E-DII-FL epitope was also created in order to reduce the potential for ADE of disease. This construct was tested for immunogenicity and pathogenicity in AG129 mice. Maximum immunogenicity required two doses of lipid nanoparticle-encapsulated mRNA 3 weeks apart. There was also a dose-dependent increase in Ab titer. C57BL/6 mice were immunized i.m. with a booster vaccination at Day 28, followed by viral challenge at eight or 18 weeks after infection. One day prior to challenge, type I interferon signaling was disrupted using an interferon alpha receptor (IFNAR)-blocking Ab. Mice were challenged with 10^6 PFU of ZIKV Dakar 41519. Control mice had a 30% survival rate compared to 100% survival in vaccinated animals. Vaccinated animals also had no measurable weight loss or viremia 5 days after challenge. The protective effects were similar at weeks 8 and 18, indicating that vaccine-induced protection was long-lived. Results indicated that the removal of the cross-reactive DII epitope reduced the production of antibodies capable of enhancing DENV infection in vitro. A third RNA-based ZIKV vaccine has been shown to elicit strong Ab and CD8+ T cell responses in C57BL/6 mice.[45] This construct is based on a modified dendrimer nanoparticle RNA replicon that has been successfully used for single-dose influenza, Ebola, and toxoplasma gondii vaccines.

The identification of a correlate of protection will be an important step forward for vaccine development. Neutralizing Ab correlates with protection from clinical diseases for other flaviviruses.[81,82] Multiple animal studies of Zika vaccine have also observed protection correlated with neutralizing Ab titer and several neutralizing epitopes have been defined.[41,83,84] Larocca et al., using a single-dose DNA vaccine, found that a serum dilution of 1:20 provided protection in mice.[42] Two doses of the same vaccine elicited a 50% virus neutralizing antibody titer of 1:100 and completely protected Rhesus macaques. Adoptive transfer of ZIKV-specific IgG into mice and rhesus macaques indicated that recipient mice with 50% microneutralization titers >60 were protected, while recipient macaques with 50% microneutralization titers >125 were also protected from viremia.[39] Two 5 μg doses of an alum-absorbed, purified inactivated ZIKV vaccine elicited 50% microneutralization titers of >2300 protected AG129 mice and provided sterile immunity following viral challenge.[77] In that same study, passive immunization of rabbit antisera into Balb/c mice yielding 50% microneutralization titers of >128 provided protection against viremia. Human data from ongoing clinical trials in immunologically naïve individuals in ZIKV-endemic areas may provide additional data necessary to define a clinically useful correlate of protection.

Several of the aforementioned vaccine candidates are currently being evaluated in clinical trials. The majority of these trials are recently initiated Phase 1 trials examining safety, tolerability, and immunogenicity. As data from these trials is collected, that information will inform larger trials that more comprehensively examine safety and efficacy. Information on these trials is provided in Table 5.1, with additional details available at www.clinicaltrials.gov.

SCIENTIFIC, REGULATORY, AND ETHICAL BARRIERS/CONSIDERATIONS IN THE DESIGN AND TESTING OF A ZIKA VACCINE

As reviewed above, continued progress is occurring in approaches toward developing Zika vaccines; however, serious scientific, ethical, and regulatory challenges lie ahead. We have previously published a discussion of some of these issues.[29,61] Below we will briefly summarize issues within each of these broad categories.

Scientific Challenges

In addition to the usual criteria of immunogenicity, efficacy, and safety, there are additional nuances to consider during Zika vaccine development. As we have outlined in previous publications, different vaccines might be developed for different situations and subpopulations.[29,61] Vaccines in immunosenescent older people, who are at most risk for subsequent neurologic complications such as GBS, may need the addition of adjuvants. Vaccines for younger healthy children might induce high titer, life-long immunity through live viral attenuated vaccines. Vaccines in pregnant women and immunocompromised individuals may require inactivated, subunit, or peptide-based vaccine approaches; therefore, we may, in fact, need to develop more than one type of vaccine product.

TABLE 5.1
ZIKV Vaccines in Clinical Trials

Trial#	Vaccine Type	Sponsor and/or Site	Type of Trial	Outcomes or Endpoints
NCT02996890	MV-ZIKA Live-attenuated vaccine Measles virus vector	Themis Bioscience GmbH; Medical University of Vienna, Center for Pathophysiology, Infectiology and Immunology, Austria; Medical University of Vienna, Department of Clinical Pharmacology, Austria	Phase 1, double-blind, randomized, placebo-controlled. Single dose versus two dose (Days 0 and 28).	Neutralizing Ab titer
NCT02952833	ZPIV Purified-inactivated vaccine	NIAID; St. Louis University Center for Vaccine Development, Missouri	Phase 1, double-blind, placebo-controlled. Prime-boost regimen (Days 1 and 29) 2.5ug, 5.0ug, and 10ug doses.	Local and systemic adverse events Binding Ab GMT Neutralizing Ab titer Seroconversion rate Response kinetics
NCT03008122	ZPIV Purified-inactivated vaccine	NIAID; Ponce School of Medicine, Puerto Rico	Phase 1, randomized, double-blind, placebo-controlled. Prime-boost regimen (Days 1 and 29) 2.5ug and 5.0ug doses.	Local and systemic adverse events Binding Ab GMT Neutralizing Ab titer Seroconversion rate Response kinetics
NCT02963909	ZPIV Purified-inactivated vaccine With or without prior vaccination (YF-VAX® or JEV IXIARO®)	NIAID; Walter Reed Army Institute of Research, Maryland	Phase 1, double-blind, randomized, placebo-controlled. Prime-boost regimen (Days 1 and 29) 5.0ug dose	Local and systemic adverse events Neutralizing Ab titer Seroconversion rate Response kinetics
NCT02937233	ZPIV Purified-inactivated vaccine	NIAID; Walter Reed Army Institute of Research, Maryland; Beth Israel Deaconess medical Center, Massachusetts	Phase 1, double-blind, randomized, placebo-controlled. Prime-boost regimen (Week 0 +/− Week 1, 2, or 4). 5ug dose	Local and systemic adverse events Binding Ab GMT Neutralizing Ab titer IFNg ELISPOT
NCT02840487	VRC-ZKADNA085−00-VP DNA vaccine	NIAID; University of Maryland Center for Vaccine Development, Maryland; Hope Clinic−Emory Vaccine Center, Georgia	Phase 1/1b, randomized Prime-boost regimen, 1st dose on Day 0 and subsequent doses at varying time-points: week 8, week 12, weeks 4 and 8, weeks 4 and 20.	Safety Tolerability Neutralizing Ab titer

NCT02996461	VRC-ZKADNA090—00-VP DNA vaccine	NIAID; NIH Clinical Center, Maryland	Phase 1, randomized Prime-boost regimen. Testing syringe versus jet injector Testing various time-points for booster	Safety Tolerability Neutralizing Ab titer
NCT03110770	VRC-ZKADNA090—00-VP DNA vaccine	NIAID; EMMES Corporation; Leidos Biomedical Research; Baylor College of Medicine, Texas; Puerto Rico Clinical and Translational Research Consortium, Puerto Rico; QPS-Miami Research Associates, Florida; Doctors Hospital at Renaissance, Texas; Hospital Civil Fray Antonio Alcalde, Mexico; Asociacion Civil Selva Amazonica, Peru; Fundación de Investigación de Diego, Puerto Rico; San Juan Hospital Research Unit, Puerto Rico	Phase 2/2b, randomized, placebo-controlled.	Safety Local and systemic adverse events Ab titer Zika infection
NCT02809443	GLS-5700 DNA plasmid	GeneOne Life Science; Inovio Pharmaceuticals; Miami Research Association, Florida University of Pennsylvania, Pennsylvania; Universite Laval hospital CHUL, Quebec	Phase 1, dose ranging Single vaccination with 1 mg or 2 mg dose	Adverse events Binding Ab titer Neutralizing Ab titer T cell response
NCT02887482	GLS-5700 DNA plasmid	GeneOne Life Science; Inovio Pharmaceuticals Clinical Research of Puerto Rico, Fundacion De Investigation, University of Puerto Rico, Puerto Rico	Phase 1, double-blind, placebo-controlled Single dose of 2 mg	Adverse events Binding Ab titer Neutralizing Ab titer T cell response
NCT03014089	mRNA-1325 RNA vaccine	Moderna Therapeutics; BARDA; San Diego, California Melbourne, Florida Peoria, Illinois	Phase 1/2, randomized, placebo-controlled	Adverse events Neutralizing Ab titer

Ab, antibody; *NIAID*, national institute of allergy and infectious diseases; *GMT*, geometric mean titer; *BARDA*, biomedical advanced research and development authority.

Other considerations also loom large. For example, in the theoretical construct of such vaccines, shall they be designed as replication-competent or replication-deficient platforms? As infection-permissive or as inducing sterilizing immunity and preventing even low-level infection? What would be the endpoints of success—prevention of infection? Prevention of viremia? Or prevention of complications? Or even, if it were possible, simply prevention of infection in the developing fetus? If Zika viral strains not associated with congenital malformations (such as the African strain) can be identified, this might facilitate the development and safety of live-attenuated vaccines. Data demonstrating a lack of adverse effects or safe sanctuary in the human testis and ovary must be presented if live viral vaccines are utilized.

From the immunity standpoint, challenges arise (particularly for specific vaccine types) in distinguishing vaccine-induced from infection-induced immunity. Concerns remain, again perhaps depending upon vaccine product type, regarding aberrant immune outcomes due to Ab-mediated enhanced disease among persons previously flavivirus-infected or the challenge of inducing immunity in previously flavivirus-infected persons (i.e., original antigenic sin). Yet other challenges include the duration of vaccine-induced immunity, the number of vaccine doses needed, and ensuring that segments of the population are not left highly vulnerable at older ages as immunity wanes. Other important challenges, particularly in less developed economies, include a need for vaccine cold chains and the cost of providing vaccines to the population. The WHO has published a TPP for ZIKV vaccines—with special emphasis on use during public health emergencies.[67]

Another challenge will be the cost of vaccine clinical trials. Currently, Zika outbreaks seem to have diminished, and one can expect they will flare up again, albeit in differing geographic locations. How shall vaccine studies and clinical efficacy trials be conducted in such an environment? Very large numbers of vaccine recipients will be needed in order to have sufficient statistical power to estimate efficacy against specific Zika complications such as GBS and congenital malformations. Similarly, clinical trials designed to estimate safety and risk among pregnant women may require very large numbers of subjects—and yet would be necessary to ensure safety before widespread use throughout the population.

Ethical Challenges

Above and beyond the ethical concerns of development, testing, and implementation of a vaccine program with any new vaccine, Zika vaccine development poses additional challenges. One area of controversy has been in human challenge studies. Should they be allowed? What are the risks? If risks exist, then in what type of selected populations do they exist?

Another significant issue is that the most immediate needs are to protect women and men of child-bearing age and their unborn children. As such, exceptional safety must be ensured and the absence of harms demonstrated. How should such vaccines be tested in pregnant women? Should they be allowed to participate in vaccine trials? The controversy and discussion about the role of pregnant women in vaccine clinical trials is ongoing. Bioethicists have lined up on both sides of the question, "should pregnant women be entered into clinical trials of Zika vaccines?" For the most part, the consensus seems to be "no," given the potential for unknown harms on two lives. Others have suggested that pregnant women have the most to gain from such research and should have the right to participate. The Ethics Working Group on ZIKV Research & Pregnancy, funded by the Wellcome Trust, has issued guidelines for the participation of pregnant women in these trials.[85] The Working Group agreed upon three key imperatives guiding Zika vaccine development in pregnant women, and the following summary is provided:

The first imperative and its recommendations address the importance of prioritizing and incentivizing development of a ZIKV vaccine that can be used by pregnant women. The second imperative and set of recommendations address the need for research specific to vaccine use in pregnancy for all ZIKV vaccines, with corresponding data collection efforts, in order to generate evidence that is critically needed to inform responsible public health policy and clinical practice affecting pregnant women. The third imperative and its recommendations address the importance of ensuring the fair inclusion of pregnant women in research studies carrying the prospect of direct benefit.[85]

Regulatory Challenges

Regulatory challenges are defined by the type of vaccine product developed. For example, live viral vaccines have specific challenges associated with them compared to inactivated vaccines. Novel vaccine platforms for which there is little in the way of experience or regulatory guidance lead to yet other challenges. No current regulatory developmental pathways are evident for DNA, adenovirus-vectored, and peptide-based vaccines.

A review of barriers to the use of Zika vaccines in pregnant women has been published.[86] These include significant knowledge gaps in understanding immune responses to viral antigens in early pregnancy, a lack of standardized definitions for outcomes in evaluating vaccines in pregnancy, inadequate experience with real-time safety assessments balanced against benefit, and even a lack of data in baseline rates of outcomes of importance in countries with poorly developed public health infrastructure. The latter is a particular issue in evaluating vaccine safety and adverse outcomes in geographic areas where other co-circulating viruses that are associated with adverse birth outcomes occur.[87]

Finally, the WHO has published recommended procedures for emergency use of investigational vaccines and listing procedures for candidate vaccines such as Zika.[88] In addition, WHO has published the results of a consultation on regulatory issues regarding Zika vaccines,[67] and the Pan American Health Organization (PAHO) has provided recommendations on important issues related to the outbreak of ZIKV.[89]

Economic Challenges

Finally, it is not clear how the considerable costs of vaccine research and development will be borne and by whom. Pharmaceutical manufacturers have recent memories of Ebola vaccine development costs and the lack of ongoing financial support for such efforts. Outside research development, financial support is critical because of the uncertain market potential, the uncertain economic markets for selling such a vaccine, and uncertainty of government support for a vaccination program. One possibility is the potential for funding through a program such as Coalition for Epidemic Pandemic Preparedness Innovations.[90] While the data are limited, Zika outbreaks thus far appear to be explosive—but short-lived—before moving on to another geographic location. The consequences of this are both increased expense and difficulty in conducting clinical trials and difficulty in understanding potential markets for selling such a vaccine.

SUMMARY

The history of Zika outbreaks thus far is one of sudden, relatively explosive outbreaks, followed by resolution of the threat over a year or two. This is followed by movement of further outbreaks to other geographic locations. The implication of this is that the outbreaks are generally not long enough to sustain human attention, interest, and funding related to vaccine research and development. ZIKV causes morbidity and occasional mortality injurious to the public health. The most significant morbidity is neurologic, which unfortunately disproportionately affects the most vulnerable—unborn children. Such effects are substantial and exist for a lifetime. In turn, this disrupts family planning

and induces significant fear in prospective parents. For this reason, the world needs vaccines effective against Zika infection and its complications.

As this chapter outlines, the need is large, and interest and opportunity are fleeting. The requirements are daunting—the recipients diverse in need—and the dollars available insufficient. Significant ethical, scientific, and regulatory obstacles remain. Yet, as discussed herein, substantial early progress has been made in demonstrating vaccine candidates that are immunogenic and efficacious in both mouse and nonhuman primate models.

Much more must be known, much more must be applied, and the world waits. Shakespeare, in his play, *Julius Caesar* (Act 4, scene 3), got it right when he has Brutus say:

> *The enemy increaseth every day … we, at the height, are ready to decline … there is a tide in the affairs of men. Which, taken at the flood, leads on to fortune; omitted, all the voyage of their life is bound in shallows and miseries. On such a full sea are we not afloat, and we must take the current when it serves, or lose our ventures.*

We are indeed on such a full sea; the currents of politics, inadequate funding by governments, and apathy must not diminish what is arguably the height in the history of mankind and of scientific knowledge to date. If research teams fail to be funded, we are indeed doomed to decline and lives will be "bound in the shallows". Perhaps only a more ancient piece of literature will do. The Book of Wisdom (Proverbs) was written circa 700 BC and in one section contrasts Wisdom and Folly. Men, it says, prefer Folly over Wisdom and, of note, Wisdom is only a fleeting visitor. How often these words seem prescient in the area of emerging infections and the world's response to them. It is our hope that this chapter may serve not only as a solid overview of ZIKV and the development of vaccines to protect against it, but also as an inducement to other scientists to apply their science to this public health threat and for governments to assist the people in what they cannot do for themselves—provide the funding and resources with which to apply science toward the control of this terrible disease. We should do no less nor tolerate the apparent apathy shown by governmental and regulatory agency oversight groups in the face of human harm.

REFERENCES

1. World Health Organization. *WHO Statement on the First Meeting of the International Health Regulations (2005) (IHR 2005) Emergency Committee on Zika Virus and Observed Increase in Neurological Disorders and Neonatal Malformations*; 2016. http://www.who.int/mediacentre/news/statements/2016/1st-emergency-committee-zika/en/.

2. Dick GW, Kitchen SF, Haddow AJ. Zika virus. I. Isolations and serological specificity. *Trans R Soc Trop Med Hyg.* 1952; 46:509–520.
3. Duffy MR, Chen TH, Hancock WT, et al. Zika virus outbreak on Yap Island, Federated States of Micronesia. *N Engl J Med.* June 11, 2009;360(24):2536–2543.
4. Cao-Lormeau VM, Blake A, Mons S, et al. Guillain-Barre Syndrome outbreak associated with Zika virus infection in French Polynesia: a case-control study. *Lancet.* April 9, 2016;387(10027):1531–1539.
5. Cao-Lormeau VM, Roche C, Teissier A, et al. Zika virus, French polynesia, South Pacific, 2013. *Emerg Infect Dis.* June 2014;20(6):1085–1086.
6. Triunfol MA. New mosquito-borne threat to pregnant women in Brazil. *Lancet Infect Dis.* February 2016;16(2): 156–157.
7. Likos A, Griffin I, Bingham AM, et al. Local mosquito-borne transmission of Zika virus — Miami-Dade and Broward Counties, Florida, June–August 2016. *MMWR.* September 30, 2016;65(38):1032–1038.
8. Deseda CC. Epidemiology of Zika. *Curr Opin Pediatr.* February 2017;29(1):97–101.
9. Ikejezie J, Shapiro CN, Kim J, et al. Zika virus transmission — region of the Americas, May 15, 2015–December 15, 2016. *MMWR.* March 31, 2017;66(12):329–334.
10. Metsky HC, Matranga CB, Wohl S, et al. Zika virus evolution and spread in the Americas. *Nature.* June 15, 2017; 546(7658):411–415.
11. Althouse BM, Vasilakis N, Sall AA, Diallo M, Weaver SC, Hanley KA. Potential for Zika virus to establish a sylvatic transmission cycle in the Americas. *PLoS Negl Trop Dis.* December 2016;10(12):e0005055.
12. Petersen LR, Jamieson DJ, Powers AM, Honein MA. Zika virus. *N Engl J Med.* April 21, 2016;374(16):1552–1563.
13. Baud D, Gubler DJ, Schaub B, Lanteri MC, Musso D. An update on Zika virus infection. *Lancet.* June 21, 2017.
14. Krow-Lucal ER, Novosad SA, Dunn AC, et al. Zika virus infection in patient with No known risk factors, Utah, USA, 2016. *Emerg Infect Dis.* August 2017;23(8):1260–1267.
15. Paz-Bailey G, Rosenberg ES, Doyle K, et al. Persistence of Zika virus in body fluids — preliminary report. *N Engl J Med.* February 14, 2017.
16. Atkinson B, Thorburn F, Petridou C, et al. Presence and persistence of Zika virus RNA in semen, United Kingdom, 2016. *Emerg Infect Dis.* April 15, 2017;23(4).
17. de Oliveira WK, de Franca GVA, Carmo EH, Duncan BB, de Souza Kuchenbecker R, Schmidt MI. Infection-related microcephaly after the 2015 and 2016 Zika virus outbreaks in Brazil: a surveillance-based analysis. *Lancet.* June 21, 2017.
18. Reagan-Steiner S, Simeone R, Simon E, et al. Evaluation of placental and fetal tissue specimens for Zika virus infection — 50 states and District of Columbia, January–December, 2016. *MMWR.* June 23, 2017;66(24):636–643.
19. Meneses JDA, Ishigami AC, de Mello LM, et al. Lessons learned at the epicenter of Brazil's congenital Zika epidemic: evidence from 87 confirmed cases. *Clin Infect Dis.* May 15, 2017;64(10):1302–1308.
20. de Araujo TV, Rodrigues LC, de Alencar Ximenes RA, et al. Association between Zika virus infection and microcephaly in Brazil, January to May, 2016: preliminary report of a case-control study. *Lancet Infect Dis.* December 2016; 16(12):1356–1363.
21. Martines RB, Bhatnagar J, de Oliveira Ramos AM, et al. Pathology of congenital Zika syndrome in Brazil: a case series. *Lancet.* August 27, 2016;388(10047):898–904.
22. Reynolds MR, Jones AM, Petersen EE, et al. Vital signs: update on Zika virus-associated birth defects and evaluation of all U.S. infants with congenital Zika virus exposure — U.S. Zika pregnancy registry, 2016. *MMWR.* April 07, 2017;66(13):366–373.
23. Dos Santos T, Rodriguez A, Almiron M, et al. Zika virus and the Guillain-Barre syndrome — case series from seven countries. *N Engl J Med.* October 20, 2016;375(16): 1598–1601.
24. da Silva IRF, Frontera JA, Bispo de Filippis AM, Nascimento O. Neurologic complications associated with the Zika virus in Brazilian adults. *JAMA Neurol.* August 14, 2017.
25. Centers for Disease Control and Prevention. *Zika Prevention;* 2017. https://www.cdc.gov/zika/prevention/index.html.
26. Centers for Disease Control and Prevention. *Integrated Mosquito Management;* 2017. https://www.cdc.gov/zika/vector/integrated_mosquito_management.html.
27. Centers for Disease Control and Prevention. *Zika Virus Testing: For Healthcare Providers;* 2017. https://www.cdc.gov/zika/hc-providers/index.html.
28. Campbell LP, Luther C, Moo-Llanes D, Ramsey JM, Danis-Lozano R, Peterson AT. Climate change influences on global distributions of dengue and chikungunya virus vectors. *Philos Trans R Soc Lond B Biol Sci.* April 5, 2015; 370(1665).
29. Palacios R, Poland GA, Kalil J. Another emerging arbovirus, another emerging vaccine: targeting Zika virus. *Vaccine.* April 29, 2016;34(20):2291–2293.
30. Lowy I. Leaking containers: success and failure in controlling the mosquito *Aedes aegypti* in Brazil. *Am J Public Health.* April 2017;107(4):517–524.
31. Marston HD, Lurie N, Borio LL, Fauci AS. Considerations for developing a Zika virus vaccine. *N Engl J Med.* September 29, 2016;375(13):1209–1212.
32. Dai L, Song J, Lu X, et al. Structures of the Zika virus envelope protein and its complex with a flavivirus broadly protective antibody. *Cell Host Microbe.* May 11, 2016;19(5): 696–704.
33. Hamel R, Dejarnac O, Wichit S, et al. Biology of Zika virus infection in human skin cells. *J Virol.* September 2015; 89(17):8880–8896.
34. Meertens L, Labeau A, Dejarnac O, et al. Axl mediates Zika virus entry in human glial cells and modulates innate immune responses. *Cell Rep.* January 10, 2017;18(2): 324–333.
35. Winkler CW, Myers LM, Woods TA, et al. Adaptive immune responses to Zika virus are important for controlling virus infection and preventing infection in brain and testes. *J Immunol.* May 01, 2017;198(9):3526–3535.

36. Grant A, Ponia SS, Tripathi S, et al. Zika virus targets human STAT2 to inhibit type I interferon signaling. *Cell Host Microbe*. June 08, 2016;19(6):882−890.
37. Aliota MT, Dudley DM, Newman CM, et al. Heterologous protection against Asian Zika virus challenge in rhesus macaques. *PLoS Negl Trop Dis*. December 2016;10(12): e0005168.
38. Dudley DM, Aliota MT, Mohr EL, et al. A rhesus macaque model of Asian-lineage Zika virus infection. *Nat Commun*. 2016;7:12204.
39. Abbink P, Larocca RA, De La Barrera RA, et al. Protective efficacy of multiple vaccine platforms against Zika virus challenge in rhesus monkeys. *Science*. August 4, 2016; 353(6304):1129−1132.
40. Sapparapu G, Fernandez E, Kose N, et al. Neutralizing human antibodies prevent Zika virus replication and fetal disease in mice. *Nature*. December 15, 2016;540(7633): 443−447.
41. Stettler K, Beltramello M, Espinosa DA, et al. Specificity, cross-reactivity, and function of antibodies elicited by Zika virus infection. *Science*. August 19, 2016;353(6301): 823−826.
42. Larocca RA, Abbink P, Peron JP, et al. Vaccine protection against Zika virus from Brazil. *Nature*. June 28, 2016; 536(7617):474−478.
43. Wang Q, Yan J, Gao GF. Monoclonal antibodies against Zika virus: Therapeutics and their implications for vaccine design. *J Virol*. October 15, 2017;91(20).
44. Dowd KA, Ko SY, Morabito KM, et al. Rapid development of a DNA vaccine for Zika virus. *Science*. October 14, 2016; 354(6309):237−240.
45. Chahal JS, Fang T, Woodham AW, et al. An RNA nanoparticle vaccine against Zika virus elicits antibody and CD8+ T cell responses in a mouse model. *Sci Rep*. March 21, 2017;7(1):252.
46. Pardi N, Hogan MJ, Pelc RS, et al. Zika virus protection by a single low-dose nucleoside-modified mRNA vaccination. *Nature*. February 02, 2017;543(7644):248−251.
47. Wang Q, Yang H, Liu X, et al. Molecular determinants of human neutralizing antibodies isolated from a patient infected with Zika virus. *Sci Transl Med*. December 14, 2016;8(369):369ra179.
48. Freire MCLC, Pol-Fachin L, Coelho D, et al. Mapping putative B-Cell Zika virus NS1 epitopes provides molecular basis for anti-NS1 antibody discrimination between Zika and dengue viruses. *ACS Omega*. 2017;2(7):3913−3920.
49. Edeling MA, Diamond MS, Fremont DH. Structural basis of Flavivirus NS1 assembly and antibody recognition. *Proc Natl Acad Sci USA*. March 18, 2014;111(11): 4285−4290.
50. Priyamvada L, Quicke KM, Hudson WH, et al. Human antibody responses after dengue virus infection are highly cross-reactive to Zika virus. *Proc Natl Acad Sci USA*. July 12, 2016;113(28):7852−7857.
51. Dejnirattisai W, Supasa P, Wongwiwat W, et al. Dengue virus sero-cross-reactivity drives antibody-dependent enhancement of infection with Zika virus. *Nat Immunol*. September 2016;17(9):1102−1108.
52. Richner JM, Himansu S, Dowd KA, et al. Modified mRNA vaccines protect against Zika virus infection. *Cell*. March 09, 2017;168(6):1114−1125 e1110.
53. Dowd KA, DeMaso CR, Pelc RS, et al. Broadly neutralizing activity of Zika virus-immune sera identifies a single viral serotype. *Cell Rep*. August 09, 2016;16(6):1485−1491.
54. Elong Ngono A, Vizcarra EA, Tang WW, et al. Mapping and role of the CD8+ T cell response during primary Zika virus infection in mice. *Cell Host Microbe*. January 11, 2017; 21(1):35−46.
55. Shrestha B, Diamond MS. Role of CD8+ T cells in control of West Nile virus infection. *J Virol*. August 2004;78(15): 8312−8321.
56. Yauch LE, Zellweger RM, Kotturi MF, et al. A protective role for dengue virus-specific CD8+ T cells. *J Immunol*. April 15, 2009;182(8):4865−4873.
57. Pardy RD, Rajah MM, Condotta SA, Taylor NG, Sagan SM, Richer MJ. Analysis of the T Cell response to Zika virus and identification of a novel CD8+ T cell epitope in immunocompetent mice. *PLoS Pathog*. February 2017;13(2): e1006184.
58. Pierson TC, Graham BS. Zika virus: immunity and vaccine development. *Cell*. October 20, 2016;167(3):625−631.
59. Zellweger RM, Eddy WE, Tang WW, Miller R, Shresta S. CD8+ T cells prevent antigen-induced antibody-dependent enhancement of dengue disease in mice. *J Immunol*. October 15, 2014;193(8):4117−4124.
60. Tripp RA, Ross TM. Development of a Zika vaccine. *Exp Rev Vaccines*. September 2016;15(9):1083−1085.
61. Poland GA, Kennedy RB, Ovsyannikova IG, Palacios R, Ho PL, Kalil J. Current development of vaccines against Zika virus. *Lancet Infect Dis*. 2018;18(7):e211−e219.
62. Barzon L, Palu G. Current views on Zika virus vaccine development. *Expert Opin Biol Ther*. June 26, 2017:1−8.
63. Gaudinski MR, Houser KV, Morabito KM, et al. Safety, tolerability, and immunogenicity of two Zika virus DNA vaccine candidates in healthy adults: randomised, open-label, phase 1 clinical trials. *Lancet*. 2018 Feb 10; 391(10120):552−562. https://doi.org/10.1016/S0140-6736(17)33106-9.
64. Modjarrad K, Lin L, George SL, et al. Preliminary aggregate safety and immunogenicity results from three trials of a purified inactivated Zika virus vaccine candidate: phase 1, randomised, double-blind, placebo-controlled clinical trials. *Lancet*. 2018 Feb 10;391(10120):563−571. https://doi.org/10.1016/S0140-6736(17)33106-9.
65. Gruber MF, Krause PR. Regulating vaccines at the FDA: development and licensure of Zika vaccines. *Exp Rev Vaccines*. June 2017;16(6):525−527.
66. Durbin AP. Vaccine development for Zika virus-timelines and strategies. *Semin Reprod Med*. September 2016;34(5):299−304.
67. Vannice KS, Giersing BK, Kaslow DC, et al. Meeting Report: WHO consultation on considerations for regulatory expectations of Zika virus vaccines for use during an emergency. *Vaccine*. December 01, 2016.
68. Shan C, Muruato AE, Nunes BTD, et al. A live-attenuated Zika virus vaccine candidate induces sterilizing immunity in mouse models. *Nat Med*. June 2017;23(6):763−767.

69. Lin HH, Yip BS, Huang LM, Wu SC. Zika virus structural biology and progress in vaccine development. *Biotechnol Adv.* September 12, 2017.

70. Wahid B, Ali A, Rafique S, Idrees M. Current status of therapeutic and vaccine approaches against Zika virus. *Eur J Intern Med.* August 07, 2017.

71. Du L, Zhou Y, Jiang S. The latest advancements in Zika virus vaccine development. *Exp Rev Vaccines.* October 2017; 16(10):951–954.

72. Xie X, Yang Y, Muruato AE, et al. Understanding Zika virus stability and developing a chimeric vaccine through functional analysis. *MBio.* February 07, 2017;8(1).

73. Kim E, Erdos G, Huang S, Kenniston T, Falo Jr LD, Gambotto A. Preventative vaccines for Zika virus outbreak: preliminary evaluation. *EBioMedicine.* November 2016;13: 315–320.

74. Betancourt D, de Queiroz NM, Xia T, Ahn J, Barber GN. Cutting edge: innate immune augmenting vesicular stomatitis virus expressing Zika virus proteins confers protective immunity. *J Immunol.* April 15, 2017;198(8):3023–3028.

75. Rosenthal KS. Immune peptide enhancement of peptide based vaccines. *Front Biosci.* 2005;10:478–482.

76. Flower DR. Designing immunogenic peptides. *Nat Chem Biol.* December 2013;9(12):749–753.

77. Sumathy K, Kulkarni B, Gondu RK, et al. Protective efficacy of Zika vaccine in AG129 mouse model. *Sci Rep.* April 12, 2017;7:46375.

78. Boigard H, Alimova A, Martin GR, Katz A, Gottlieb P, Galarza JM. Zika virus-like particle (VLP) based vaccine. *PLoS Negl Trop Dis.* May 2017;11(5):e0005608.

79. Muthumani K, Griffin BD, Agarwal S, et al. *In Vivo Protection against ZIKV Infection and Pathogenesis through Passive Antibody Transfer and Active Immunisation with a PrMEnv DNA Vaccine.* Vol. 1. 2016:16021.

80. Tebas P, Roberts CC, Muthumani K, et al. Safety and immunogenicity of an anti-Zika virus DNA vaccine — preliminary report. *N Engl J Med.* October 4, 2017.

81. Ishikawa T, Yamanaka A, Konishi E. A review of successful flavivirus vaccines and the problems with those flaviviruses for which vaccines are not yet available. *Vaccine.* March 10, 2014;32(12):1326–1337.

82. Nybakken GE, Oliphant T, Johnson S, Burke S, Diamond MS, Fremont DH. Structural basis of West Nile virus neutralization by a therapeutic antibody. *Nature.* September 29, 2005;437(7059):764–769.

83. Zhao H, Fernandez E, Dowd KA, et al. Structural basis of Zika virus-specific antibody protection. *Cell.* August 11, 2016;166(4):1016–1027.

84. Swanstrom JA, Plante JA, Plante KS, et al. Dengue virus envelope dimer epitope monoclonal antibodies isolated from dengue patients are protective against Zika virus. *MBio.* July 19, 2016;7(4).

85. Ethics Working Group on ZIKV Research, Pregnancy. *Pregnant Women & the Zika Virus Vaccine Research Agenda: Ethics Guidance on Priorities, Inclusion, and Evidence Generation*; June 2017. Baltimore, MD http://guidance. zikapregnancyethics.org/wp-content/uploads/2017/08/ Full+Guidance-Pregnant-Women-the-Zika-Virus-Vaccine-Research-Agenda_optimized.pdf.

86. *NIH Begins Testing Investigational Zika Vaccine in Humans*; 2016. https://www.niaid.nih.gov/news/newsreleases/ 2016/Pages/Zika-Investigational-Vaccine.aspx.

87. *Inovio Launches Zika Vaccine Trial in Midst of Puerto Rico Epidemic to Explore Early Signals of Vaccine Efficacy*; 2016. http://ir.inovio.com/news/news-releases/news-releases-details/2016/Inovio-Launches-Zika-Vaccine-Trial-in-Midst-of-Puerto-Rico-Epidemic-to-Explore-Early-Signals-of-Vaccine-Efficacy/default.aspx.

88. World Health Organization. *Emergency Use Assessment and Listing Procedure (EUAL) for Candidate Vaccines for Use in the Context of a Public Health Emergency*; 2015. http://www. who.int/medicines/news/EUAL-vaccines_7July2015_MS. pdf.

89. Pan American Health Organization. Zika Ethics Consultation: Ethics Guidance on Key Issues Raised by the Outbreak. http://iris.paho.org/xmlui/bitstream/handle/ 123456789/28425/PAHOKBR16002_eng.pdf? sequence=11&isAllowed=y.

90. Coalition for Epidemic Pandemic Preparedness Innovations. www.cepi.net.

CHAPTER 6

Influenza Vaccines—Are They Efficacious or Not?

BIAO WANG, PHD • MARK LOEB, MD, MSC, FRCPC

HUMAN INFLUENZA VIRUSES

Influenza is a significant cause of morbidity and mortality worldwide.[1-3] There are three types of influenza viruses—influenza A, B, and C—that can infect human beings, with influenza types A and B causing annual epidemics.[4]

Influenza A viruses can be further divided into subtypes based on two proteins on their surface: hemagglutinin (H) and neuraminidase (N).[5] So far, 18 types of hemagglutinin protein (H1 through H18) and 11 types of neuraminidases (N1 through N11) have been discovered. Two subtypes of influenza A viruses found in human population are influenza A (H1N1) and influenza A (H3N2). Besides human hosts, influenza A virus can also cause infection in various wild and domesticated birds and mammalian hosts.[5,6] Through the combination of a high mutation rate and the reassortment of segmented genomes, influenza A viruses have the ability to change rapidly and adapt to new hosts. Therefore, influenza A viruses can cause both epidemics and pandemics.[5] In the last century, there were four influenza pandemics, and all were caused by influenza A viruses, including the 1918 pandemic (H1N1), the 1957 pandemic (H2N2), the 1968 pandemic (H3N2), and the 2009 pandemic (H1N1).[7,8]

Influenza B viruses are not divided by subtypes but by lineages. Currently, there are two influenza B lineages[9]: B/Yamagata and B/Victoria. Influenza B viruses are known to only infect human beings and seals.[10] Also, influenza B viruses mutate slower than influenza A viruses do and do not cause pandemics.[9,11] As a result, they do not cause pandemics as influenza A viruses do.[9]

Influenza C virus infections are less common and cause mild diseases compared with influenza A and B viruses.[12,13] Therefore, no vaccines against influenza C viruses are developed for human beings.

THE TYPES OF INFLUENZA VACCINES

Although there have been new types of vaccines in the progress of development,[14,15] two major types of vaccines are adapted commercially for production: inactivated influenza vaccines (IIVs) and live-attenuated vaccines (LAIVs).[16-18]

IIVs are made of killed influenza viruses. They may contain either the entire whole inactivated viruses (whole virus vaccines), viruses disrupted by detergents or solvents (split vaccines),[19,20] or purified HA and NA (subunit vaccines).[18,21-23] The first generation IIVs were based on whole virions inactivated by formalin or β-propiolactone.[24] Since the 1970s, most vaccines have been split vaccines or subunit vaccines.[25] IIVs induce a strain-specific serum IgG antibody response, and they are licensed for individuals aged over 6 months.[14]

LAIVs are made from weakened influenza viruses. They are developed through serial passages of influenza viruses in specific pathogen-free cells at certain conditions to achieve attenuation of the viruses.[26-28] The development of stable, immunogenic, and safe cold-adapted temperature-sensitive LAIV was considered as an important achievement. Vaccination with LAIVs will induce strain-specific serum IgG as well as mucosal IgA and T cell responses. LAIVs are licensed in some countries for healthy individuals aged between 2 and 49 years,[14] although their recommended use in these countries by public health authorities is in children. Notably, in the US, the use of LAIV has not been recommended in the last several seasons but will be reinstated in 2018–19.

The production of IIV and LAIV uses either egg-based or cell-based manufacturing processes, with the vast majority of them produced by egg-based processes.[16,17] Cell-based influenza vaccine production does not require chicken eggs because the vaccine viruses used to make vaccine are grown in animal cells. Cell culture technology has the potential for a faster start-up of the flu vaccine manufacturing process. Therefore, they have the potential to give fast response to pandemics.[29–31] In addition, intradermal and recombinant hemagglutinin vaccines have been licensed in the United States.

FORMULATION OF INFLUENZA VACCINES

Since the isolation of the first influenza virus, the development of influenza vaccine has evolved for more than 80 years with more understanding on influenza viruses.[32]

In 1936 the first influenza vaccine was developed against A/PR8 (H1N1) in Russia shortly after its isolation.[33] This vaccine was an LAIV and was in wide use in Russia.[34,35] In 1940, the first influenza B virus—B/Lee—was discovered.[36] Shortly after its discovery, in 1942 a bivalent vaccine against both A/PR8 and B/Lee was developed by the US army to protect the America troops primarily during the Second World War and civilians later in 1945.[37,38] This vaccine was the first IIV.[28]

In 1958, following the identification of influenza H2N2 virus, the need for trivalent influenza vaccines was recognized.[39,40] Starting from 1973, the World Health Organization (WHO) has issued recommendations annually for the compositions of seasonal influenza vaccines based on global surveillance results. Since 1992, two recommendations have been issued separately for the northern hemisphere and southern hemisphere. Until 2012, all WHO recommendations were for a trivalent composition, including two strains of influenza A (i.e., H1N1 and H3N2) and one strain of influenza B (either B/Victoria or B/Yamagata lineage). Since 2013, quadrivalent influenza vaccine composition has been annually recommended by the WHO with the addition of a second strain of influenza B due to the recognition of poor predictability of influenza B circulation in the past.[28]

VACCINE EFFICACY AND EFFECTIVENESS STUDY DESIGN

The protectiveness of a vaccine is an important parameter to be considered in public health policy-making and in clinical practices.[41] Vaccine protectiveness is often measured by vaccine efficacy and vaccine effectiveness. Vaccine efficacy typically refers to the effect of the vaccine as demonstrated in randomized controlled trials while vaccine effectiveness refers to the effect of the vaccine as assessed in observational studies.[41–43] Efficacy studies of influenza vaccines

through randomized control trials (RCTs), although more rigorous, have a number of limitations, including only one or two season enrollment periods, enrollment of only healthy individuals, low power to measure efficacy by subtype, and the inapplicability of results from the previous season to subsequent seasons. Therefore, effectiveness studies of influenza vaccine are more common.[44]

Although several study designs might be used to measure influenza vaccine effectiveness,[45–48] the test-negative study design has emerged as the preferred method for the evaluation of influenza vaccine effectiveness.[49] Test-negative studies are a modification of traditional case-control studies where cases and controls are not identified at the time of enrollment. In a test-negative study, patients seeking healthcare for an acute respiratory illness are recruited into the study and are tested for influenza infection by reverse transcript polymerase chain reaction (RT-PCR). Cases are those who test positive for influenza infection, and controls are those who test negative. Influenza vaccine effectiveness is then estimated from the ratio of the odds of vaccination among subjects testing positive for influenza to the odds of vaccination among subjects testing negative.[49–53]

A number of test-negative studies for estimating influenza vaccine effectiveness have been conducted.[44] The popularity of this method has primarily arisen from its ease of implementation. Also, studies have shown that vaccine effectiveness estimated from test-negative studies is valid and unbiased under a wide range of assumptions.[50]

OUTCOME OF INFLUENZA VACCINE EFFICACY AND EFFECTIVENESS STUDIES

Studies of influenza vaccine efficacy and effectiveness have included a number of outcomes. Outcomes can be classified by two properties: the specificity for influenza infection and the severity of the illness. A typical highly specific outcome is laboratory-confirmed influenza illness, whereas influenza-like illness is a typical nonspecific outcome. Highly specific outcomes are often associated higher relative risk reductions. Influenza outcomes are sometimes also classified by severity of the diseases. Typical outcomes used include (1) sever acute respiratory infections; (2) all cause pneumonia requiring hospitalization; and (3) all-cause mortality. These outcomes are nonspecific but often used because they provide important information on the burden of influenza diseases for policy-makers.[48,54]

A large body of literature exists about the efficacy and effectiveness of influenza vaccine in various populations, including healthy children, healthy adults, elderly adults, and people with various conditions. A number of systematic review and meta-analysis studies have also been published trying to summarize the body of literature regarding efficacy and effectiveness of influenza vaccine.[55] Wherever possible, in this chapter, we draw data primarily from these systematic review and meta-analysis studies.

As summarized by Remschmidt et al., systematic review and meta-analysis studies on influenza vaccine efficacy and effectiveness have significant heterogeneity.[55] In order to achieve comparable results, we primarily extracted two types of data stratified by the two major vaccine types (i.e., IIV and LAIV): (1) influenza vaccine efficacy derived from RCTs against laboratory-confirmed influenza infection, including confirmation by culture or RT-PCR and (2) influenza vaccine effectiveness derived from observational studies against clinically defined influenza cases (i.e., influenza-like illness).

DIRECT EFFECT IN DIFFERENT POPULATION
Healthy Children
Ten systematic review or meta-analyses were found from the literature with the first one published in 2004 and the latest published in 2013 (Table 6.1).[43,56–64] Among them, there were three systematic reviews conducted by Cochrane. The first Cochrane systematic review appeared in 2005, and it was updated in 2008 and 2012 with similar results.[57,61,63]

As suggested by these 10 studies, the efficacy of IIV against laboratory-confirmed influenza infection ranged from 59% to 67%, and effectiveness of IIV against clinically defined influenza cases ranged from 28% to 45%. As a comparison for LAIV, the two ranges were from 72% to 87% for vaccine efficacy and from 31% to 38% for vaccine effectiveness, respectively. Such reports suggest that LAIVs had both higher efficacy and effectiveness than IIVs did. However, we must be cautious about this observation, as these differences were not derived from direct comparison between LAIV and IIV in the same studies.[64] In fact, a recent cluster randomized clinical trial (cRCT) by Loeb et al. suggested that there was no difference between LAIV and IIV in term of vaccine efficacy.[65]

It is worth noting that these data only apply to children aged between 2 and 17 years. There are limited data for children younger than 2 years. In fact, only one study was found in the literature that studied this population. Considering IIVs were recommended by

public health agencies for children aged 6–24 months in several countries including the United States and Canada, more studies on this population are urgently needed.[63]

Another notable result suggested by the data is that a significant gap exists between efficacy and effectiveness for both IIV and LAIV, with the efficacy being consistently larger than effectiveness even when both studies use laboratory-confirmed influenza as an outcome. Many factors could contribute to this discrepancy. One important contributor is that efficacy studies are often performed through RCTs with less bias, while effectiveness studies are conducted through observational study designs that are more prone to bias.[41] Nevertheless, the remarkable difference highlights challenges of developing practical effective vaccines against influenza viruses.

The difference between vaccine and circulating virus matching or mismatching was not reported in most of the meta-analysis studies in this population. Studies that considered the matching difference were all for LAIV, and vaccine efficacy was slightly better with vaccine matching.[60,62]

In summary, influenza vaccines have modest vaccine efficacy but considerably lower vaccine effectiveness in practice for both LAIV and IIV in healthy children aged between 2 and 17 years. There are lack of data on vaccine efficacy and vaccine effectiveness for children younger than 2 years, although IIVs have been recommended for children between 6 months and 2 years.

Healthy Young Adults
Five systematic review or meta-analyses were found on healthy young adults aged between 15 and 65 years with slight variation on the lower age limit (Table 6.2).[43,66–69] The first review was published in 2004 by Villari et al. with no mention on the types of vaccine reviewed.[66]

Among the five reviews, there were three systematic reviews conducted by Cochrane and the latest update was in 2014.[67–69] The Cochrane reviews conducted distinguish on LAIV, IIV-parenteral, and IIV-aerosol and also considered the difference between vaccine match and mismatch.

As suggested by the studies, the vaccine efficacy of parental IIV against laboratory-confirmed influenza infection ranged from 73% to 85% with vaccine match and from 44% to 56% with vaccine mismatch or unknown. The pooled vaccine efficacy regardless of vaccine match or mismatch is 62% (56%–67%) in the latest update, which is comparable to the widely cited results (59% [51%–67%]) by Osterholm et al.[43,69]

TABLE 6.1
Influenza Vaccine Efficacy and Effectiveness in Healthy Children from Meta-analyses

Article	Year of Publication	Search End Date	Vaccine Type	Age Group	Strain Match	Efficacy Against Laboratory-Confirmed Influenza		Effectiveness Against Influenza Like Illness	
						Effect Size	# of Studies	Effect Size	# of Studies
Zangwill and Belshe[56]	2004	NA	IIV	≤9	NA	63% (45%–70%)	5		
Jefferson et al.[57]	2005	May, 2004	LAIV	≤18	NA	79% (48%–92%)	4	38% (33%–43%)	12
			IIV	≤18	NA	65% (47%–76%)	8	28% (22%–33%)	6
Negri et al.[58]	2005	December, 2003	LAIV	≤18	NA	80% (53%–91%)	6	34% (31%–38%)	10
			IIV	≤18	NA	65% (45%–77%)	6	33% (22%–42%)	8
Manzoli et al.[59]	2007	May, 2005	LAIV	≤18	NA	72% (38%–87%)	7	35% (30%–40%)	10
			IIV	≤18	NA	62% (45%–75%)	11	45% (33%–55%)	9
Rhorer et al.[60]	2009	NA	LAIV—year 1, one dose	≤17	Match	60% (51%–68%)	4		
			LAIV—year 1, two doses		Match	77% (72%–80%)	6		
			LAIV—year 2, revaccination		Match	87% (81%–90%)	4		
Jefferson et al.[61]	2008	December, 2007	LAIV	≤17	NA	82% (71%–89%)	5	33% (28%–38%)	8
			IIV	≤17	NA	59% (41%–71%)	5	36% (24%–46%)	5
Ambrose et al.[62]	2012	NA	LAIV—year 1, one dose	≤17	Pooled	79% (73%–83%)	5		
			LAIV—year 1, two doses		Match	83% (78%–87%)	5		
			LAIV—year 2, revaccination	≤17	Pooled	78% (72%–82%)	4		
					Match	87% (82%–91%)	4		
Jefferson et al.[63]	2012	November, 2011	LAIV	≤17	NA	80% (68%–87%)	7	33% (28%–38%)	13
			IIV	≤17	NA	59% (41%–71%)	7	36% (24%–46%)	7
Osterholm et al.[43]	2012	February, 2011	LAIV	2–7 years	Pooled	83% (69%–91%)	7		
Luksic et al.[64]	2013	NA	LIAV	≤18	Match	83% (78%–89%)	NA	31% (25%–40%)	NA
			IIV	≤18	Pooled	67% (58%–78%)	NA	33% (20%–53%)	NA

LAIV, live-attenuated influenza vaccine; *IIV*, inactivated influenza vaccine; *NA*, not available.

TABLE 6.2
Influenza Vaccine Efficacy and Effectiveness in Healthy Young Adults from Meta-analyses

Article	Year of Publication	Search End Date	Age Group	Type of Vaccine	Strain Match	EFFICACY AGAINST LABORATORY-CONFIRMED INFLUENZA		EFFECTIVENESS AGAINST CLINICAL INFLUENZA CASES	
						Effect Size	# of Studies	Effect Size	# of Studies
Villari et al.[66]	2004	December, 2002	15–65	NA		63% (53%–71%)	25	22% (16%–28%)	49
Demicheli et al.[67]	2007	January, 2006	16–65	LAIV	Pooled	62% (45%–73%)	6	10% (4%–16%)	6
					Match	56% (19%–76%)	2	8% (−12% to 24%)	2
					Not match	64% (18%–84%)	2	11% (3%–18%)	3
				IIV-parenteral	Pooled	65% (51%–75%)	15	23% (13%–32%)	20
					Match	80% (56%–91%)	7	30% (17%–41%)	10
					Not match	50% (27%–65%)	5	12% (−8% to 28%)	8
				IIV-aerosol	Pooled			42% (17%–60%)	4
					Match			53% (−13% to 81%)	2
					Not match			37% (−7% to 63%)	2
Jefferson et al.[68]	2010	June, 2010	16–65	LAIV	Pooled	62% (45%–73%)	6	10% (4%–16%)	6
					Match	56% (19%–76%)	2	8% (−12% to 24%)	2
					Not match	64% (18%–84%)	2	11% (3%–18%)	3
				IIV-parenteral	Pooled	61% (48%–70%)	17	20% (11%–29%)	22
					Match	73% (54%–84%)	8	30% (17%–41%)	10
					Not match	44% (23%–59%)	6	7% (−9% to 21%)	9
				IIV-aerosol	Pooled			42% (17%–60%)	4
					Match			53% (−13% to 81%)	2
					Not match			37% (−7% to 63%)	2

Continued

TABLE 6.2
Influenza Vaccine Efficacy and Effectiveness in Healthy Young Adults from Meta-analyses—cont'd

Article	Year of Publication	Search End Date	Age Group	Type of Vaccine	Strain Match	EFFICACY AGAINST LABORATORY-CONFIRMED INFLUENZA		EFFECTIVENESS AGAINST CLINICAL INFLUENZA CASES	
						Effect Size	# of Studies	Effect Size	# of Studies
Osterholm et al.[43]	2012	February, 2011	18–64	IIV	Pooled	59% (51%–67%)	8		
Demicheli et al.[69]	2014	May, 2013	16–65	LAIV	Pooled	53% (38%–65%)	9	10% (4%–16%)	6
					Match	45% (18%–63%)	4	8% (−12% to 24%)	2
					Not match	57% (32%–73%)	3	11% (3%–18%)	3
				IIV-parenteral	Pooled	62% (56%–67%)	22	17% (13%–22%)	16
					Match	63% (55%–69%)	12	17% (11%–23%)	7
					Not match	56% (44%–65%)	7	18% (10%–25%)	7
				IIV-aerosol	Pooled	62% (−2% to 86%)	1		
					Match				
					Not match				

aCochrane review.
LAIV, live-attenuated influenza vaccine; *IIV*, inactivated influenza vaccine; *NA*, not available.

The vaccine effectiveness of parenteral IIV against clinically defined influenza cases ranged from 17% to 30% with vaccine match and from 7% to 18% with vaccine mismatch. The pooled vaccine effectiveness regardless of vaccine match or mismatch is 17% (13%−22%) in the latest update. Vaccine match or mismatch has a strong impact on vaccine efficacy and effectiveness for parenteral IIV.

For LAIV, the vaccine efficacy against laboratory-confirmed influenza infection in the latest update was 45% with vaccine match and from 57% with vaccine mismatch with a pooled result of 53%. The vaccine effectiveness against clinically defined influenza cases in the latest update was 8% with vaccine match and from 11% with vaccine mismatch with a pooled result of 10%. These results were counterintuitive, as LAIV had higher efficacy when there was vaccine mismatch.[69]

A similar gap between efficacy and effectiveness for both IIV and LAIV was observed in this population as in children. However, the efficacy and effectiveness in this population were both lower than in healthy children population.

Also as suggested by the reviews, there was no strong difference between LAIV and IIV in both vaccine efficacy and effectiveness in healthy adults.

Elderly Adults

Seven systematic review or meta-analyses studies were identified that focused on the elderly population aged 65 years or above with the first one published in 1995 and the latest published in 2017 (Table 6.3).[70−77] Among them, there were two systematic reviews conducted by Cochrane with the first one in 2005 and updated in 2010 subsequently.[72,73] All the vaccines studied were IIV. One review focused on IIV-MF59 and another focused on IIV-high dose specifically.[75,76] Only the lasted Cochrane review had data in both vaccine efficacy and effectiveness.[73] Other six studies just had one of the items.

In total, there were two reviews that had information about vaccine efficacy, one by Jefferson et al.[73] and the other by Wilksion et al.[76] Jefferson review had a result of 58% (34%−73%). This result was for IIV in general and was derived from three studies. Wilkinson review was for high-dose IIV and had a reduction of 24% (10%−35%) compared with standard dose based on two RCTs by DiazGranados et al.[78,79] With such a small number of studies, authors from both studies concluded that they were unable to reach a conclusion on the vaccine efficacy on elderly population.[73,76]

There were six studies that had information about vaccine effectiveness.[70−75] Among them, five reviews studied IIV in general with a result ranging from 23% to 56%. However, the most recent one was conducted in 2014 by Darvishiar et al. and showed that IIV had no significant reduction against clinically defined influenza cases.[74] One study by Domnich et al. looked at IIV-MF59 specifically, and the result was a 94% reduction of clinically defined influenza cases in institutionalized elderly.[75]

In summary, there is a lack of evidence on vaccine efficacy and vaccine effectiveness in the elderly in general. Adjuvant IIV appears to be effective of preventing clinically defined influenza cases in institutionalized elderly population.

Pregnant Women

Since the 1918 influenza pandemic, influenza virus infections have been felt to be an important cause of severe disease in pregnant women[80−82] and in their newborns.[83−85] A recent review study shows that there was a higher risk for hospitalization in pregnant versus nonpregnant patients infected with influenza (odds ratio: 2.44, 95% confidence interval: 1.22−4.87).[86] Infants aged <6 months infected with influenza have the highest risk for hospitalization than any other age groups.[87] Although the reasons for more severe influenza disease in pregnancy remain unclear, it is believed that physiologic changes associated with pregnancy might be a major contributor.[88] Research has shown that influenza vaccination of women during pregnancy may afford direct protection to pregnant women as well as their infants through transfer of antibodies from their mother.[89,90]

Although pregnant women have been recognized as a high-risk group to be prioritized for annual influenza vaccination in many countries, the study of vaccine efficacy and vaccine effectiveness in this high-risk group is limited.[88,91,92] A recent review found that there were only three clinical trials available up to year 2016 (Table 6.4).[88] None of the three trials were from developed countries. The first trial was conducted in Bangladesh with 340 pregnant women.[92] The results show that vaccine efficacy and effectiveness in infants <6 months were 63% and 29%, respectively. While for mothers, the vaccine effectiveness was 36%, and there was no vaccine efficacy data reported. All the reported results were statistically significant. The second trial was conducted in South Africa with 2116 HIV uninfected and 194 HIV infected pregnant women.[93] The results showed that vaccine efficacy was significant in both infants <6 months and mothers with the effect size of 49% and 50%, respectively, in HIV uninfected group. However, vaccine effectiveness against clinically

TABLE 6.3
Influenza Vaccine Efficacy and Effectiveness in the Elderly from Meta-analyses

Article	Year of Publication	Search End Date	Type of Vaccine	Age Group	Strain Match	EFFICACY AGAINST LABORATORY-CONFIRMED INFLUENZA		EFFECTIVENESS AGAINST CLINICAL INFLUENZA CASES	
						Effect Size	# of Studies	Effect Size	# of Studies
Gross et al.[70]	1995	NA	IIV	≥65 years	NA			56% (39%–68%)	20
Vu et al.[71]	2002	December, 2000	IIV	≥65 years	NA			35% (19%–47%)	3
Jefferson et al.[72]	2005	December, 2004	IIV	≥65 years	Match			23% (6%–36%)	16
Jefferson et al.[73]	2010	October, 2009	IIV	≥65 years	Pooled	58% (34%–73%)	3	25% (13%–35%)	25
Darvishian et al.[74]	2014	September, 2011	IIV	≥60 years	NA			36% (−29% to 68%)	4
Domnich et al.[75]	2016	April, 2016	IIV-MF59	≥65 years	NA			94% (47%–100%)	11
Wilkinson et al.[76]	2017	NA	IIV-high dose	≥65 years	NA	24% (10%–35%)[c]	2		

IIV, inactivated influenza vaccine; *NA*, not available.

TABLE 6.4
Vaccine Efficacy and Effectiveness in Pregnant Women and Their Infant from Recent RCTs

ARTICLE	ZAMA ET AL.[92]	MADHI ET AL.[93]		STENIHOFF ET AL.[94]
		SOUTH AFRICA		
Study Location	Bangladesh	HIV Uninfected	HIV Infected	Nepal
Sample size	340	2116	194	3693
Maternal Outcome				
Efficacy against laboratory-confirmed influenza infection	NA	50% (15%−71%)	58% (0%−82%)	31% (−11% to 56%)
Effectiveness against clinically defined influenza illness	36% (4%−57%)	4% (−16% to 21%)	0% (−64% to 38%)	NA
Infant Outcome				
Efficacy against laboratory-confirmed influenza infection	63% (5%−85%)	49% (12%−70%)	27% (−132% to 77%)	30% (5%−49%)
Effectiveness against clinically defined influenza illness	29% (7%−46%)	−2% (−10% to 6%)	−2% (−26% to 17%)	NA

NA, not available.

defined influenza illness in both infants and mothers were not significant and closed 0%. In HIV infected group, influenza vaccination had neither efficacy against laboratory-confirmed influenza nor effectiveness against clinically defined influenza illness. The lasted trial reported was conducted in Nepal with a large sample size of 3693.[94] The vaccine efficacy in infants is statistically significant with an effect size of 30%. The vaccine efficacy in mothers is 30% but not statistically significant.

In summary, the evidence from these trials supports that a moderate protective effect of influenza vaccination in pregnant women can be achieved in both mothers and infants.

INDIRECT PROTECTION AND HERD IMMUNITY

Besides direct protection for the vaccinated individuals, vaccines also offer indirect protection to those who are not vaccinated.[95,96] This indirect protection is called herd protection, which is defined as "the resistance of a group to attach by a disease to which a large proportion of the members are immune, thus lessening the likelihood of a patient with disease coming into contact with a susceptible individual".[97]

In recent years, increasing attention has been given to vaccination strategies that exploit herd protection

against influenza in the most vulnerable population such as the elderly aged over 65 years and young children because of limitations of direct vaccination in these populations.[98,99]

For example, in the elderly, influenza is one of the leading causes of mortality and is related to between 250 000 and 500 000 deaths worldwide annually.[100] Direct vaccination has shown limited ability to improve the situation in this population, as the elderly with a waning of the immune system have limited immunologic response to vaccines.[73]

Young children have similar hospitalization rates as the elderly for laboratory-confirmed influenza and have higher outpatient visits for influenza than any other age group do. Direct vaccination against influenza in this population is also less optimal. For example, there are no vaccines available for infants <6 months. For children <9 years who have never been vaccinated, IIVs are administered 4 weeks apart and therefore protection may be reduced during this period of time.

Indirect Effects of Vaccinating Children

Owing to high intensity of social contact, long virus shedding period, and high influenza attack rate, school-aged children import influenza virus transmitters in community settings. Therefore, vaccinating children is thought to be able to create indirect protection for other community members. In recent decades, evaluating the indirect protectiveness of vaccinating children with influenza vaccines has attracted considerable interest in research community.[101-103]

There are two systematic review or meta-analyses on indirect benefits to the community of vaccinating children against influenza with the first one published in 2006 by Jordan et al.,[104] which included 11 studies up to 2004. The latest one was published in 2017 by Yin et al.,[105] which included 19 additional studies that conducted in recent years. Of the 30 studies in this topic so far, nine were cluster RCT (cRCT) in different community settings with one study not fully randomized. The rest of 30 studies were observational studies or ecological studies, which were considered inferior to provide best evidence.

Pooled results from the eight fully randomized cRCT showed that (1) indirect protectiveness to community from vaccinating school-age children is 60% (41%–72%); (2) indirect protectiveness to household members from vaccinating school-age children is 8% (−46% to 35%); and (3) indirect protectiveness to household members from vaccinating preschool children is 22% (1%–38%). These available evidence suggests that vaccinating children with influenza afford indirect protection in some but not all settings. This leads to a number of questions that still need to be answered, including what are the settings that herd protection is likely to be achieved? What is the minimal vaccine coverage to achieve herd protection in these settings? What is the cost-effectiveness trade-off of this approach? More research is needed to answer these questions.[99]

Indirect Effects of Vaccinating Healthcare Workers

There are substantial rates of clinical and subclinical rates of influenza infection in healthcare workers such as nurse, doctors, and porters in influenza season. Owing to the nature of their work, healthcare workers have the potential to transmit influenza viruses to high-risk populations such as elderly in nursing home and long stay patients in hospitals. Therefore, healthcare workers are another group who been targeted by policy-makers for influenza vaccination to provide indirect protection to high-risk populations.

There are six systematic reviews or meta-analyses that summarized the indirect effect of influenza vaccination of healthcare workers on morbidity and mortality among patients with the first one published in 2006 and the latest one published in 2016.[106-111]

As suggested by these reviews, up to 2016, there were four cRCTs conducted in long-term care or hospital settings. In the systematic review by Ahmed et al.,[109]

results from these four cRCTs were pooled and showed that (1) indirect protectiveness for all-cause mortality is 29% (15%–41%); (2) indirect protectiveness for influenza-like illness is 42% (27%–54%); and (3) indirect protectiveness for all-cause hospitalization and laboratory-confirmed influenza are not statistically significant. However, the quality of these results were considered low to moderate due to limitations of studies including risk of bias, indirectness, and imprecision. In fact a recent detailed analysis of these four cRCTs found that the results of these studies had violated the basic mathematical principle of dilution and attributed implausibly large reductions in patient risk to Healthcare worker (HCW) vaccination.[112] The validity of these studies has been seriously challenged.

Despite the fact that >40 countries have recommended influenza vaccination for healthcare workers, there is a paucity of research on the effect of this policy, particularly on morbidity and mortality among patients. Considering the quantity and quality of the existing studies on this topic, the effect of influenza vaccination of healthcare worker on morbidity and mortality among patients is inconclusive.

ISSUE OF REPEATED VACCINATION

Annual influenza vaccination is recommended in many parts of the world including Canada and United States. However, there is limited understanding on the effect of repeated influenza vaccination.[113]

The concern that repeated influenza vaccination could have negative impact on vaccine performance was raised in the 1970s. In a study of three outbreaks of influenza A in boys at a British boarding school in 1972 (A/England/42/72), in 1974 (A/Port Chalmers), and in 1976 (A/Victoria), Hoskins et al. demonstrated that vaccination in early seasons can have impact on the risk of influenza infection in future seasons.[114] Another study from Australia over the same period of time showed that significant protection by IIV against A/Victoria/75 (H3N2) existed among healthcare workers with little or no prior vaccination, but no effect among those that had prior vaccination.[115]

The results from these two studies raised concerns on the policy of annual vaccination in the United States, which led to a 5-year trial (1983–88) by Keitel et al. to assess the effects of repeated annual influenza vaccinations of adults on serum antibody responses and efficacy against infection and illness.[116,117] The results of the trial showed that there was "no consistent differences in efficacy of primary influenza vaccination versus sequential annual revaccination". However, this conclusion might be undermined by several limitations of the study, including partial randomization of the participants, the use of seroconversion as the primary end point, and small number of influenza cases in each of the vaccination group.

The observed variation in Hoskins and Keitel studies on the efficacy of repeated vaccination stimulated the formulation of "antigenic distance hypothesis" by Smith et al., which was simulated through a computer model.[118] The antigenic distance hypothesis stated that variation in repeated vaccine efficacy is due to differences in antigenic distances among vaccine strains and between the vaccine strains and the epidemic strain. The model accurately predicted the observed vaccine efficacies in Hoskins and Keitel studies. The antigenic distance hypothesis has been a major theoretic framework to explain the variation of repeated influenza vaccination. However, it also has several limitations including (1) the framework only takes into account the prior season vaccination, therefore it is unclear whether a longer history will also have impact and (2) the hypothesis is purely based on HI antibody response, and the impact of other immune response components is unknown.

Concerns regarding impact of repeated influenza vaccination have been raised again in recent years.[113,119–121] A recent meta-analysis showed that repeat vaccination may negatively have impact on vaccine effectiveness particularly for H3N2.[122–124] There have been only observational studies on repeated vaccination since the 5-year trial in the 1980s. The immunologic mechanism and clinical significance of repeated influenza vaccination are still poorly understood.

CONCLUSION

Although a large number of studies including RCTs and reviews have been conducted to evaluate the performance of influenza vaccines, many limitations make it challenging to draw conclusions. Both IIVs and LAIVs have shown vaccine efficacy in healthy children (aged over 2 years) and adults. However, there is great discrepancy between vaccine efficacy and vaccine effectiveness even when considering confirmed influenza with the latter often being significantly lower than the former.

Although many countries have national policies recommending annual vaccination for high-risk groups such as young children aged 6 months to 2 years, elderly aged over 65 years, and pregnant women, there is surprisingly little evidence of high quality (i.e., RCTs) to support these policies. Another issue about annual vaccination is the negative impact of repeated vaccination. Almost four decades have passed since the issue

was first raised in 1970s; it was still poorly understood in terms of immunologic mechanism and clinical significance. There is an urgent need to conduct adequate studies to address these problems.

Recent studies have shown indirect protectiveness of influenza vaccination in children and in healthcare workers in some but not all settings. More research is needed to understand how indirect protectiveness could be achieved. In addition, cost-effectiveness analysis of influenza vaccination programs should also take indirect benefits into account.

REFERENCES

1. Nair H, Brooks WA, Katz M, et al. Global burden of respiratory infections due to seasonal influenza in young children: a systematic review and meta-analysis. *Lancet.* 2011;378(9807):1917–1930.
2. Descalzo MA, Clara W, Guzmán G, et al. Estimating the burden of influenza-associated hospitalizations and deaths in Central America. *Influenza Other Respiratory Viruses.* 2016;10(4):340–345.
3. Thompson WW, Comanor L, Shay DK. Epidemiology of seasonal influenza: use of surveillance data and statistical models to estimate the burden of disease. *J Infectious Diseases.* 2006;194(Supplement_2):S82–S91.
4. Zambon MC. Epidemiology and pathogenesis of influenza. *J Antimicrob Chemother.* 1999;44(Suppl 2):3–9.
5. Suarez DL. Influenza A virus. *Anim Influenza.* 2008:1–30.
6. Olsen B, Munster VJ, Wallensten A, Waldenström J, Osterhaus AD, Fouchier RA. Global patterns of influenza A virus in wild birds. *Science.* 2006;312(5772):384–388.
7. Belshe RB. The origins of pandemic influenza—lessons from the 1918 virus. *New Engl J Med.* 2005;353(21):2209–2211.
8. Girard MP, Tam JS, Assossou OM, Kieny MP. The 2009 A (H1N1) influenza virus pandemic: a review. *Vaccine.* 2010;28(31):4895–4902.
9. Hay AJ, Gregory V, Douglas AR, Lin YP. The evolution of human influenza viruses. *Philosophical Trans R Soc Lond Ser B.* 2001;356(1416):1861.
10. Osterhaus A, Rimmelzwaan G, Martina B, Bestebroer T, Fouchier R. Influenza B virus in seals. *Science.* 2000;288(5468):1051–1053.
11. Nobusawa E, Sato K. Comparison of the mutation rates of human influenza A and B viruses. *J Virol.* 2006;80(7):3675–3678.
12. Elliott RM, Yuanji G, Desselberger U. Protein and nucleic acid analyses of influenza C viruses isolated from pigs and man. *Vaccine.* 1985;3(3):182–188.
13. Speranskaya A, Melnikova N, Belenikin M, Dmitriev A, Oparina NY, Kudryavtseva A. Genetic diversity and evolution of the influenza C virus. *Russ J Genetics.* 2012;48(7):671–678.

14. Houser K, Subbarao K. Influenza vaccines: challenges and solutions. *Cell Host Microbe*. 2015;17(3):295−300.

15. Lambert LC, Fauci AS. Influenza vaccines for the future. *New Engl J Med*. 2010;363(21):2036−2044.

16. Del Giudice G, Rappuoli R. *Inactivated and Adjuvanted Influenza Vaccines. Influenza Pathogenesis and Control*. Vol. II. Springer; 2014:151−180.

17. Jin H, Subbarao K. *Live Attenuated Influenza Vaccine. Influenza Pathogenesis and Control*. Vol. II. Springer; 2014: 181−204.

18. Dormitzer PR, Galli G, Castellino F, et al. Influenza vaccine immunology. *Immunol Rev*. 2011;239(1):167−177.

19. Duxbury A, Hampson A, Sievers J. Antibody response in humans to deoxycholate-treated influenza virus vaccine. *J Immunol*. 1968;101(1):62−67.

20. Laver W, Webster R. Preparation and immunogenicity of an influenza virus hemagglutinin and neuraminidase subunit vaccine. *Virology*. 1976;69(2):511−522.

21. Bachmayer H, Liehl E, Schmidt G. Preparation and properties of a novel influenza subunit vaccine. *Postgrad Med J*. 1976;52(608):360.

22. Brady MI, Furminger I. A surface antigen influenza vaccine: 2. Pyrogenicity and antigenicity. *Epidemiol Infect*. 1976;77(2):173−180.

23. Brady MI, Furminger I. A surface antigen influenza vaccine. 1. Purification of haemagglutinin and neuraminidase proteins. *Epidemiol Infect*. 1976;77(2):161−172.

24. Stanley W. The preparation and properties of influenza virus vaccines concentrated and purified by differential centrifugation. *J Exp Med*. 1945;81(2):193−218.

25. Wong S-S, Webby RJ. Traditional and new influenza vaccines. *Clin Microbiol Rev*. 2013;26(3):476−492.

26. Wareing M, Tannock G. Live attenuated vaccines against influenza; an historical review. *Vaccine*. 2001;19(25): 3320−3330.

27. Ambrose CS, Luke C, Coelingh K. Current status of live attenuated influenza vaccine in the United States for seasonal and pandemic influenza. *Influenza Other Respiratory Viruses*. 2008;2(6):193−202.

28. Hannoun C. The evolving history of influenza viruses and influenza vaccines. *Exp Rev Vaccines*. 2013;12(9): 1085−1094.

29. Liu J, Shi X, Schwartz R, Kemble G. Use of MDCK cells for production of live attenuated influenza vaccine. *Vaccine*. 2009;27(46):6460−6463.

30. Kon TC, Onu A, Berbecila L, et al. Influenza vaccine manufacturing: effect of inactivation, splitting and site of manufacturing. comparison of influenza vaccine production processes. *PLoS One*. 2016;11(3):e0150700.

31. McLean KA, Nannei C, Sparrow E, Torelli G. The 2015 global production capacity of seasonal and pandemic influenza vaccine. *Vaccine*. 2016;34(45):5410−5413.

32. Smith W, Andrewes C, Laidlaw P. A virus obtained from influenza patients. *Lancet*, ii. 1933;66.

33. Smorodintseff A, Tushinsky M, Drobyshevskaya A, Korovin A, Osetroff A. Investigation on volunteers infected with the influenza virus. *Am J Med Sci*. 1937; 194:159−170.

34. Kendal AP. Cold-adapted live attenuated influenza vaccines developed in Russia: can they contribute to meeting the needs for influenza control in other countries? *Eur J Epidemiol*. 1997;13(5):591−609.

35. Zhdanov V. Live influenza vaccines in USSR: development of studies and practical application. *Options Control Influenza NY Alan R Liss*. 1986:193−205.

36. Sharp D, Taylor A, McLean I, et al. *Isolation and Characterization of Influenza Virus B (Lee Strain)*. 1943.

37. Francis Jr T, Salk JE, Pearson HE, Brown PN. Protective effect of vaccination against induced influenza A. *J Clin Invest*. 1945;24(4):536.

38. Salk JE, Pearson HE, Brown PN, Francis Jr T. Protective effect of vaccination against induced influenza B. *J Clin Invest*. 1945;24(4):547.

39. Scholtissek C, Wv R, Von Hoyningen V, Rott R. On the origin of the human influenza virus subtypes H2N2 and H3N2. *Virology*. 1978;87(1):13−20.

40. Joseph U, Linster M, Suzuki Y, et al. Adaptation of pandemic H2N2 influenza A viruses in humans. *J Virol*. 2015;89(4):2442−2447.

41. Weinberg GA, Szilagyi PG. Vaccine epidemiology: efficacy, effectiveness, and the translational research roadmap. *J Infect Dis*. 2010;201(11):1607−1610.

42. Fedson D. Measuring protection: efficacy versus effectiveness. *Dev Biol Standard*. 1998;95:195−201.

43. Osterholm MT, Kelley NS, Sommer A, Belongia EA. Efficacy and effectiveness of influenza vaccines: a systematic review and meta-analysis. *Lancet Infect Dis*. 2012;12(1): 36−44.

44. Belongia EA, Simpson MD, King JP, et al. Variable influenza vaccine effectiveness by subtype: a systematic review and meta-analysis of test-negative design studies. *Lancet Infect Dis*. 2016;16(8):942−951.

45. COMSTOCK GW. *Vaccine Evaluation by Case-control or Prospective Studies*. Oxford University Press; 1990.

46. Moulton LH, Wolff MC, Brenneman G, Santosham M. Case-cohort analysis of case-coverage studies of vaccine effectiveness. *Am J Epidemiol*. 1995;142(9): 1000−1006.

47. Clemens J, Brenner R, Rao M, Tafari N, Lowe C. Evaluating new vaccines for developing countries: efficacy or effectiveness? *JAMA*. 1996;275(5):390−397.

48. Organization WH. *Evaluation of Influenza Vaccine Effectiveness: A Guide to the Design and Interpretation of Observational Studies*. 2017.

49. Jackson ML, Nelson JC. The test-negative design for estimating influenza vaccine effectiveness. *Vaccine*. 2013; 31(17):2165−2168.

50. Foppa IM, Haber M, Ferdinands JM, Shay DK. The case test-negative design for studies of the effectiveness of influenza vaccine. *Vaccine*. 2013;31(30):3104−3109.

51. Feng S, Cowling BJ, Sullivan SG. Influenza vaccine effectiveness by test-negative design—Comparison of inpatient and outpatient settings. *Vaccine*. 2016;34(14): 1672−1679.

52. Sullivan SG, Tchetgen Tchetgen EJ, Cowling BJ. Theoretical basis of the test-negative study design for assessment

of influenza vaccine effectiveness. *Am J Epidemiol.* 2016; 184(5):345−353.

53. Talbot HK, Nian H, Chen Q, Zhu Y, Edwards KM, Griffin MR. Evaluating the case-positive, control test-negative study design for influenza vaccine effectiveness for the frailty bias. *Vaccine.* 2016;34(15):1806−1809.

54. Nichol KL. Heterogeneity of influenza case definitions and implications for interpreting and comparing study results. *Vaccine.* 2006;24(44):6726−6728.

55. Remschmidt C, Wichmann O, Harder T. Methodological quality of systematic reviews on influenza vaccination. *Vaccine.* 2014;32(15):1678−1684.

56. Zangwill KM, Belshe RB. Safety and efficacy of trivalent inactivated influenza vaccine in young children: a summary for the new era of routine vaccination. *Pediatr Infect Dis J.* 2004;23(3):189−197.

57. Jefferson T, Smith S, Demicheli V, Harnden A, Rivetti A, Di Pietrantonj C. Assessment of the efficacy and effectiveness of influenza vaccines in healthy children: systematic review. *Lancet.* 2005;365(9461):773−780.

58. Negri E, Colombo C, Giordano L, Groth N, Apolone G, La Vecchia C. Influenza vaccine in healthy children: a meta-analysis. *Vaccine.* 2005;23(22):2851−2861.

59. Manzoli L, Schioppa F, Boccia A, Villari P. The efficacy of influenza vaccine for healthy children: a meta-analysis evaluating potential sources of variation in efficacy estimates including study quality. *Pediatr Infectious Dis J.* 2007;26(2):97−106.

60. Rhorer J, Ambrose CS, Dickinson S, et al. Efficacy of live attenuated influenza vaccine in children: a meta-analysis of nine randomized clinical trials. *Vaccine.* 2009;27(7): 1101−1110.

61. Jefferson T, Rivetti A, Harnden A, Di Pietrantonj C, Demicheli V. Vaccines for preventing influenza in healthy children. *Cochrane Database Syst Rev.* 2008;2(2).

62. Ambrose CS, Wu X, Knuf M, Wutzler P. The efficacy of intranasal live attenuated influenza vaccine in children 2 through 17 years of age: a meta-analysis of 8 randomized controlled studies. *Vaccine.* 2012;30(5): 886−892.

63. Jefferson T, Rivetti A, Di Pietrantonj C, Demicheli V, Ferroni E. Vaccines for preventing influenza in healthy children. *Cochrane Libr.* 2012.

64. Lukšić I, Clay S, Falconer R, et al. Effectiveness of seasonal influenza vaccines in children—a systematic review and metaanalysis. *Croat Med J.* 2013;54(2):135−145.

65. Loeb M, Russell ML, Manning V, et al. Live attenuated versus inactivated influenza vaccine in Hutterite ChildrenA cluster randomized blinded TrialLive attenuated versus inactivated influenza vaccine in Hutterite children. *Ann Intern Med.* 2016;165(9):617−624.

66. Villari P, Manzoli L, Boccia A. Methodological quality of studies and patient age as major sources of variation in efficacy estimates of influenza vaccination in healthy adults: a meta-analysis. *Vaccine.* 2004;22(25):3475−3486.

67. Demicheli V, Di Pietrantonj C, Jefferson T, Rivetti A, Rivetti D. Vaccines for preventing influenza in healthy adults. *Cochrane Database Syst Rev.* 2007;2.

68. Jefferson T, Di Pietrantonj C, Rivetti A, Bawazeer GA, Al-Ansary LA, Ferroni E. Vaccines for preventing influenza in healthy adults. *Cochrane Libr.* 2010.

69. Demicheli V, Jefferson T, Al-Ansary LA, Ferroni E, Rivetti A, Di Pietrantonj C. Vaccines for preventing influenza in healthy adults. *Cochrane Libr.* 2014.

70. Gross PA, Hermogenes AW, Sacks HS, Lau J, Levandowski RA. The efficacy of influenza vaccine in elderly personsa meta-analysis and review of the literature. *Ann Intern Med.* 1995;123(7):518−527.

71. Vu T, Farish S, Jenkins M, Kelly H. A meta-analysis of effectiveness of influenza vaccine in persons aged 65 years and over living in the community. *Vaccine.* 2002; 20(13):1831−1836.

72. Jefferson T, Rivetti D, Rivetti A, Rudin M, Di Pietrantonj C, Demicheli V. Efficacy and effectiveness of influenza vaccines in elderly people: a systematic review. *Lancet.* 2005;366(9492):1165−1174.

73. Jefferson T, Di Pietrantonj C, Al-Ansary LA, Ferroni E, Thomas R. Vaccines for preventing influenza in the elderly. *Cochrane Database Syst Rev.* 2010;2(2).

74. Darvishian M, Gefenaite G, Turner RM, et al. After adjusting for bias in meta-analysis seasonal influenza vaccine remains effective in community-dwelling elderly. *J Clin Epidemiol.* 2014;67(7):734−744.

75. Domnich A, Arata L, Amicizia D, Puig-Barberà J, Gasparini R, Panatto D. Effectiveness of MF59-adjuvanted seasonal influenza vaccine in the elderly: a systematic review and meta-analysis. *Vaccine.* 2016.

76. Wilkinson K, Wei Y, Szwajcer A, et al. Efficacy and safety of high-dose influenza vaccine in elderly adults: a systematic review and meta-analysis. *Vaccine.* 2017.

77. Darvishian M, Bijlsma MJ, Hak E, van den Heuvel ER. Effectiveness of seasonal influenza vaccine in community-dwelling elderly people: a meta-analysis of test-negative design case-control studies. *Lancet Infect Dis.* 2014;14(12):1228−1239.

78. DiazGranados CA, Dunning AJ, Jordanov E, Landolfi V, Denis M, Talbot HK. High-dose trivalent influenza vaccine compared to standard dose vaccine in elderly adults: safety, immunogenicity and relative efficacy during the 2009−2010 season. *Vaccine.* 2013;31(6):861−866.

79. DiazGranados CA, Dunning AJ, Kimmel M, et al. Efficacy of high-dose versus standard-dose influenza vaccine in older adults. *N Engl J Med.* 2014;371(7):635−645.

80. Neuzil KM, Reed GW, Mitchel EF, Simonsen L, Griffin MR. Impact of influenza on acute cardiopulmonary hospitalizations in pregnant women. *Am J Epidemiol.* 1998;148(11):1094−1102.

81. Hartert TV, Neuzil KM, Shintani AK, et al. Maternal morbidity and perinatal outcomes among pregnant women with respiratory hospitalizations during influenza season. *Am J Obstet Gynecol.* 2003;189(6):1705−1712.

82. Lindsay L, Jackson LA, Savitz DA, et al. Community influenza activity and risk of acute influenza-like illness episodes among healthy unvaccinated pregnant and postpartum women. *Am J Epidemiol.* 2006;163(9): 838−848.

83. Glezen WP, Taber LH, Frank AL, Gruber WC, Piedra PA. Influenza virus infections in infants. *Pediatr Infect Dis J.* 1997;16(11):1065–1068.

84. Izurieta HS, Thompson WW, Kramarz P, et al. Influenza and the rates of hospitalization for respiratory disease among infants and young children. *N Engl J Med.* 2000; 342(4):232–239.

85. Munoz FM. Influenza virus infection in infancy and early childhood. *Paediatr Respiratory Rev.* 2003;4(2): 99–104.

86. Mertz D, Geraci J, Winkup J, Gessner BD, Ortiz JR, Loeb M. Pregnancy as a risk factor for severe outcomes from influenza virus infection: a systematic review and meta-analysis of observational studies. *Vaccine.* 2016.

87. Benowitz I, Esposito DB, Gracey KD, Shapiro ED, Vázquez M. Influenza vaccine given to pregnant women reduces hospitalization due to influenza in their infants. *Clin Infect Dis.* 2010;51(12):1355–1361.

88. Phadke VK, Omer SB. Maternal vaccination for the prevention of influenza: current status and hopes for the future. *Exp Rev Vaccines.* 2016;15(10):1255–1280.

89. Esposito S, Bosis S, Morlacchi L, Baggi E, Sabatini C, Principi N. Can infants be protected by means of maternal vaccination? *Clin Microbiol Infect.* 2012;18(s5): 85–92.

90. Esposito S, Tagliabue C, Tagliaferri L, Semino M, Longo M, Principi N. Preventing influenza in younger children. *Clin Microbiol Infect.* 2012;18(s5):42–49.

91. Mak TK, Mangtani P, Leese J, Watson JM, Pfeifer D. Influenza vaccination in pregnancy: current evidence and selected national policies. *Lancet Infect Dis.* 2008;8(1): 44–52.

92. Zaman K, Roy E, Arifeen SE, et al. Effectiveness of maternal influenza immunization in mothers and infants. *N Engl J Med.* 2008;359(15):1555–1564.

93. Madhi SA, Cutland CL, Kuwanda L, et al. Influenza vaccination of pregnant women and protection of their infants. *N Engl J Med.* 2014;371(10):918–931.

94. Steinhoff M, Tielsch J, Katz J, et al. Evaluation of year-round maternal influenza immunization in tropical SE Asia: a placebo-controlled randomized trial. *Pap Presented A. T Open Forum Infect Dis.* 2015.

95. Fine PE. Herd immunity: history, theory, practice. *Epidemiol Rev.* 1993;15(2):265–302.

96. Rashid H, Khandaker G, Booy R. Vaccination and herd immunity: what more do we know? *Curr Opinion Infect Dis.* 2012;25(3):243–249.

97. Fox JP, Elveback L, Scott W, Gatewood L, Ackerman E. Herd immunity: basic concept and relevance to public health immunization practices. *Am J Epidemiol.* 1971; 94(3):179–189.

98. Glezen WP. Herd protection against influenza. *J Clin Virol.* 2006;37(4):237–243.

99. Kim TH, Johnstone J, Loeb M. Vaccine herd effect. *Scand J Infectious Diseases.* 2011;43(9):683–689.

100. Haq K, McElhaney JE. Immunosenescence: influenza vaccination and the elderly. *Curr Opinion Immunol.* 2014;29:38–42.

101. Grijalva CG, Zhu Y, Simonsen L, Mitchel E, Griffin MR. The population impact of a large school-based influenza vaccination campaign. *PLoS One.* 2010;5(11):e15097.

102. Piedra PA, Gaglani MJ, Kozinetz CA, et al. Herd immunity in adults against influenza-related illnesses with use of the trivalent-live attenuated influenza vaccine (CAIV-T) in children. *Vaccine.* 2005;23(13):1540–1548.

103. Weycker D, Edelsberg J, Halloran ME, et al. Population-wide benefits of routine vaccination of children against influenza. *Vaccine.* 2005;23(10):1284–1293.

104. Jordan R, Connock M, Albon E, et al. Universal vaccination of children against influenza: are there indirect benefits to the community?: a systematic review of the evidence. *Vaccine.* 2006;24(8):1047–1062.

105. Yin JK, Heywood AE, Georgousakis M, et al. Systematic review and meta-analysis of indirect protection afforded by vaccinating children against seasonal influenza: implications for policy. *Clin Infect Dis.* 2017.

106. Burls A, Jordan R, Barton P, et al. Vaccinating healthcare workers against influenza to protect the vulnerable—is it a good use of healthcare resources?: a systematic review of the evidence and an economic evaluation. *Vaccine.* 2006;24(19):4212–4221.

107. Thomas R, Jefferson T, Demicheli V, Rivetti D. Influenza vaccination for health-care workers who work with elderly people in institutions: a systematic review. *Lancet Infect Dis.* 2006;6(5):273–279.

108. Thomas RE, Jefferson T, Lasserson TJ. Influenza vaccination for healthcare workers who work with the elderly: systematic review. *Vaccine.* 2010;29(2):344–356.

109. Ahmed F, Lindley MC, Allred N, Weinbaum CM, Grohskopf L. Effect of influenza vaccination of healthcare personnel on morbidity and mortality among patients: systematic review and grading of evidence. *Clin Infect Dis.* 2013;58(1):50–57.

110. Thomas RE, Jefferson T, Lasserson TJ. Influenza vaccination for healthcare workers who care for people aged 60 or older living in long-term care institutions. *Cochrane Libr.* 2013.

111. Thomas RE, Jefferson T, Lasserson TJ. Influenza vaccination for healthcare workers who care for people aged 60 or older living in long-term care institutions. *Cochrane Libr.* 2016.

112. De Serres G, Skowronski DM, Ward BJ, et al. Influenza vaccination of healthcare workers: critical analysis of the evidence for patient benefit underpinning policies of enforcement. *PLoS One.* 2017;12(1):e0163586.

113. Belongia EA, Skowronski DM, McLean HQ, Chambers C, Sundaram ME, De Serres G. Repeated annual influenza vaccination and vaccine effectiveness: review of evidence. *Exp Rev Vaccines.* 2017 (just-accepted).

114. Hoskins T, Davies J, Smith A, Miller C, Allchin A. Assessment of inactivated influenza-A vaccine after three outbreaks of influenza A at Christ's Hospital. *Lancet.* 1979; 313(8106):33–35.

115. Feery BJ, Evered MG, Morrison EI. Different protection rates in various groups of volunteers given subunit influenza virus vaccine in 1976. *J Infect Dis.* 1979;139(2): 237–241.

116. Keitel W, Cate T, Couch RB. Efficacy of sequential annual vaccination with inactivated influenza virus vaccine. *Am J Epidemiol.* 1988;127(2):353–364.

117. Keitel WA, Cate TR, Couch RB, Huggins LL, Hess KR. Efficacy of repeated annual immunization with inactivated influenza virus vaccines over a five year period. *Vaccine.* 1997;15(10):1114–1122.

118. Smith DJ, Forrest S, Ackley DH, Perelson AS. Variable efficacy of repeated annual influenza vaccination. *Proc Natl Acad Sci.* 1999;96(24):14001–14006.

119. Caspard H, Heikkinen T, Belshe RB, Ambrose CS. A systematic review of the efficacy of live attenuated influenza vaccine upon revaccination of children. *Hum Vaccines Immunotherapeut.* 2016;12(7):1721–1727.

120. Höpping AM, McElhaney J, Fonville JM, Powers DC, Beyer WE, Smith DJ. The confounded effects of age and exposure history in response to influenza vaccination. *Vaccine.* 2016;34(4):540–546.

121. Treanor J. Flu vaccine—too much of a good thing? *J Infect Dis.* 2017;215(7):1017–1019.

122. McLean HQ, Thompson MG, Sundaram ME, et al. Impact of repeated vaccination on vaccine effectiveness against influenza A (H3N2) and B during 8 seasons. *Clin Infect Dis.* 2014;59(10):1375–1385.

123. Skowronski DM, Chambers C, Sabaiduc S, et al. A perfect storm: impact of genomic variation and serial vaccination on low influenza vaccine effectiveness during the 2014–2015 season. *Clin Infect Dis.* 2016;63(1):21–32.

124. Thompson MG, Naleway A, Fry AM, et al. Effects of repeated annual inactivated influenza vaccination among healthcare personnel on serum hemagglutinin inhibition antibody response to A/Perth/16/2009 (H3N2)-like virus during 2010-11. *Vaccine.* 2016;34(7):981–988.

CHAPTER 7

Practical Use of Meningococcal Vaccines—Whom and When to Vaccinate

LEE H. HARRISON, MD

INTRODUCTION

During the past 10—15 years the field of meningococcal immunization has seen a remarkable increase in the development and utilization of new vaccines. This has resulted in drastic changes in meningococcal disease epidemiology in many parts of the world. For many years, vaccine prevention relied on purified polysaccharide vaccines that, because of the immunologic limitations of polysaccharide vaccines in general, were used primarily in response to outbreaks and epidemics and for use in high-risk individuals. Beginning in the late 1990s, monovalent capsular group C meningococcal polysaccharide-protein conjugate vaccines were developed and incorporated into national immunization programs in several countries outside of the United States. Postlicensure studies of these vaccines demonstrated high vaccine effectiveness, including in infants, and enormous herd protection effects that are characteristic of conjugate vaccines. This success was subsequently followed by development and introduction of a group A conjugate vaccine that has resulted in one of the biggest public health accomplishments of the past few decades: the virtual elimination of the devastating group A epidemics that have plagued the meningitis belt of Sub-Saharan Africa.[1,2] Given the diversity of meningococcal capsular groups in some geographic regions such as the U.S., quadrivalent conjugate vaccines that cover capsular groups A, C, W, and Y were developed and introduced into routine use in a variety of countries, including the U.S.

In the U.S. two concomitant phenomena have greatly influenced meningococcal vaccine policy: (1) licensure of a variety of new meningococcal vaccines and (2) a dramatic decline in meningococcal disease incidence to historically low levels. In this chapter, I will review clinical aspects, epidemiology, and vaccine prevention of meningococcal disease. Although the focus of this chapter is the U.S., some relevant global aspects of meningococcal disease and vaccines are included to provide an overview of this highly dynamic field. This chapter is meant to be a practical guide primarily for practitioners in the U.S. who provide care to adults. However, because much of the data on meningococcal vaccines have been generated in children, information in persons aged below 18 years will also be presented. More comprehensive reviews of meningococcal disease and vaccines for healthcare providers for all age groups, public health officials, and researchers have recently been published elsewhere.[3,4]

Meningococcal Disease in the United States

The first description in the U.S. of apparent epidemic meningococcal disease came from Medfield, Massachusetts in 1806.[5,6] The authors vividly described the clinical and autopsy features of a sample of nine fatal cases that occurred over a 23-day period in March of 1806: "The…examination…on the body of a girl of 5 years old…whose case was…strongly marked. Between the dura and pia matter was effused a fluid resembling pus, both over the cerebrum and cerebellum, the veins of the brain turgid with blood…". The causative organism, *Neisseria meningitidis*, was first isolated in culture in 1887.[7] Meningococcal epidemics continued to occur in the U.S. until near the end of World War II.[8]

Meningococcal disease remains a major cause of serious bacterial infection in the U.S. The organism, *Neisseria meningitis*, is exclusively a human pathogen. Clinical syndromes include meningitis, septicemia, purpura fulminans, pneumonia, and other less common infections. Meningococcal urethritis, a previously uncommon infection, has recently emerged in several areas of the U.S. and is caused by clonal expansion of

Vaccinations. https://doi.org/10.1016/B978-0-323-55435-0.00007-0

an unencapsulated strain of *N. meningitidis*.[9–11] Despite major advances in healthcare, the case fatality rate of invasive meningococcal disease, generally defined as the isolation of the organism from a normally sterile body fluid, remains around 15%.[12] Permanent sequelae among survivors of meningococcal disease are common and include loss of toes and/or extremities through amputation, skin necrosis, focal neurologic deficits, cognitive deficits, seizures, and hearing loss.[13,14]

Definitive diagnosis of meningococcal disease requires laboratory confirmation. This is most commonly achieved through the isolation of *N. meningitidis* in culture from a normally sterile body site, such as blood or cerebrospinal fluid. However, the diagnosis is increasingly being made through culture-independent diagnostic tests, such as PCR.[15]

Intravenous penicillin has traditionally been considered to be the treatment of choice for confirmed meningococcal disease. However, intermediate susceptibility to penicillin is common among U.S. meningococcal isolates.[16] Intravenous ceftriaxone is a reasonable alternative given the unknown clinical significance of intermediate susceptibility to penicillin, as well the convenient dosing schedule and reasonable cost of this agent. In the United Kingdom, ceftriaxone or cefotaxime are recommended as the antibiotics of choice for treatment of meningococcal disease.[17] Meningococcal isolates with reduced susceptibility to third-generation cephalosporins (minimum inhibitory concentration of 0.125 mg/L to cefotaxime) have recently been reported in France, although this has not been reported in the U.S. and the clinical significance is unknown.[18]

Adjunctive dexamethasone given before or at the same time as the first dose of antibiotics has been shown to be of benefit in some patients with bacterial meningitis. In one study of bacterial meningitis in adults, dexamethasone administration was associated with decreased mortality. Although the benefit was only seen in patients with meningitis due to *Streptococcus pneumoniae*, the study did not have sufficient statistical power for *N. meningitidis*.[19] The use of low-dose corticosteroids for adjunctive therapy for septic shock remains controversial.

Antibiotic chemoprophylaxis for prevention of secondary cases is recommended for persons who are close contacts of a patient with meningococcal disease, including household members, daycare center contacts, and anyone with exposure to oral secretions.[20] There have been many reported cases of meningococcal disease among microbiology laboratory workers, with the major risk being the processing of liquid cultures

on an open laboratory bench. In one series, half of reported laboratory-acquired cases had a fatal outcome.[21] The risk is low among other types of healthcare workers, except in the setting of direct contact with respiratory secretions, such as can occur during mouth-to-mouth resuscitation and unprotected exposure during insertion and management of endotracheal tubes.[22] The main regimens that are recommended for eradication of meningococcal pharyngeal carriage and therefore prevention of secondary cases are rifampin, ciprofloxacin, and ceftriaxone.[20] Although not considered to be a first-line chemoprophylactic agent, azithromycin has also been recommended in some settings. Following acquisition of carriage, the risk of disease is highest in the first week [23] so prophylaxis should be given as soon as possible, preferably within 24 h. Prophylaxis should be given following a high-risk exposure even in immunized persons given the potentially severe consequences of infection and incomplete protection from meningococcal vaccines.

Risk Factors for Meningococcal Disease and Carriage

N. meningitidis frequently colonizes the pharynx asymptomatically as a normal commensal bacterium. Transmission is most commonly from carriers who are asymptomatically colonized. The issue of meningococcal carriage is important for immunization policy because in general, conjugate vaccines reduce acquisition of meningococcal carriage. This reduction in carriage among immunized individuals leads to decreased transmission and therefore disease prevention in unimmunized persons, a phenomenon known as herd protection. Although infants have the highest rate of disease, carriage prevalence in infants is relatively low. Rates of carriage peak in adolescence and young adulthood.[24]

Person-to-person transmission occurs via respiratory droplets, and in general, transmission generally requires close contact through respiratory secretions. Risk factors for meningococcal carriage and/or disease include age, lack of serum bactericidal activity, viral upper respiratory infections, tobacco smoke exposure, exposure to bars and discothèques, and binge drinking.[24] HIV infection and deficiencies of some proteins involved in the complement cascade are associated with a markedly increased risk of meningococcal disease. Eculizumab (Soliris; Alexion Pharmaceuticals), which is used for treatment of atypical hemolytic uremic syndrome or paroxysmal nocturnal hemoglobinuria, increases the risk of meningococcal disease by inhibiting the terminal complement pathway.[25–29] Numerous cases of invasive meningococcal disease despite immunization with meningococcal vaccine have been reported among patients receiving eculizumab, in part because a substantial proportion of cases are caused by nongroupable *N. meningitidis* and are therefore not preventable with meningococcal conjugate vaccines.[30] There are numerous genetic polymorphisms that are also associated with an increased risk.

Current Epidemiology

Much of what is known about meningococcal disease epidemiology in the U.S. comes from the National Notifiable Diseases Surveillance System, a passive public health surveillance system and, for the past several decades, from active, laboratory-based surveillance performed by the CDC-funded Active Bacterial Core surveillance (ABCs) network.[12,31]

For a period of around 50 years after the end of World War II, the annual incidence of invasive meningococcal disease in the U.S. tended to fluctuate between 0.5 and 1.5 cases per 100,000 population. Since the mid-1990s, there has been a dramatic change in meningococcal disease epidemiology, with a greater than 90% decline to a rate of 0.11−0.12 in 2015 (Fig. 7.1).[32,33] By

2015 the estimated annual number of meningococcal diseases cases and deaths, respectively, had declined to 370 and 60.[33] In contrast, before introduction of *Haemophilus influenzae* type b (Hib) conjugate vaccines at 2 months of age in 1990, one child in 200 developed invasive Hib by the age of 5 years, which translated into an estimated 20,000 annual cases of invasive Hib infection, including 12,000 cases of meningitis.[34] The burden of invasive pneumococcal disease before the introduction of the first pneumococcal conjugate vaccine in 2000 was estimated to be 3000 cases of meningitis and 50,000 cases of bacteremia.[35]

The introduction of meningococcal conjugate vaccines in 2005[36] is responsible for some of the decline in invasive meningococcal disease.[12] However, there is evidence that much of the decrease occurred naturally because the overall trajectory of the decline was not greatly impacted by vaccines (Fig. 7.1). In addition, the beginning of the decline preceded the introduction of conjugate vaccines by about a decade, and group B cases have also declined despite the lack of group B vaccines until very recently. This natural reduction in meningococcal disease incidence has had a major impact on immunization policy because the extremely

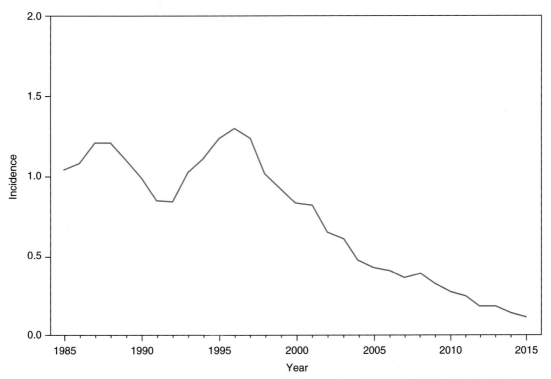

FIG. 7.1   Meningococcal disease incidence, per 100,000 population, in the U.S., 1985−2015 (Ref. 32).

low disease burden in the U.S. has made it difficult to justify vaccine use in some age groups that previously had substantially higher rates of disease.

Meningococcal disease incidence is highest in infants, peaks slightly during adolescence and young adulthood, and then increases again in the elderly (Fig. 7.2).[12] Capsular group distribution varies by age with group B predominating for most age groups and group Y predominating in the elderly. The importance of groups C and Y has diminished in adolescents and young adults since the introduction of the quadrivalent meningococcal conjugate vaccines. For the period of 2006–15 the meningococcal capsular group distribution for 599 groupable isolates for all age groups was B, 38%; C, 24%; W, 7%; and Y, 30%.[12] Among 62 meningococcal disease cases in persons with HIV infection during 1999–2014, the distribution was B, 21%; C, 37%; W, 5%; Y, 27%; and other or unknown group, 10%.[37]

With few exceptions, group A infection has not been a cause of meningococcal infection in the U.S. for decades despite its documented introduction into the U.S.[38] Group B infection causes infection at all ages but is particularly prominent in infants. Group B strains are responsible for most of the outbreaks in U.S.

colleges and universities over the past decade. Group C organisms are responsible for recent outbreaks among men who have sex with men and other settings.[39] Group Y strains are associated with the elderly and with pneumonia but cause infection in all age groups and can cause all of the meningococcal syndromes. Group W is responsible for a small proportion of disease in the U.S., although outbreaks have been reported, and for major epidemics in the African meningitis belt.[40,41] Recently group W infection has been associated with gastrointestinal symptoms including nausea, vomiting, and diarrhea, as well as a high case fatality rate, in Chile and England.[42,43]

Most meningococcal disease is sporadic, but outbreaks are responsible for a small proportion of cases. Since the introduction of quadrivalent conjugate vaccines in the U.S., there has been a change in the epidemiology of meningococcal outbreaks in the U.S. Before vaccine introduction, most outbreaks were caused by capsular group C strains, with a minority being caused by groups B (25%) and Y (13%).[44] Outbreaks occur both in the community and associated with institutions, including colleges and universities. Currently most college/university outbreaks are caused by capsular group B strains. Since 2008 there have been

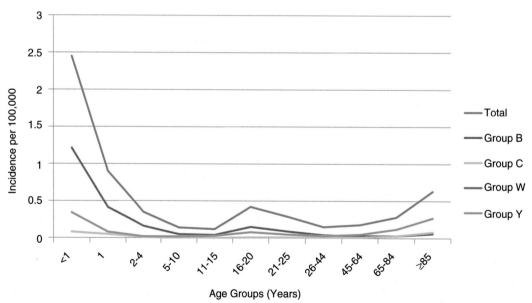

FIG. 7.2 Average annual age-specific incidence of meningococcal disease, by age group and capsular group, 2006–15. Data are from the National Notifiable Diseases Surveillance System (NNDSS). Totals rates are higher than the sum of the individual group rates because the total includes those without group information (19%), other groups, and nongroupables (6.0% combined) (Ref. 12). Data used with permission of Oxford University Press on behalf of the Infectious Diseases Society of America.

TABLE 7.1
Capsular Group B Outbreaks on US College Campuses, 2008 Through September 2017

Institution (Reference)	Time Period	No. cases	No. fatalities
Ohio University (Ref. 45)	January 2008–November 2010	13	1
University of Pennsylvania	February–March 2009	4	0
Lehigh University	November 2011	2	0
Princeton University (Refs. 46,47)	March 2013–March 2014	9	1
University of California, Santa Barbara (Ref. 47)	November 2013–May 2015	6	0
University of Oregon (Ref. 48)	January–May 2015	7	1
Providence College (Ref. 49)	January–February 2015	2	0
Santa Clara University (Ref. 50)	January–February 2016	2	0
Rutgers University (Ref. 51)	March–April 2016	2	0
University of Wisconsin–Madison	October 2016	3	0
Oregon State University	November 2016–February 2017	3	0
TOTAL		**53**	**3**

11 reported capsular group B outbreaks at institutions of higher education involving 53 cases and 3 deaths (Table 7.1). Despite the relatively small number of cases, meningococcal disease outbreaks are highly disruptive to college campuses and generally require expensive and labor-intensive immunization campaigns that target a large numbers of students.[52,53] In addition, there have been five outbreaks of capsular group C meningococcal disease among men who have sex with men. Some of these clusters have been prolonged, lasting up to 2.5 years and have involved 5–22 cases. Meningococcal conjugate vaccines were used to control all of these outbreaks.

Characterization of *N. meningitidis*

The meningococcal polysaccharide is a major virulence factor, and therefore the vast majority of meningococcal strains that cause invasive disease are encapsulated. The biochemical composition of the polysaccharide capsule determines the capsular group, of which there are 12: A, B, C, W (previously referred to as W-135), X, and Y, which collectively cause almost all invasive disease, and E (previously referred to as 29E), H, I, K, L, and Z, which are uncommon causes of infection. Group D *N. meningitidis* was recently found to be an unencapsulated variant of a group C strain and therefore is no longer considered to be a meningococcal capsular group.[54] Most asymptomatic pharyngeal colonization is due to unencapsulated, commensal strains that are

incapable of causing invasive disease in normal hosts.[55] The distribution of meningococcal capsular groups among isolates that cause invasive disease is highly dynamic and varies widely by geographic location and time.[56]

In addition to capsular group, meningococci can be broadly classified genetically according to multilocus sequencing typing, which uses DNA sequencing of portions of seven housekeeping genes to determine the sequence type (ST). Based on this classification, most invasive meningococcal isolates belong to a limited number of so-called hypervirulent lineages; carriage isolates are genetically much more diverse. Additional strain characterization schemata involve the use of outer membrane protein (OMP) genotyping, sometimes referred to as fine typing. More recently molecular characterization of meningococcal strains has increasingly used whole-genome sequencing, which allows for a much more efficient and comprehensive view of important meningococcal genes (including those that are used to determine ST and fine type) as well as detailed phylogenetic analysis.[57]

Because meningococcal factor H binding protein (FHbp) is a major component of both vaccines that are licensed for prevention of capsular group B infection, two classification systems have been developed to characterize variants of this protein. As of November 2017 there are more than 1100 FHbp amino acid sequence variants in the public database in which these variants are curated and housed (http://pubmlst.org/neisseria/fHbp/). Each variant is assigned a unique FHbp peptide identification (ID) number. Based on the amino acid sequence similarity, these variants can be, depending on the classification system, subclassified into three variant groups (1, 2, or 3) [58] or two subfamilies (A and B).[59] Variant group 1 corresponds to subfamily B, and variant groups 2 and 3 correspond to subfamily A. Within each subfamily, the identity of FHbp amino acid sequences ranges from 88% to 99%, and between subfamilies, the sequence identity is around 60%. In general, antibodies directed at one subfamily have greater serum bactericidal activity than the other subfamily.[58,60,61]

BACKGROUND ON MENINGOCOCCAL VACCINES

Measurement of Meningococcal Vaccine Immunogenicity

The licensure of all meningococcal conjugate vaccines in the U.S. since 2005 has been based primarily on immunogenicity and safety. Randomized, controlled efficacy trials have not been feasible because of the relatively low incidence of infection in the U.S. Therefore an understanding of the basis of meningococcal vaccine licensure requires an introduction on how immunogenicity is assessed.

Measurement of serum bactericidal activity (SBA) is the primary assay used for determining the immunogenicity of meningococcal vaccines. The rationale is the historic observation of a correlation between naturally acquired SBA and protection against invasive meningococcal disease.[62] SBA assays measure the ability of test serum with an exogenous complement source to kill *N. meningitidis* in vitro. Although rabbit serum is a more readily available source of exogenous complement than human complement, the U.S. Food and Drug Administration (FDA) requires the use of human complement for SBA assays (hSBA) to support licensure because of uncertainty in inferring protection from rabbit complement-based SBA assays (rSBA). This is because of species specificity in binding of certain complement components to *N. meningitidis*.[63,64]

As discussed in the following, an important attribute of meningococcal conjugate vaccines is the induction of immunologic B-cell memory, one of the major advantages of polysaccharide-protein conjugate vaccines over polysaccharide vaccines. Methods that are used to measure immunologic memory include measurement of maturation of antibody avidity,[65–67] booster antibody responses to a subsequent administration of conjugate vaccine, and measurement of postimmunization antigen-specific peripheral blood memory B-cell responses.[68–70] A previous practice of using a dose of polysaccharide vaccine to measure booster responses to a previous dose of conjugate vaccine is generally no longer used because of the immunologic phenomenon of hyporesponsiveness, which results in decreasing antibody response after repeated doses of meningococcal polysaccharide.

Measurement of Vaccine-Induced Strain Coverage

Vaccine-induced strain coverage refers to the proportion of meningococcal strains that cause invasive disease in a population that would be expected to be prevented by an effective vaccine. The polysaccharide-based conjugate vaccines theoretically cover all strains expressing one of the polysaccharide capsular groups that are included in the vaccine. However, the story is much more complex for the vaccines that were developed to prevent capsular group B infection because they are based on antigenically variable, surface-exposed proteins. Whether a particular meningococcal strain is covered by a protein-based vaccine depends on (1) the presence in the meningococcal genome of the gene encoding for the protein antigen or antigens included in the vaccine, (2) the expression of the protein, and (3) immunologic reactivity or cross-reactivity of the protein variant in the vaccine with the protein expressed in the strain in question.

The main assay used to estimate MenB-4C (Bexsero; GlaxoSmithKline) strain coverage is the meningococcal antigen typing system (MATS) that provides a measure of expression of the tested antigen and cross-reactivity between the variant of the antigen in the test strain and the vaccine.[71] This assay has been used to predict strain coverage in various geographic regions. For example, MATS predicted that 78% of European group B strains would be killed by the sera of immunized individuals.[72]

For predicting coverage by MenB-FHbp (Trumenba; Pfizer), hSBA is used to determine the ability of sera from immunized individuals to kill an antigenically diverse and epidemiologically relevant group of group B isolates; using this approach, strain coverage has been estimated to be approximately 80%.[73–75]

POLYSACCHARIDE VACCINES

For many years the only meningococcal vaccines that were available in the U.S. and globally were purified polysaccharide products. In the U.S. a single quadrivalent polysaccharide vaccine that covers capsular groups

A, C, W, and Y (Menomune; Sanofi Pasteur) was available for more than 30 years. However, because of the immunologic limitations of polysaccharide vaccines, its use was limited to persons at high risk of meningococcal disease and for control of outbreaks, a practice that continues in some parts of the world.[76] These limitations included poor immunogenicity and lack of efficacy in infants, hyporesponsiveness with repeated doses rather than induction of a booster response through immunologic memory, and lack of impact on pharyngeal carriage and therefore absence of herd protection. Given these limitations and the increasing availability of meningococcal polysaccharide-protein conjugate vaccines, Menomune is no longer produced in the U.S., with all remaining lots having expired by September 2017. Therefore meningococcal polysaccharide vaccines will not be further discussed in this chapter but have been comprehensively reviewed elsewhere.[77]

POLYSACCHARIDE-PROTEIN CONJUGATE VACCINES

Conjugate vaccines differ from polysaccharide vaccines in that they use a protein carrier that is covalently linked to the polysaccharide. Purified polysaccharides induce an antibody response primarily without the assistance of T-cells.[78,79] In contrast, the conjugation of a protein carrier to the polysaccharide leads to T cell–dependent properties, which confers major immunologic advantages over polysaccharide vaccines, including immunogenicity and efficacy in infants, immunologic memory, and impact on pharyngeal carriage (and therefore herd protection). The development of conjugate vaccines has revolutionized the prevention of invasive disease caused by encapsulated bacteria, starting with the introduction of Hib conjugate vaccines more than 25 years ago. Hib used to be responsible for around 95% of the 20,000 yearly invasive *H. influenzae* infections in the U.S. Hib vaccines demonstrated that conjugate vaccines could (1) protect infants,[80] who had the highest rates of disease, (2) provide substantial herd protection through reductions in acquisition of pharyngeal carriage,[81] and (3) through a combination of direct and indirect protection, lead to near disappearance of invasive Hib disease.[82] This initial success in the prevention of infectious caused by encapsulated bacteria was followed by the introduction of a 7-valent pneumococcal conjugate vaccine (PCV7) in 2000 and, a decade later, a 13-valent pneumococcal conjugate vaccine (PCV13). PCV7 and PCV13 have led to near elimination of vaccine-type invasive pneumococcal infections although substantial disease remains because there are more than 80 pneumococcal serotypes that are not covered by the vaccines.

The first experience with meningococcal conjugate vaccines occurred in the United Kingdom in the late 1990's, during which the incidence of group C meningococcal disease had increased substantially. The increase was associated with severe disease in adolescents and young adults. In response, vaccine manufacturers produced three monovalent C conjugate vaccines, two of which used CRM_{197} as the protein carrier and another that used tetanus toxoid. These vaccines were used in a campaign that was characterized by very rapid attainment of high vaccine coverage in the target population and extensive prelicensure and postlicensure studies that allowed for a comprehensive assessment of program impact. The campaign and the introduction of the vaccines into the infant and childhood immunization schedule led to the near elimination of group C infection, with around 90% of remaining meningococcal infection in the U.K. being caused by group B strains. Numerous studies revolving around this campaign led to a number of important findings, some that were reminiscent of the Hib experience, including (1) high vaccine effectiveness in infants, (2) dramatic impact on group C pharyngeal carriage, which resulted in substantial herd protection, (3) protection of vulnerable infants through the immunization of adolescents through herd protection, (4) the realization that immunologic memory in the absence of circulating serum bactericidal antibodies is insufficient to protect infants from invasive infection,[23,83] and (5) that the emergence of infection caused by other meningococcal capsular groups can complicate immunization programs that use vaccines that do not cover all capsular groups.[84]

The first meningococcal conjugate vaccine was licensed in the U.S. in 2005 and the second in 2010. The vaccines are quadrivalent products that cover capsular groups A, C, W, and Y (MCV4). Monovalent C vaccines are not licensed in the U.S. in part because a substantial proportion of US disease is caused by group Y strains. The inclusion of group A allows the vaccine to be used for persons traveling to countries with ongoing group A infection, and the inclusion of group W is because of the occurrence, albeit as a small proportion, of this capsular group in the U.S.

The two licensed MCV4s in the U.S. are Menactra (Sanofi Pasteur, or MCV4-DT) and Menveo (GlaxoSmithKline Vaccines, or MCV4-CRM).[85,86] The carrier proteins are diphtheria toxoid and CRM_{197}. MCV4-DT is provided in 0.5-mL single-dose vials with natural latex rubber stoppers and single-dose, prefilled syringes. MCV4-CRM is provided in a single-dose vial with the group A component in lyophilized form and another single-dose vial with remaining components as a liquid. The group A component needs to be reconstituted with the solution containing the other capsular groups immediately before administration.

Immunogenicity of MCV4-DT and MCV4-CRM

As mentioned previously, the low burden of meningococcal disease in the U.S. makes it impractical to conduct randomized clinical trials that use meningococcal disease as the outcome. This is because the number of participants required for such a trial given the current low burden would be enormous. Accordingly the FDA has licensed meningococcal vaccines in the U.S. based on immunogenicity and safety.

Unlike pneumococcal and Hib conjugate vaccines, MCV4-DT was not sufficiently immunogenic in infants <6 months old using a 2-, 4-, and 6-month schedule for the primary series.[87] However, the vaccine is immunogenic when given as a two-dose schedule to infants at 9 and 12 months of age, which is the rationale for FDA licensure starting at 9 months of age.[88] MCV4-DT has also been shown to be immunogenic in children aged 2–11 years and adolescents.[89,90]

There is evidence of immunologic interference between MCV4-DT and several other pediatric vaccines.[88] Meningococcal antibody titers were lower in children who received MCV4-DT at the same time as PCV7 than in children who received MCV4-DT by itself. In addition, pneumococcal IgG geometric mean titers were lower for three PCV7 serotypes (4, 6B, and 18C), although no data have been published on simultaneous use of MCV4-DT and PCV13, the pneumococcal conjugate vaccine that is currently used in the US pediatric immunization schedule. Immunologic interference was also demonstrated between MCV4-DT and diphtheria, tetanus, and pertussis vaccine (DTaP. Dapatcel, Sanofi Pasteur) among children aged 4–6 years. Noninferiority criteria for antibody responses to all four meningococcal capsular groups were not fulfilled in children who received MCV4-DT 30 days after DTaP, a phenomenon that was not observed when the vaccines were given concomitantly.[88]

MCV4-CRM was found to be immunogenic in infants when given at 2, 4, and 6 months of age and a booster dose at 12 months and toddlers given two doses at 12 and 18 months of age.[91,92] There have been several head-to-head comparisons of MCV4-CRM with MCV4-DT. In children aged 2–10 years

immunogenicity was similar for both vaccines 1 month after a single dose of for groups A and C but around twofold higher for MCV-CRM for groups W and Y.[93] MCV4-CRM met preestablished noninferiority criteria against capsular groups C, Y, and W, whereas the responses to group A did not satisfy noninferiority criteria.[94] In a comparison of immunogenicity of MCV4-CRM and MCV4-DT in 2180 11- to 18-year-olds, MCV4-CRM was superior to MCV4-DT for groups A, W, and Y and also met noninferiority criteria for group C. MCV4-CRM was also shown to be immunologically superior for groups C, W, and Y in adults aged 19–55 years.[95]

Some chronic medical conditions are associated with both an increased risk of meningococcal disease and a suboptimal response to meningococcal conjugate vaccines, which has led to studies of a two-dose primary series. Two doses have been shown to increase the antibody response in patients with asplenia (monovalent capsular group C vaccine) and in adolescents with HIV infection and CD4$^+$ lymphocyte percentage $\geq$15% (MCV4-DT).[96,97] Among subjects with HIV infection and CD4+ lymphocyte percentage <15%, responses to two doses were generally poor.

Persistence of Serum Antibody

There is evidence that persistence of hSBA antibody titers is needed for protection against meningococcal disease. The immunologic memory that is seen with the conjugate vaccines is insufficient to confer protection after exposure most likely because the increase in antibody after exposure to the organism does not occur rapidly enough given the short incubation period,[83] which underscores the importance of antibody persistence studies.

There are several studies that have examined antibody persistence after MCV4-DT. Among children aged 2–11 years who were given one dose of MCV4-DT or the recently discontinued quadrivalent meningococcal polysaccharide vaccine, hSBA titers 6 months later had declined in both groups, but more rapidly in the polysaccharide vaccine group.[98] Among 2-year-old children who had received MCV4-DT 2.4 years earlier, 15% (group A), 33% (group Y), and 45% (group W) had hSBA titers of at least 1:4.[99] In teenagers a substantial proportion of subjects who had been immunized with a single dose 3 years earlier did not have protective hSBA titers to capsular groups C, W, and Y.[100] Another study compared serum antibody persistence among adolescents who had been immunized with MCV4-CRM or MCV4-DT 22 months earlier.[101] The proportions of subjects with protective hSBA titers, defined as $\geq$ 1:8, were, respectively, 36% versus 25% for group A, 62% versus 58% for group C, 84% versus 74% for group W, and 67% versus 54% for group Y; the differences were statistically significant for groups A, Y, and W.

Antibody persistence after a booster dose with MCV4-CRM was assessed among adolescents who had had initial immunization with either MCV4-DT or MCV-CRM. Two years after the booster dose, 77% −100% of individuals had hSBA titers >1:8.[102]

Vaccine Effectiveness

As stated previously, there were no prelicensure efficacy trials for either MCV4-CRM or MCV4-DT. Postlicensure observational studies are often used to estimate questions about vaccine effectiveness after licensure. A postlicensure case-control vaccine effectiveness study that was conducted among adolescents for MCV4-DT was consistent with the aforementioned antibody persistence data.[103] Overall vaccine effectiveness for all capsular groups for 0−8 years after vaccination was estimated to be 69%. There was evidence for substantial waning of effectiveness over time with estimates of 79% during the first year after vaccination, 69% at 1−3 years, and 61% at 3−8 years. No effectiveness data are available for MCV4-CRM. Based on these antibody persistence and effectiveness data for MCV4-DT, the ACIP recommended the addition of a booster dose of MCV4-DT or MCV4-CRM (see "ACIP recommendations and rationale" in the following).[104] Although the clinical significance of the differences in immunogenicity between MCV4-CRM and MCV4-DT that are described previously is not known, one might expect less rapid waning of effectiveness over time for MCV4-CRM.

Safety

MCV4-DT was found to be safe and well tolerated among the approximately 7000 persons who received it before licensure.[36,89] Temperature $\geq$38°C occurred in 5.1% of adolescents and 0.5% of adults. Serious systemic reactions, such as high fever, headache, fatigue, malaise, chills, arthralgia, anorexia, vomiting, diarrhea, or rash or seizures, occurred in <5% of subjects. Moderate pain at the injection site, moderate swelling, severe pain resulting in inability to move the arm and severe injection-site swelling occurred in 16.7%, 2.5%, 0.7%, and 9.7%, respectively.[89] Local reactions generally resolved within 2−3 days and were similar to those observed after Td vaccination. Rates of local reactions were lower in adults than in adolescents. A concern about an association between MCV4-DT immunization

and Guillain-Barré syndrome that was raised soon after licensure in 2005[105] was not confirmed in subsequent studies.[106] Safety and tolerability of MCV4-CRM have been assessed in comparison with MCV4-DT. In 2- to 5-year olds, 6- to 10-year olds, and 11- to 18-year olds, local and systemic reactions were similar for both vaccines.[93,107]

Impact on Pharyngeal Carriage

One of the major benefits of conjugate vaccines is, through reductions in asymptomatic pharyngeal carriage, herd protection. Monovalent group C conjugate vaccines led to both decreased group C carriage and substantial herd protection in the U.K.[108−110] A study comparing the impact of MCV4-CRM and MenB-4C on carriage was conducted in the U.K. When compared to a control group that received two doses of Japanese encephalitis vaccine, the MCV4-CRM group had a 39.0% lower carriage prevalence of capsular group Y strains and 36.2% lower carriage prevalence of capsular groups C, W, and Y combined during the period of 2−12 months after immunization; the study did not address any longer term impact on carriage.[111] There are no data on the impact of MCV4-DT on pharyngeal carriage of vaccine capsular groups.[55]

CAPSULAR GROUP B VACCINES

With the success of the meningococcal conjugate vaccines, a high proportion of meningococcal disease in many countries has been caused by group B strains.[112] Capsular B polysaccharide cross-reacts with fetal neural tissue and is a poor antigen,[113,114] which led to a major delay in the development of vaccines to prevent group B disease. Give this barrier to the development of a group B vaccine using capsular polysaccharide, focus turned on identifying immunogenic OMPs. Proof of concept for potential clinical protection provided by protein-based vaccines was demonstrated through the use of outer membrane vesicle vaccines with a single variant of PorA as the primary antigen for control of clonal capsular group B outbreaks caused by strains that expressed that PorA variant.[115,116] Although this success was promising, endemic group B disease differs from outbreaks in that the former is caused by a population of strains that is antigenically very variable in terms or PorA. This meant that many PorA variants would need to be included to cover the majority of endemic group B strains, an impractical approach.[117] Thus a search was initiated to identify immunogenic meningococcal OMPs that were relatively antigenically conserved.

After decades of lagging behind the conjugate vaccines, protein-based meningococcal vaccines were finally developed for prevention of group B disease. There are two vaccines in the U.S., both licensed by the FDA for persons aged 10−25 years. The first, MenB-FHbp (Trumenba, Pfizer), was licensed in October 2014 and is composed of 60 µg each of two lipidated variants of factor H−binding protein, one each from subfamily A and B, that are absorbed with Al^{+3} as aluminum phosphate. The lipids serve as an adjuvant and may also contribute to the vaccine's reactogenicity.[118] The second, MenB-4C (Bexsero, Glaxo SmithKline), is composed of a single variant of FHbp that is fused with a protein called GNA 2019, neisserial heparin binding antigen (NHBA) (fused with GNA 1030), and neisserial adhesin A (NadA), as well as the outer membrane vesicle (which contains a single variant of PorA) that was used to control a capsular group B outbreak in New Zealand.[115] The antigens are absorbed with Al^{3+} as aluminum hydroxide.

The antigens included in MenB-4C were identified through the process of reverse vaccinology, by which the whole-genome sequence of a capsular group strains was mined to identify the antigens included in the vaccine.[119,120] FHbp was independently identified using traditional biochemical and immunologic approaches.[60] Although MenB-FHbp and MenB-4C were developed for prevention of group B infection, the vaccine antigens are capsular group independent and therefore are likely to provide some clinical protection against all meningococcal capsular groups.[121−124]

As with the meningococcal conjugate vaccines that are licensed in the U.S., no prelicensure efficacy trials were performed for the new group B vaccines because of the low disease burden. Therefore licensure was based on safety and immunogenicity, with efficacy being inferred from the hSBA responses. The manufacturers of both vaccines tested hSBA against a panel of three or four selected strains. There are no studies that directly compare the immunogenicity or safety of MenB-4C and MenB-FHbp. However, the reported rates of adverse events are similar for the two vaccines.

Immunogenicity of MenB-4C and MenB-FHbp

Determining the immunogenicity of MenB-4C has been challenging because of its multiple components. To assess the immunogenicity of each antigen, reference strains were selected which were each mismatched for three of the four antigens in the vaccine and had high expression of the antigen of interest. In infants, MenB-4C elicited hSBA against the majority of the strain panel. In addition, the data indicated that the OMV component served as an adjuvant that enhanced the immune response to the vaccine antigens.[125]

When given at 2, 4, 6, and 12 months of each, >90% of infants developed protective titers against three reference strains and most also developed protective titers against three of four disease-causing test isolates. In larger studies, a two- or three-dose schedule of MenB-4C given to infants and toddlers led to protective antibody levels against three reference antigen-specific strains.[126,127] Antibody levels measured at an age of 40 months in infants who were immunized using the same schedule [128] were higher than unimmunized children for some but not all test strains.

In a Chilean study 92%−97% of adolescents given a single dose of MenB-4C developed hSBA titers of ≥1:4 for NadA, PorA, and FHbp; 99%−100% had protective titers after two or three doses.[129] In a study of European laboratory workers aged 18−50 years who were administered MenB-4C and also a separate injection of MCV4-CRM, 61%−80% had ≥fourfold increases in serum bactericidal titers after a single dose of MenB-4C; 69%−100% had protective responses after three doses.[130]

In a study of Canadian and Australian adolescents aged 11−17 years at 1 month postdose 2, nearly all participants developed responses to FHbp or NadA, but the response to PorA strain was only 39%.[131] In a study of UK university students, responses to the three antigens ranged from 67% to 94%.

The immunogenicity of MenB-4C has also been studied in the setting of college outbreaks. Eight weeks after a two-dose schedule of MenB-4C, a third of students who had been immunized in response to the outbreak at Princeton University did not have an hSBA ≥1:4. This was despite the fact that coverage was predicted by the FHbp and NHBA variants expressed by the outbreak strain and that the vast majority of students had protective titers against two group B reference strains. No meningococcal disease cases occurred among immunized students.

Concomitant administration of MenB-4C with other infant vaccines has been studied for antigens in DTaP-HBV-IPV/Hib and heptavalent pneumococcal conjugate vaccine (PCV7).[126] Interference by MenB-4C was demonstrated for the pertactin component of pertussis vaccine and pneumococcal serotype 6B antigen in PCV7. In another study[127] of concomitant administration of MenB-4C and DTaP-HBV-IPV/Hib, lack of interference was demonstrated for diphtheria and tetanus toxoids, Hib polysaccharide, HBV, pertussis toxin, filamentous hemagglutinin, pertactin, and polio virus types 1 and 3; noninferiority was not demonstrated for type 2 polio virus. The clinical importance of these minor decreases in immunogenicity, if any, is not known.

In healthy Australian adults aged 18–40 years given MenB-FHbp with a 0-, 1-, and 6-month schedule, a hSBA titer ≥1:4 was observed in 94.3% against a strain expressing the same FHbp antigen as in the vaccine and 70.0%–94.7% against four heterologous strains.[132] The immunogenicity of MenB-FHbp was also studied in adolescents and young adults aged 10–25 years in the U.S., Canada, and Europe who were administered the vaccine on a 0-, 2-, and 6-month schedule.[133] Immunogenicity was determined against four group B strains with FHbp variants that were selected to be representative of disease-causing isolates, two each in subfamilies A and B. The proportion of subjects who developed at ≥fourfold rise in hSBA titer ranged from 79.3% to 92.0% against the four test strains.

In another study of European 11- to 18-year olds, immunogenicity using four reference strains of five different MenB-FHbp vaccination schedules were assessed: 0, 1, 6 month; 0, 2, 6 month; 0 and 2 month; 0 and 4 month; and 0 and 6 month.[134] For the three-dose schedules, the proportion of subjects with an hSBA titer ≥ 1:8 to all four strains was 83.1% of subjects in the 0-, 1-, and 6-month group and 81.7% in the 0-, 2-, and 6-month group. The values for the two-dose schedules were 73.5% (0- and 6-month schedule), 58.9% (0- and 4-month schedule), and 56.8% (0- and 2-month schedule). Thus response rates were highest for the three-dose schedules, and among the two-dose schedules, the optimal interval was 0 and 6 months.

Immunogenicity of MenB-FHbp has also been demonstrated in adolescents and young adults against an expanded panel of strains with 14 FHbp variants.[75]

Data on coadministration of MenB-FHbp with adolescent vaccines are available for 4vHPV (Gardasil, Merck), MCV-4-DT (Menactra, Sanofi Pasteur), Tdap (Adacel, Sanofi Pasteur), or dTaP/IPV (Repevax, Sanofi Pasteur).[135–138] There was evidence of interference of MenB-FHbp with human papillomavirus (HPV) type 18 antigen, although the clinical significance of this finding is unknown.

Persistence of Serum Antibody

Persistence of bactericidal activity after administration of MenB-4C has been studied in adolescents. In Chile antibody levels 18–24 months after MenB-4C immunization varied according to the number of doses in the original schedule.[139] For a single dose of vaccine the proportion with hSBA titers ≥1:4 after 18–24 months

against the three antigens ranged from 62% to 73% and 75% to 93% for adolescents immunized with two or three doses, respectively. Short-term persistence has also been evaluated after immunization in response to four university outbreaks and is highly dependent on the outbreak strain.[140] The proportion of students with protective titers ≥1:4 7 months after immunization against the four outbreak strains was 31%, 38%, 57%, and 86%. Data on concomitant administration of MenB-4C with adolescent vaccines are not available.[135]

Antibody levels at 60 months of age of a booster dose at 40 months of age in children immunized at 2, 4, 6, and 12 months or 6, 8, and 12 months of age were also assessed.[141] hSBA titers ≥1:4 ranged from 44% to 100% for the FHbp, NadA, NHba, and PorA components. Additional studies are needed to determine the timing of any additional booster doses to maintain clinical protection through, for example, adolescence.

In studies of the kinetics of antibody persistence for MenB-FHbp, antibody levels decline substantially by 12 months after a two- or three-dose schedule, with the majority of 11- to 18-year olds not having protective antibody titers by that time and then remain relatively stable through 48 months.[142] A booster dose given at 48 months after the primary series led to protective antibody titers in nearly all subjects. In a study of 17 healthcare and laboratory workers given two or three doses of Trumenba, hSBA responses against diverse capsular group B isolates were determined 9–11 months after immunization: less than half had protective antibody titers for four of nine capsular group B isolates tested.[143] Taken together, these data suggest that booster vaccination will be needed to sustain protective immunity in adolescents and adults.

Vaccine Effectiveness

As mentioned, no efficacy trials were conducted for the group B meningococcal vaccines. Therefore, postlicensure assessments of protection using observational methods have been used to determine vaccine effectiveness of MenB-4C. Because of high rates of endemic group B disease caused by strain with an FHbp variant that was antigenically closely related to the variant in Bexsero in the Saguenay—Lac-Saint Jean region of Quebec, in May 2014, a mass MenB-4C immunization campaign targeting the age group of 2 months to 20 years was implemented. Using several approaches for estimating protection, the effectiveness of the campaign in decreasing the overall incidence of invasive meningococcal disease was estimated to be around 40%–75%.[144,145]

The United Kingdom incorporated MenB-4C into the pediatric immunization schedule with doses at 2, 4, and 12 months of age. This schedule is considered to be reduced because the vaccine was licensed for a primary series of three doses for infants aged 2–5 months followed by a booster at 12–15 months of age. The introduction of MenB-4C into the UK schedule offered an excellent opportunity to assess vaccine effectiveness.[146] Vaccine uptake was high with 89% of eligible infants receiving two doses. Using the screening method, two-dose vaccine effectiveness was estimated to be 82.9%, and there was a 50% reduction in the number of group B cases after introduction of routine immunization. Taken together, the results provide strong evidence for short-term protection against group B disease in infants; the duration of protection provided by this schedule is unknown. No data were provided on the meningococcal strains that caused invasive disease in immunized children to determine whether they were the result of vaccine failure or lack of coverage by the vaccine in part because 73% of the cases were confirmed only by PCR, and therefore many strains were unavailable for characterization. The vaccine has also been introduced into other countries for use in infants.[147]

No vaccine effectiveness data are available for MenB-FHbp.

Safety

High fever, irritability, severe crying, and local injection-site reactions occurred more commonly when MenB-4C was administered to infants at the same visit as other childhood vaccines.[126,127] In studies of persons aged 10–25 years, there were high rates of injection-site reactions. The rates of serious adverse events (SAEs) were similar for vaccinated and placebo (either saline or containing aluminum hydroxide) recipients.[111,129,148] In teenagers and young adults, local reactions were common, including erythema and pain at the injection site. For SAEs the rates among the vaccinated were similar to unvaccinated controls.[135]

Several postlicensure studies assessing adverse events in the UK have confirmed that MenB-4C has substantial reactogenicity in infants. Among Scottish infants, who received MenB-4C at 8 and 16 weeks of age, there was an increased risk of hospitalization for fever within 3 days of immunization which was believed to be due to the introduction of MenB-4C into the immunization schedule.[149] Similarly there was an increase in emergency department visits and intravenous antibiotic use among infants in Oxford, U.K., after MenB-4C immunization.[150] Finally, in a study in a regional hospital in Northern Ireland, 35 infants (0.8% of the vaccinated population in the study catchment area) were seen at the pediatric emergency department within 4 days of receipt of MenB-4C.[151] Eighty percent presented with fever, and other common symptoms included irritability and reduced feeding. Among the children who were tested, 73% had leukocytosis of >15,000 cells/µL. Among infants who had culture of blood (19 children) or cerebrospinal fluid (CSF) (6 children), all were negative, and no child with CSF taken had CSF pleocytosis. Half of the children were admitted to the hospital, and in all cases the final diagnosis was vaccine related.

There has also been postlicensure adverse event experience with MenB-4C in the control of college outbreaks in the U.S. and a community outbreak in Quebec.[46,135] Among nearly 60,000 vaccinated persons there were three SAEs related or possibly related to vaccination: anaphylaxis within half an hour of vaccine administration, rhabdomyolysis, and fever.

The manufacturer of MenB-FHbp did not pursue licensure for infants because of a high rate of febrile reactions.[152] Safety in more than 4000 persons aged 10–26 years was assessed in controlled trials.[153] Pain at the injection site, fatigue, headache, any muscle pain, chills, and joint pain were common but mostly nonsevere, with rates that were slightly higher than those of in person who received other vaccines (e.g., HPV vaccine). For adolescents the rates of severe injection-site pain (8.2%) or redness >10 cm (2.2%) at the injection were higher among those who had received the first dose of MenB-FHbp than in control subjects who received saline (0.2% and 0%, respectively). Severe systemic reactions such as headache (1.4%), fatigue (4.3%), chills (1.3%), generalized myalgia (3.1%), or joint pain (0.9%) occurred with rates higher than were reported for control subjects who were immunized with HPV vaccine. For subsequent doses of MenB-FHbp the trend was for a lower incidence of these reactions.

Among more than 2500 persons who participated in four clinical trials, there were no SAEs considered to be related or possibly related to MenB-FHbp vaccine.[132,135] In additional unpublished studies of more than 7200 persons who received at least one dose of MenB-FHbp, there were seven self-limited SAEs that were reported in four persons which were considered to be related or possibly related to the vaccine: anaphylaxis, chills, fever, headache, neutropenia, vertigo, and vomiting.[135]

Among students who received MenB-FHbp in response to a college outbreak, injection-site pain was reported after the first dose of vaccine in 77.6%; 4.0% were characterized as severe.[154] After the third dose, the reported rates of injection-site pain were 71.1% and 1.8%, respectively. Depending on the dose, 31.3%—38.9% reported fatigue, 11.3%—16.1% reported headache, 15.8%—47.1% reported myalgia, and 4.4%—6.1% had confirmed fever.

In a study of more than 5000 healthy adolescents and young adults in Europe and the U.S., adverse events were more common in the group that received MenB-FHbp than in that received hepatitis A vaccine, with the excess appearing to be mainly due to events related to reactogenicity.[155]

In summary, MenB-4C and MenB-FHbp are both associated with substantial rates of both local and systemic reactions.

Impact on Pharyngeal Carriage

As indicated previously, the herd protection provided by the conjugate vaccine provides huge public health benefit through protection of unimmunized persons. Therefore whether there is any impact on carriage of group B vaccines has been of intense interest. Among 2954 UK university students aged 18—24 years who received two doses of MenB-4C, MCV-CRM, or a Japanese encephalitis vaccine, MenB-4C was associated with a 26% reduction in carriage of combined capsular groups B, C, W, and Y 2—12 months after vaccination.[111] There was a similar, but not statistically significant, reduction in carriage of capsular group B strains alone. There was no statistically significant impact on acquisition of carriage of any capsular group.

A carriage study was performed in the setting of an immunization campaign to control an ST-9069 capsular group B outbreak.[156] MenB-FHbp was recommended to be given as three doses over 6 months. Overall meningococcal carriage rates were approximately 20%, with group B carriage being around 4%. Despite immunization, carriage rates did not decrease over the course of 13 months, and 10 students acquired group B carriage: three, four, and three students acquired group B carriage, respectively, after one, two, and three doses of MenB-FHbp.

Based on the relatively limited information from these studies, it appears likely that group B vaccines will provide substantially less herd protection, if any, than that provided by conjugate vaccines.[116] Despite the fact that the current group B vaccines will likely prevent infection caused by capsular groups other than B, it is unlikely that they will supplant the meningococcal conjugate vaccines.

ADVISORY COMMITTEE FOR IMMUNIZATION PRACTICES RECOMMENDATIONS AND RATIONALE

The Centers for Disease Control and Prevention's (CDC) Advisory Committee for Immunization Practices (ACIP) is responsible for making recommendations on use of meningococcal vaccines for both children and adults. Meningococcal vaccine recommendations are somewhat complex and have changed substantially over time because of the sequential addition of a variety of new vaccines with different immunologic properties (i.e., quadrivalent conjugate vaccines that use different protein carriers and protein-based vaccines for prevention of capsular group B disease) over the past dozen years, the marked changes in the epidemiology of meningococcal disease in the U.S., and the availability of new data over time on the licensed vaccines. Current ACIP recommendations are shown in Tables 7.2 (MCV4) and 7.3 (group B vaccines) and are also available on the ACIP website (www.cdc.gov/vaccines/hcp/acip-recs/vacc-specific/mening.html).

The ACIP has the option to recommend licensed vaccines (1) for all persons in an age- or risk factor—based group (which is commonly referred to as a "routine use" recommendation,[159]) (2) to make a recommendation for "individual clinical decision-making" (generally based on discussions between the healthcare provider and the patient and/or the patient's family), or (3) to make no recommendation. Recommendations for "individual clinical decision-making" are often made when the ACIP believes that the evidence or disease burden is insufficient to support a routine use recommendation. Both "routine use" and "individual clinical decision-making" recommendations appear on the ACIP immunization schedule and are required to be covered by commercial insurance under the Affordable Care Act. Given that any FDA-licensed vaccine is available for use independent of ACIP recommendations, the important distinction between an "individual clinical decision-making" recommendation and no recommendation is that the former is covered by commercial insurance, whereas the latter is not required to be. In addition, both types of recommendations generally lead to coverage by the Vaccines for Children Program, which assures that children aged <19 years receive recommended vaccines regardless of the ability to pay.

Meningococcal Conjugate Vaccines

Conjugate vaccines are generally preferred over unconjugated polysaccharide vaccines because of the superior

TABLE 7.2

Recommendations for Use of Meningococcal Conjugate Vaccines (MCV4-DT [Menactra], MCV4-CRM [Menveo]) to Prevent Groups A, C, W, and Y Infection in the United States.

Risk Group	Primary Series	Booster Doses
Healthy persons aged 11–18 years	1 dose of MCV4-CRM or MCV4-DT, preferably at age 11–12 years	At age 16 years if primary series at age 11 or 12 years
		At age 16–18 years if primary dose at age 13–15 years
		No booster needed if primary dose on or after age 16 years
Persons aged 2–23 months with complement component deficiency (deficiency in C3, C5-9, properdin, factor D, factor H, or taking eculizumab [Solaris]), human immunodeficiency virus infection, functional/anatomic asplenia, or increased risk of exposure (for example, because of a community outbreak caused by a vaccine capsular group and travelers to or residents of countries where meningococcal disease is hyperendemic or epidemic)	MCV4-CRM at 2, 4, 6, and 12–15 months OR (only if ≥ 9 months of age) 2 doses of MCV4-DT at least 12 weeks apart In children with asplenia or HIV infection, **do not use** MCV4-DT until age 24 months (see below) If starting schedule at 7–23 months, 2 doses of MCV4-CRM with the second dose over 12 months of age and at least 3 months after the first dose.	If previous dose at age <7 years, after 3 years. If previous dose at age ≥7 years, after 5 years. If continued risk, additional boosters every 5 years
Persons aged ≥24 months with complement component deficiency (deficiency in C3, C5-9, properdin, factor D, factor H, or taking eculizumab [Solaris]), human immunodeficiency virus infection, or functional or anatomic asplenia	2 doses of MCV4-CRM or MCV4-DT at least 8 weeks apart In children with asplenia or HIV infection, **do not use** MCV4-DT until the age of 24 months **and** administer at least 4 weeks after administration of all PCV13 doses	If previous dose at age <7 years, after 3 years. If previous dose at age ≥7 years, after 5 years. If continued risk, additional boosters every 5 years
Persons aged 24 months–55 years with increased risk of exposure (for example, microbiologists routinely working with *Neisseria meningitidis*, because of a community outbreak caused by a vaccine capsular group, and travelers to or residents of countries where meningococcal disease is hyperendemic or epidemic)	1 dose of MCV4-CRM or MCV4-DT	If previous dose at age <7 years and who remain at increased risk of exposure, after 3 years If previous dose at age ≥7 years, after 5 years. If continued risk, additional boosters every 5 years

Note: For all high-risk children if MCV4-DT used, it should be given either before or at the same time as DTaP (Ref. 88)

Modified from recommendations of the Advisory Committee on Immunization Practices (Refs. 20,37,157)

immunologic properties of the conjugates. However, this issue has become moot in the U.S. with the recent discontinuation of the only polysaccharide vaccine, a quadrivalent capsular group ACWY product (Menomune, Sanofi Pasteur), which was licensed for persons aged 2 years and above.[77] Given that neither MCV4-DT nor MCV4-CRM is licensed for persons aged above 55 years, off-label use of MCV4 is needed for protection of persons in this age category.

ROUTINE USE IMMUNIZATION
Persons Aged 11–18 Years

The ACIP recommends routine immunization for all persons aged 11–18 years with one of the two ACWY conjugate vaccines, with a preference for immunization beginning at 11–12 years of age (Table 7.2). The focus on adolescents is because of studies that were conducted during a time that the incidence of invasive meningococcal infection was much higher than it is

TABLE 7.3
Recommendations for Use of Vaccines (MenB-4C [Bexsero] or MenB-FHbp [Trumenba] to Prevent Capsular Group B Meningococcal Infection in the United States. Bexero and Trumenba are Not Interchangeable Because the Composition of the Vaccines are Substantially Different. The Same Vaccine Should be Used for all Doses

	VACCINE	
Risk group	MenB-4C (Bexsero, GSK)	MenB-FHbp (Trumenba, Pfizer)
Persons aged ≥10 years at increased risk of group B infection (a "routine use" recommendation): complement component deficiency (deficiency in C3, C5-9, properdin, factor D, factor H, or taking eculizumab [Solaris]), functional/anatomic asplenia, or increased risk of exposure during a capsular group B outbreak or work as a microbiologist with routine exposure to live *N. meningitidis* (a "routine use" recommendation)	2 doses, with doses at least 1 month apart	3 doses, with the second dose at least 1–2 months after the first dose and the third dose at least 6 months after the first
Persons aged 16–23 years who are not at increased risk of group B infection, preferably at age 16–18 years (an "individual clinical decision-making" recommendation)	2 doses, administered at 0 and ≥ 1 months	2 doses, administered at 0 and 6 months. If the second dose of Men-FHbp is given at an interval of <6 months, a third dose should be given at least 6 months after the first dose. The minimum interval between the second and third doses is 4 weeks

Recommendations regarding any booster doses will be forthcoming from ACIP as new data become available. Note: 1. FDA licensure for both vaccines is for ages 10–25 years. Vaccine use outside of this age range is considered to be off-label.
Modified from recommendations of the Advisory Committee on Immunization Practices Refs. (135,142,158)

currently.[160–162] Given the evidence for rapid waning of immunity and vaccine effectiveness of MCV4-DT that was discussed previously, the ACIP recommendation was revised to indicate that children immunized at 11–12 years should receive a booster dose at 16 years and 16–18 years if the first dose was given at 13–15 years.[20] A single dose is recommended for those who received the primary dose on or after 16 years of age.

Groups at Increased Risk of Disease or Exposure

Age 2–23 months: A four-dose schedule of MCV4-CRM is recommended at 2, 4, 6, and 12–15 months of age for infants who are at increased risk of meningococcal disease.[157] High-risk conditions include those with persistent complement component deficiencies, HIV infection, functional or anatomic asplenia, exposure to an outbreak for which the vaccine is recommended, and those traveling to areas where meningococcal

disease caused by vaccine capsular groups is hyperendemic or epidemic. The recommendation for persons with HIV infection is recent and based on studies demonstrating an increased risk of infection.[37,163,164] High-risk infants aged 7–23 months should receive two doses of MCV4-CRM, with the second dose over 12 months of age and at least 3 months after the first dose. MCV4-DT, which is licensed for those aged 9 months–55 years, can be used as an alternative for infants older than 9 months (except those with functional or anatomic asplenia or HIV infection).

If MCV4-DT or MCV4-CRM has been used to initiate immunization at 2–23 months, the first booster should be given 3 years later with a quadrivalent vaccine and subsequent boosters every 5 years.

Infants and toddlers with functional or anatomic asplenia or HIV infection should receive MCV4-CRM starting at 2 months of age. The less preferable option is to wait until 2 years of age, because this vaccine interferes with PCV13-CRM responses, and administer MCV4-DT.

For all high-risk children if MCV4-DT used, it should be given either before or at the same time as DTaP.[88]

Age 24 months and above with increased risk: A two-dose primary series of MCV4-DT or MCV4-CRM 8–12 weeks apart is recommended for individuals with complement deficiency, HIV infection, or functional or anatomic asplenia. A single dose of MCV4 is recommended for persons without these conditions but who are at increased risk of exposure: travelers to regions with epidemic or hyperendemic meningococcal disease, college freshmen living in dormitories (below 22 years), and microbiologists with routine exposure to *N. meningitidis* and during an outbreak due to a vaccine preventable strain. For those at ongoing risk of disease, initial booster doses are recommended after 3 years among those who were immunized below 7 years of age and at 5 years for older children and adults. Further boosters are recommended every 5 years.

There are no published data on the use of quadrivalent meningococcal conjugate vaccines in persons aged 55 years or above. However, off-label use of one of the conjugate vaccines is reasonable for persons in this age group who are at increased risk of disease or exposure.

As mentioned previously, for all high-risk children if MCV4-DT used, it should be given either before or at the same time as DTaP.[88]

NO RECOMMENDATION

MCV4-CRM is FDA approved for infants as young as 6 weeks old; MCV4-DT is licensed beginning as young as 9 month of age. Historically it was anticipated that there would be a routine recommendation for use of meningococcal conjugate vaccines in all infants. However, there is no recommendation for immunization of infants without increased risk for several reasons, including historically low disease burden, the predominance of capsular group B disease in infants, the high cost of the vaccines, and concerns about the addition of the vaccines to a crowded infant vaccination schedule.[165]

GROUP B VACCINES

Because the composition of the two group B vaccines is substantially different, MenB-4C and MenB-FHbp are not interchangeable. Accordingly the same vaccine should be used for all doses.

ROUTINE USE IMMUNIZATION

Group B vaccination is recommended for persons at high risk, such as microbiologists with exposure to live *N. meningitidis*, persons with functional or anatomic asplenia or complement deficiency, including those being treated eculizumab[30] (Table 7.3). Both capsular group B vaccines are licensed for only persons aged 10–25 years. However, there is no reason to believe that safety would be substantially different for persons aged >25 years, and therefore ACIP recommends off-label use of group B vaccines in individuals at increased risk of group B meningococcal disease in this age group.[135]

Unlike the recommendations for meningococcal polysaccharide-protein conjugate vaccines, the group B vaccine recommendation excludes persons traveling or residing in countries where meningococcal disease is hyperendemic or epidemic (unless the epidemic strain is known to be capsular group B), first-year college students living in residence halls, military recruits, and all adolescents. In addition, children aged <10 years are excluded from the current ACIP recommendations, even those at high risk. However, given the high risk of developing invasive meningococcal disease in children aged <10 years with complement deficiencies or functional or anatomic asplenia, off-label immunization with MenB-4C should be strongly considered. As discussed previously, this vaccine has been incorporated into the routine infant immunization schedule in the U.K. and has been shown to be safe and effective, albeit reactogenic.[146]

BASED ON CLINICAL DECISION-MAKING

The ACIP also recommends that a group B vaccine may be administered to adolescents and adults aged 16–23 years in the general population to provide short-term protection against most strains causing capsular group B disease.[158] The preferred age is 16–18 years because the majority of cases in adolescents and young adults occur after age 15 years (Fig. 7.2). The ACIP did not make a routine-use recommendation for this age group despite the current recommendation for MCV4 for 11–18 year olds because of the lower burden of capsular group B meningococcal disease, uncertainty about vaccine effectiveness and the durability of protection, as well as other scientific unknowns about these vaccines.[116]

No Recommendation

There is no recommendation for use of capsular group B vaccines in infants. Although MenB-4C is licensed and used routinely in infants in the U.K.,[146] neither of the meningococcal group B vaccines is licensed in the U.S. for persons aged below 10 years.

PRECAUTIONS AND CONTRAINDICATIONS

Owing to a lack of SAEs reported among women vaccinated with MCV4 during pregnancy or their newborns, MCV4 can be administered during pregnancy if indicated. There are no data on safety of either MenB-4C or MenB-FHbp in pregnancy, and therefore the vaccines should be used in pregnancy with caution and only if clearly indicated based on a careful assessment of risk. The vaccines can be administered during a minor acute illness, including presence of low-grade fever, but should be deferred in the setting of moderate-to-severe illness.

All meningococcal vaccines can be safely administered to persons who are immunocompromised but are contraindicated in persons with known hypersensitivity to any vaccine component or severe reaction to a previous dose. The caps of the prefilled syringes for MenB-4C and the single-dose vials of MCV-DT both contain latex, which may result in allergic reactions in persons with latex allergy.

In addition to MCV4, vaccines that are routinely recommended for adolescents and adults include Tdap, HPV, and influenza vaccines. Coadministration of MCV4-DT with diphtheria combined with tetanus toxoid (dT) with the Vi polysaccharide typhoid vaccine is immunogenic and safe. MCV4-CRM can be safely coadministered with HPV vaccine and Tdap.

Conjugate vaccines can generally be safely and effectively given together with live attenuated viral vaccines or purified subcomponent vaccines. The risk of syncope after immunization is of concern particularly in adolescents[166]; thus after vaccine administration ACIP recommends patient observation for 15 minutes.[167]

CONTROL OF MENINGOCOCCAL OUTBREAKS

Multiple outbreaks of meningococcal disease have occurred in institutions and in the community. Given the recent shift to capsular group B strains as a major cause of outbreaks, the recent advent of capsular group B meningococcal vaccines has dramatically expanded the vaccine preventability of outbreaks. Even if a vaccination campaign is mounted in response to an outbreak, it is still important to provide antibiotic chemoprophylaxis to close contacts as outlined previously.

The CDC has recently issued new guidance on public health management of meningococcal outbreaks.[168] The decision to vaccinate in response to an outbreak can be complicated and needs to be made on an outbreak-by-outbreak basis. In general, all isolates from the institution or community that is experiencing the outbreak should have determination of the capsular group. Strains of the same capsular group should be considered to be part of the outbreak unless molecular characterization refutes that assumption. For institutions such as colleges and universities, 2—3 cases caused by the same capsular group over a 3-month period are considered to be an outbreak. For the community an increase in the incidence of disease over a 3-month period caused by the same capsular group is considered to be an outbreak.

For outbreaks involving one of the four capsular groups in the quadrivalent meningococcal vaccines, either MCV-DT or MCV4-CRM can be used. The vaccination schedule should be according to age as shown in Table 7.2. For capsular group B outbreaks, the CDC recommends vaccination for persons aged 10 years and above using either MenB-4C (2-dose schedule over 1 month) or Trumenba (3-dose schedule over 6 months) (Table 7.3). For outbreaks involving persons outside of the licensed age range for licensure, off-label use is reasonable.

In situations in which vaccination is not possible, expanded chemoprophylaxis can be considered and in some situations can be used in conjunction with vaccination.

Vaccine Coverage and Evidence for Impact of ACIP Recommendations

MCV4 vaccine coverage among US 13- to 17-year olds has steadily increased over time, from 11% in 2006 to 82% in 2016. However, only 39% of 17-year olds had received at least two doses as recommended by the ACIP.[169,170]

Although there is strong evidence that the bulk of the decline meningococcal disease incidence in the U.S. is not due to use of meningococcal vaccines as mentioned previously (Fig. 7.1), there is evidence for impact of MCV4 in adolescents and young adults. For the period of 2011—15 as compared to 2006—10 there were declines in both group B disease and groups A, C, W, and Y disease combined, but the declines were much more marked for the latter than for the former (Fig. 7.3).

There are no data on the impact of capsular group B meningococcal vaccines in the U.S. because (1) the vaccines were only recently licensed, (2) the vaccines are not universally recommended for any age group in the U.S., and (3) the rate of capsular group B infection is very low.

Prospects for the Future

Advances in meningococcal vaccine development over the past 10—15 years have been impressive, both in

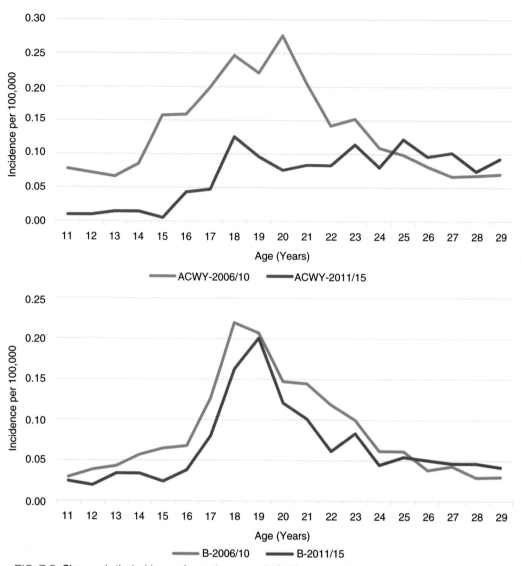

FIG. 7.3 Changes in the incidence of capsular groups A, C, W, and Y combined (panel a) and capsular group B (panel b) among US adolescents and young adults, from 2006 to 2010 and 2011 to 15 (Ref. 12). (Data are from the NNDSS. Reproduced with permission of Oxford University Press on behalf of the Infectious Diseases Society of America.)

the U.S. and globally. In the U.S. we now have both conjugate vaccines that can be given to infants and novel capsular group B vaccines. However, there are opportunities for improved meningococcal vaccines for the U.S. First, the holy grail of meningococcal vaccines in the U.S. is a product that covers all relevant capsular groups, namely a pentavalent product for groups A, B, C, W, and Y, and can be given to infants, the group with the highest risk of meningococcal infection; such vaccines are currently being studied. In addition, data on immunogenicity and antibody persistence suggest that improved capsular group B vaccines could be developed. One approach is mutant FHbp that binds less to human factor H yet retains its key epitopes,[171] which has the potential to enhance the immunogenicity and hopefully the duration of protection of the capsular group B vaccines. That said, the future of meningococcal vaccine development and utilization in the U.S. will ultimately depend at least in part on the ever-changing epidemiology of this highly dynamic disease.

REFERENCES

1. Trotter CL, Lingani C, Fernandez K, et al. Impact of MenAfriVac in nine countries of the African meningitis belt, 2010−15: an analysis of surveillance data. *Lancet Infect Dis.* 2017;17:867−872.
2. Mustapha MM, Harrison LH. Vaccine prevention of meningococcal disease in Africa: major advances but remaining challenges. *Hum Vaccin Immunother.* 2018;14: 1107−1115.
3. Harrison LH, Granoff DM, Pollard AJ. Meningococcal capsular group A, C, W, and Y Conjugate vaccines. In: Plotkin SA, Orenstein WA, Offit PA, Edwards KM, eds. *Vaccines.* 7th ed. Philadelphia: Elsevier; 2018:619−643.
4. Granoff DM, Pollard AJ, Harrison LH. Meningococcal capsular group B vaccines. In: Plotkin SA, Orenstein WA, Offit PA, Edwards KM, eds. *Vaccines.* 7th ed. Philadelphia: Elsevier; 2018:644−662.
5. Danielson L, Mann E. The history of a singular and very mortal disease, which lately made its appearance in Medfield. *Med Agric Reg.* 1806;1:65−69.
6. Danielson L, Mann E. Classics in infectious diseases: the first American account of cerebrospinal meningitis. *Rev Infect Dis.* 1983;5:969−972.
7. Weichselbaum A. Ueber die Aetiologie der akuten Meningitis Cerebrospinalis. *Fortschr Med.* 1887;5:573.
8. Harrison LH, Broome CV. The epidemiology of meningococcal meningitis in the U.S. civilian population. In: Vedros NA, ed. *Evolution of Meningococcal Disease.* Boca Raton, Fla: CRC Press; 1987:27−45.
9. Bazan JA, Turner AN, Kirkcaldy RD, et al. Large cluster of *Neisseria meningitidis* urethritis in Columbus, Ohio, 2015. *Clin Infect Dis.* 2017;65(1).
10. Tzeng YL, Bazan JA, Turner AN, et al. Emergence of a new *Neisseria meningitidis* clonal complex 11 lineage 11.2 clade as an effective urogenital pathogen. *Proc Natl Acad Sci USA.* 2017;114:4237−4242. PMCID: 5402416.
11. Bazan JA, Peterson AS, Kirkcaldy RD, et al. Notes from the field: increase in *Neisseria meningitidis*-Associated urethritis among men at two sentinel clinics - columbus, Ohio, and Oakland county, Michigan, 2015. *MMWR Morb Mortal Wkly Rep.* 2016;65:550−552. PMCID: 5390329.
12. MacNeil JR, Blain AE, Wang X, Cohn AC. Current epidemiology and trends in meningococcal disease-United States, 1996-2015. *Clin Infect Dis.* 2017.
13. Kaplan SL, Schutze GE, Leake JA, et al. Multicenter surveillance of invasive meningococcal infections in children. *Pediatrics.* 2006;118:e979−984.
14. Viner RM, Booy R, Johnson H, et al. Outcomes of invasive meningococcal serogroup B disease in children and adolescents (MOSAIC): a case-control study. *Lancet Neurol.* 2012;11:774−783.
15. Langley G, Besser J, Iwamoto M, et al. Effect of culture-independent diagnostic tests on future emerging infections program surveillance. *Emerg Infect Dis.* 2015;21: 1582−1588.
16. Harcourt BH, Anderson RD, Wu HM, et al. Population-based surveillance of *Neisseria meningitidis* antimicrobial resistance in the United States. *Open Forum Infect Dis.* 2015;2:ofv117. PMCID: 4561371.
17. McGill F, Heyderman RS, Michael BD, et al. The UK joint specialist societies guideline on the diagnosis and management of acute meningitis and meningococcal sepsis in immunocompetent adults. *J Infect.* 2016;72:405−438.
18. Deghmane AE, Hong E, Taha MK. Emergence of meningococci with reduced susceptibility to third-generation cephalosporins. *J Antimicrob Chemother.* 2017;72:95−98.
19. de Gans J, van de Beek D. Dexamethasone in adults with bacterial meningitis. *N Engl J Med.* 2002;347:1549−1556.
20. Cohn AC, MacNeil JR, Clark TA, et al. Prevention and control of meningococcal disease: recommendations of the Advisory Committee on Immunization Practices (ACIP). *MMWR Recomm Rep.* 2013;62:1−28.
21. Sejvar JJ, Johnson D, Popovic T, et al. Assessing the risk of laboratory-acquired meningococcal disease. *J Clin Microbiol.* 2005;43:4811−4814.
22. Centers for Disease Control, Prevention. Prevention and control of meningococcal disease. Recommendations of the Advisory Committee on Immunization Practices (ACIP). *MMWR Recomm Rep.* 2000;49:1−10.
23. Edwards EA, Devine LF, Sengbusch GH, Ward HW. Immunological investigations of meningococcal disease. III. Brevity of group C acquisition prior to disease occurrence. *Scand J Infect Dis.* 1977;9:105−110.
24. Christensen H, May M, Bowen L, Hickman M, Trotter CL. Meningococcal carriage by age: a systematic review and meta-analysis. *Lancet Infect Dis.* 2010;10:853−861.
25. Hublikar S, Maher WE, Bazan JA. Disseminated gonococcal infection and eculizumab—a "high risk" connection? *Sex Transm Dis.* 2014;41:747−748.
26. Zlamy M, Hofer J, Elias J, et al. Immunogenicity of meningococcus C vaccination in a patient with atypical hemolytic uremic syndrome (aHUS) on eculizumab therapy. *Pediatr Transpl.* 2012;16:E246−E250.
27. Gleesing J, Chiwane S, Rongkavilit C. Gonococcal septic shock associated with eculizumab treatment. *Pediatr Infect Dis J.* 2012;31:543.
28. Bouts A, Monnens L, Davin JC, Struijk G, Spanjaard L. Insufficient protection by *Neisseria meningitidis* vaccination alone during eculizumab therapy. *Pediatr Nephrol.* 2011;26:1919−1920. PMCID: PMC3163808.
29. McNamara LA, Topaz N, Wang X, Hariri S, Fox L, MacNeil JR. High risk for invasive meningococcal disease among patients receiving eculizumab (Soliris) despite receipt of meningococcal vaccine. *Am J Transpl.* 2017; 17:2481−2484.

30. McNamara LA, Topaz N, Wang X, Hariri S, Fox L, MacNeil JR. High risk for invasive meningococcal disease among patients receiving eculizumab (Soliris) despite receipt of meningococcal vaccine. *MMWR Morb Mortal Wkly Rep.* 2017;66:734–737.

31. Langley G, Schaffner W, Farley MM, et al. Twenty years of active bacterial core surveillance. *Emerg Infect Dis.* 2015; 21:1520–1528.

32. Adams DA, Thomas KR, Jajosky RA, et al. Summary of notifiable infectious diseases and conditions - United States, 2015. *MMWR Morb Mortal Wkly Rep.* 2017;64: 1–143.

33. Centers for Disease Control, Prevention. *Active Bacterial Core Surveillance (ABCs) Report, Emerging Infections Program Network,* Neisseria meningitidis; 2015. https://www. cdc.gov/abcs/reports-findings/survreports/mening15.pdf.

34. Haemophilus b conjugate vaccines for prevention of *haemophilus influenzae* type b disease among infants and children two months of age and older. Recommendations of the Immunization Practices Advisory Committee (ACIP). *MMWR Recomm Rep.* 1991;40:1–7.

35. Prevention of pneumococcal disease: recommendations of the Advisory Committee on Immunization Practices (ACIP). *MMWR Recomm Rep.* 1997;46:1–24.

36. Bilukha OO, Rosenstein N. Prevention and control of meningococcal disease. Recommendations of the Advisory Committee on Immunization Practices (ACIP). *MMWR Recomm Rep.* 2005;54:1–21.

37. MacNeil JR, Rubin LG, Patton M, Ortega-Sanchez IR, Martin SW. Recommendations for use of meningococcal conjugate vaccines in HIV-infected persons - advisory committee on immunization practices, 2016. *MMWR Morb Mortal Wkly Rep.* 2016;65:1189–1194.

38. Moore PS, Harrison LH, Telzak EE, Ajello GW, Broome CV. Group A meningococcal carriage in travelers returning from Saudi Arabia. *JAMA.* 1988;260:2686–2689.

39. Outbreak of meningococcal disease associated with an elementary school – Oklahoma, March 2010. *MMWR Morb Mortal Wkly Rep.* 2012;61:217–221.

40. Doyle TJ, Mejia-Echeverry A, Fiorella P, et al. Cluster of serogroup W135 meningococci, southeastern Florida, 2008–2009. *Emerg Infect Dis.* 2010;16:113–115. PMCID: 2874373.

41. Mustapha MM, Marsh JW, Harrison LH. Global epidemiology of capsular group W meningococcal disease (1970-2015): multifocal emergence and persistence of hypervirulent sequence type (ST)-11 clonal complex. *Vaccine.* 2016;34:1515–1523.

42. Moreno G, Lopez D, Vergara N, Gallegos D, Advis MF, Loayza S. Clinical characterization of cases with meningococcal disease by W135 group in Chile, 2012. *Rev Chilena Infectol.* 2013;30:350–360.

43. Campbell H, Parikh SR, Borrow R, Kaczmarski E, Ramsay ME, Ladhani SN. Presentation with gastrointestinal symptoms and high case fatality associated with group W meningococcal disease (MenW) in teenagers, England, July 2015 to January 2016. *Euro Surveill.* 2016;21.

44. Brooks R, Woods CW, Benjamin Jr DK, Rosenstein NE. Increased case-fatality rate associated with outbreaks of *Neisseria meningitidis* infection, compared with sporadic meningococcal disease, in the United States, 1994–2002. *Clin Infect Dis.* 2006;43:49–54.

45. Mandal S, Wu HM, MacNeil JR, et al. Prolonged university outbreak of meningococcal disease associated with a serogroup B strain rarely seen in the United States. *Clin Infect Dis.* 2013;57:344–348.

46. McNamara LA, Shumate AM, Johnsen P, et al. First use of a serogroup B meningococcal vaccine in the US in response to a university outbreak. *Pediatrics.* 2015;135: 798–804.

47. Rossi R, Beernink PT, Giuntini S, Granoff DM. Susceptibility of meningococcal strains responsible for two Serogroup B outbreaks on U.S. university campuses to serum bactericidal activity elicited by the MenB-4C Vaccine. *Clin Vaccine Immunol.* 2015;22. https://doi.org/ 10.1128/CVI.00474-00415.

48. McNamara LA, Thomas JD, MacNeil J, et al. Meningococcal carriage following a university serogroup B meningococcal disease outbreak and vaccination campaign with MenB-4C and MenB-FHbp - Oregon, 2015–2016. *J Infect Dis.* 2017.

49. Soeters HM, McNamara LA, Whaley M, et al. Serogroup B meningococcal disease outbreak and carriage evaluation at a college - Rhode Island, 2015. *MMWR Morb Mortal Wkly Rep.* 2015;64:606–607.

50. Biswas HH, Han GS, Wendorf K, et al. Notes from the field: outbreak of serogroup B meningococcal disease at a university - California, 2016. *MMWR Morb Mortal Wkly Rep.* 2016;65:520–521.

51. Soeters HM, Dinitz-Sklar J, Kulkarni PA, et al. Serogroup B meningococcal disease vaccine recommendations at a university, New Jersey, USA, 2016. *Emerg Infect Dis.* 2017;23:867–869. PMCID: 5403061.

52. Duffy J, Johnsen P, Ferris M, et al. Safety of a meningococcal group B vaccine used in response to two university outbreaks. *J Am Coll Health.* 2017:1–8.

53. Fiorito TM, Bornschein S, Mihalakos A, et al. Rapid response to a college outbreak of meningococcal serogroup B disease: nation's first widespread use of bivalent rLP2086 vaccine. *J Am Coll Health.* 2017;65: 294–296.

54. Harrison OB, Claus H, Jiang Y, et al. Description and nomenclature of *Neisseria meningitidis* capsule locus. *Emerg Infect Dis.* 2013;19:566–573. PMCID: 3647402.

55. Harrison LH, Shutt KA, Arnold KE, et al. Meningococcal carriage among Georgia and Maryland high school students. *J Infect Dis.* 2015;211:1761–1768.

56. Harrison LH, Trotter CL, Ramsay ME. Global epidemiology of meningococcal disease. *Vaccine.* 2009;27(suppl 2):B51–B63.

57. Mustapha MM, Marsh JW, Krauland MG, et al. Genomic epidemiology of hypervirulent serogroup W, ST-11 *Neisseria meningitidis.* *EBioMedicine.* 2015;2:1447–1455. PMCID: 4634745.

58. Masignani V, Comanducci M, Giuliani MM, et al. Vaccination against *Neisseria meningitidis* using three variants of the lipoprotein GNA1870. *J Exp Med*. 2003;197:789–799.

59. Murphy E, Andrew L, Lee KL, et al. Sequence diversity of the factor H binding protein vaccine candidate in epidemiologically relevant strains of serogroup B *Neisseria meningitidis*. *J Infect Dis*. 2009;200:379–389.

60. Fletcher LD, Bernfield L, Barniak V, et al. Vaccine potential of the *Neisseria meningitidis* 2086 lipoprotein. *Infect Immun*. 2004;72:2088–2100.

61. Beernink PT, Granoff DM. Bactericidal antibody responses induced by meningococcal recombinant chimeric factor H-binding protein vaccines. *Infect Immun*. 2008;76:2568–2575.

62. Goldschneider I, Gotschlich EC, Artenstein MS. Human immunity to the meningococcus. I. The role of humoral antibodies. *J Exp Med*. 1969;129:1307–1326.

63. Santos GF, Deck RR, Donnelly J, Blackwelder W, Granoff DM. Importance of complement source in measuring meningococcal bactericidal titers. *Clin Diagn Lab Immunol*. 2001;8:616–623.

64. Schneider MC, Exley RM, Chan H, et al. Functional significance of factor H binding to *Neisseria meningitidis*. *J Immunol*. 2006;176:7566–7575.

65. Goldblatt D, Vaz AR, Miller E. Antibody avidity as a surrogate marker of successful priming by *Haemophilus influenzae* type b conjugate vaccines following infant immunization. *J Infect Dis*. 1998;177:1112–1115.

66. Borrow R, Goldblatt D, Andrews N, et al. Antibody persistence and immunological memory at age 4 years after meningococcal group C conjugate vaccination in children in the United Kingdom. *J Infect Dis*. 2002;186:1353–1357.

67. Goldblatt D, Borrow R, Miller E. Natural and vaccine-induced immunity and immunologic memory to *Neisseria meningitidis* serogroup C in young adults. *J Infect Dis*. 2002;185:397–400.

68. Snape MD, Maclennan JM, Lockhart S, et al. Demonstration of immunologic memory using serogroup C meningococcal glycoconjugate vaccine. *Pediatr Infect Dis J*. 2009;28:92–97.

69. Kelly DF, Snape M, Clutterbuck EC, et al. CRM197-conjugated serogroup C meningococcal capsular polysaccharide, but not the native polysaccharide, induces persistent antigen specific memory B cells. *Blood*. 2006.

70. Blanchard Rohner G, Snape MD, Kelly DF, et al. The magnitude of the antibody and memory B cell responses during priming with a protein-polysaccharide conjugate vaccine in human infants is associated with the persistence of antibody and the intensity of booster response. *J Immunol*. 2008;180:2165–2173.

71. Donnelly J, Medini D, Boccadifuoco G, et al. Qualitative and quantitative assessment of meningococcal antigens to evaluate the potential strain coverage of protein-based vaccines. *Proc Natl Acad Sci USA*. 2010;107:19490–19495. PMCID: 2984153.

72. Vogel U, Taha MK, Vazquez JA, et al. Predicted strain coverage of a meningococcal multicomponent vaccine (4CMenB) in Europe: a qualitative and quantitative assessment. *Lancet Infect Dis*. 2013;13:416–425.

73. Jiang HQ, Hoiseth SK, Harris SL, et al. Broad vaccine coverage predicted for a bivalent recombinant factor H binding protein based vaccine to prevent serogroup B meningococcal disease. *Vaccine*. 2010;28:6086–6093.

74. Donald RG, Hawkins JC, Hao L, et al. Meningococcal serogroup B vaccines: estimating breadth of coverage. *Hum Vaccin Immunother*. 2017;13:255–265. PMCID: 5328210.

75. Harris SL, Donald RG, Hawkins JC, et al. *Neisseria meningitidis* serogroup B vaccine, bivalent rLP2086, induces broad serum bactericidal activity against diverse invasive disease strains including outbreak strains. *Pediatr Infect Dis J*. 2017;36:216–223.

76. Aku FY, Lessa FC, Asiedu-Bekoe F, et al. Meningitis outbreak caused by vaccine-preventable bacterial pathogens - northern Ghana, 2016. *MMWR Morb Mortal Wkly Rep*. 2017;66:806–810.

77. Granoff DM, Pelton S, Harrison LH. Meningococcal vaccines. In: Plotkin S, Orenstein WA, Offit PA, eds. *Vaccines*. 6th ed. Philadelphia: Saunders Elsevier; 2013:388–418.

78. Pollard AJ, Perrett KP, Beverley PC. Maintaining protection against invasive bacteria with protein-polysaccharide conjugate vaccines. *Nat Rev Immunol*. 2009;9:213–220.

79. Granoff DM, Pollard AJ. Reconsideration of the use of meningococcal polysaccharide vaccine. *Pediatr Infect Dis J*. 2007;26:716–722.

80. Santosham M, Wolff M, Reid R, et al. The efficacy in Navajo infants of a conjugate vaccine consisting of *Haemophilus influenzae* type b polysaccharide and *Neisseria meningitidis* outer-membrane protein complex. *N Engl J Med*. 1991;324:1767–1772.

81. Adams WG, Deaver KA, Cochi SL, et al. Decline of childhood *Haemophilus influenzae* type b (Hib) disease in the Hib vaccine era. *JAMA*. 1993;269:221–226.

82. Livorsi DJ, Macneil JR, Cohn AC, et al. Invasive *Haemophilus influenzae* in the United States, 1999–2008: epidemiology and outcomes. *J Infect*. 2012;65:496–504.

83. Snape MD, Kelly DF, Salt P, et al. Serogroup C meningococcal glycoconjugate vaccine in adolescents: persistence of bactericidal antibodies and kinetics of the immune response to a booster vaccine more than 3 years after immunization. *Clin Infect Dis*. 2006;43:1387–1394.

84. Campbell H, Edelstein M, Andrews N, Borrow R, Ramsay M, Ladhani S. Emergency meningococcal ACWY vaccination program for teenagers to control group W meningococcal disease, England, 2015–2016. *Emerg Infect Dis*. 2017;23.

85. Advisory Committee on Immunization Practices Centers for Disease C. Prevention. Report from the Advisory Committee on Immunization Practices (ACIP): decision not to recommend routine vaccination of all children aged 2–10 years with quadrivalent meningococcal

conjugate vaccine (MCV4). MMWR. *Morb Mortality Weekly Report*. 2008;57:462–465.

86. Centers for Disease C, Prevention. Licensure of a meningococcal conjugate vaccine (Menveo) and guidance for use - advisory committee on immunization practices (ACIP), 2010. *MMWR Morb Mortal Wkly Rep*. 2010;59: 273.

87. Rennels M, King Jr J, Ryall R, Papa T, Froeschle J. Dosage escalation, safety and immunogenicity study of four dosages of a tetravalent meninogococcal polysaccharide diphtheria toxoid conjugate vaccine in infants. *Pediatr Infect Dis J*. 2004;23:429–435.

88. Sanofi Pasteur Inc. *Menactra Prescribing Information*; September 16, 2016. Available at: http://www.fda.gov/ downloads/biologicsbloodvaccines/vaccines/approved products/ucm131170.pdf.

89. Keyserling H, Papa T, Koranyi K, et al. Safety, immunogenicity, and immune memory of a novel meningococcal (groups A, C, Y, and W-135) polysaccharide diphtheria toxoid conjugate vaccine (MCV-4) in healthy adolescents. *Arch Pediatr Adolesc Med*. 2005;159: 907–913.

90. Pichichero M, Casey J, Blatter M, et al. Comparative trial of the safety and immunogenicity of quadrivalent (A, C, Y, W-135) meningococcal polysaccharide-diphtheria conjugate vaccine versus quadrivalent polysaccharide vaccine in two- to ten-year-old children. *Pediatr Infect Dis J*. 2005;24:57–62.

91. Snape MD, Perrett KP, Ford KJ, et al. Immunogenicity of a tetravalent meningococcal glycoconjugate vaccine in infants: a randomized controlled trial. *JAMA*. 2008;299: 173–184.

92. Halperin SA, Diaz-Mitoma F, Dull P, Anemona A, Ceddia F. Safety and immunogenicity of an investigational quadrivalent meningococcal conjugate vaccine after one or two doses given to infants and toddlers. *Eur J Clin Microbiol Infect Dis*. 2010;29:259–267.

93. Halperin SA, Gupta A, Jeanfreau R, et al. Comparison of the safety and immunogenicity of an investigational and a licensed quadrivalent meningococcal conjugate vaccine in children 2-10 years of age. *Vaccine*. 2010;28: 7865–7872.

94. Food and Drug Adminstration. Menveo prescribing information. https://www.fda.gov/downloads/biologicsblood vaccines/vaccines/approvedproducts/ucm201349.pdf.

95. Reisinger KS, Baxter R, Block SL, Shah J, Bedell L, Dull PM. Quadrivalent meningococcal vaccination of adults: phase III comparison of an investigational conjugate vaccine, MenACWY-CRM, with the licensed vaccine, Menactra. *Clin Vaccine Immunol*. 2009;16:1810–1815. PMCID: 2786376.

96. Lujan-Zilbermann J, Warshaw MG, Williams PL, et al. Immunogenicity and safety of 1 vs 2 doses of quadrivalent meningococcal conjugate vaccine in youth infected with human immunodeficiency virus. *J Pediatr*. 2012; 161:676–681. PMCID: 3434315.

97. Balmer P, Falconer M, McDonald P, et al. Immune response to meningococcal serogroup C conjugate vaccine in asplenic individuals. *Infect Immun*. 2004;72: 332–337.

98. Granoff DM, Harris SL. Protective activity of group C anticapsular antibodies elicited in two-year-olds by an investigational quadrivalent *Neisseria meningitidis*-diphtheria toxoid conjugate vaccine. *Pediatr Infect Dis J*. 2004;23:490–497.

99. Granoff DM, Morgan A, Welsch JA. Immunogenicity of an investigational quadrivalent *Neisseria meningitidis*-diphtheria toxoid conjugate vaccine in 2-year old children. *Vaccine*. 2005;23:4307–4314.

100. Vu DM, Welsch JA, Zuno-Mitchell P, Dela Cruz JV, Granoff DM. Antibody persistence 3 years after immunization of adolescents with quadrivalent meningococcal conjugate vaccine. *J Infect Dis*. 2006;193:821–828.

101. Gill CJ, Baxter R, Anemona A, Ciavarro G, Dull P. Persistence of immune responses after a single dose of Novartis meningococcal serogroup A, C, W-135 and Y CRM-197 conjugate vaccine (Menveo(R)) or Menactra(R) among healthy adolescents. *Hum Vaccin*. 2010;6: 881–887.

102. Baxter R, Reisinger K, Block SL, et al. Antibody persistence after primary and booster doses of a quadrivalent meningococcal conjugate vaccine in adolescents. *Pediatr Infect Dis J*. 2014;33:1169–1176.

103. Cohn AC, MacNeil JR, Harrison LH, et al. Effectiveness and duration of protection of one dose of a meningococcal conjugate vaccine. *Pediatrics*. 2017;139.

104. Centers for Disease C, Prevention. Updated recommendations for use of meningococcal conjugate vaccines – Advisory Committee on Immunization Practices (ACIP), 2010. *MMWR Morb Mortal Wkly Rep*. 2011;60:72–76.

105. Centers for Disease C, Prevention. Guillain-Barré syndrome among recipients of Menactra meningococcal conjugate vaccine—United States, June-July 2005. *MMWR Morb Mortal Wkly Rep*. 2005;54:1023–1025.

106. Velentgas P, Amato AA, Bohn RL, et al. Risk of Guillain-Barré syndrome after meningococcal conjugate vaccination. *Pharmacoepidemiol Drug Saf*. 2012;21: 1350–1358.

107. Jackson LA, Baxter R, Reisinger K, et al. Phase III comparison of an investigational quadrivalent meningococcal conjugate vaccine with the licensed meningococcal ACWY conjugate vaccine in adolescents. *Clin Infect Dis*. 2009;49:e1–10.

108. Maiden MC, Ibarz-Pavon AB, Urwin R, et al. Impact of meningococcal serogroup C conjugate vaccines on carriage and herd immunity. *J Infect Dis*. 2008;197: 737–743.

109. Maiden MC, Stuart JM. Carriage of serogroup C meningococci 1 year after meningococcal C conjugate polysaccharide vaccination. *Lancet*. 2002;359:1829–1831.

110. Ramsay ME, Andrews NJ, Trotter CL, Kaczmarski EB, Miller E. Herd immunity from meningococcal serogroup C conjugate vaccination in England: database analysis. *BMJ*. 2003;326:365–366.

111. Read RC, Baxter D, Chadwick DR, et al. Effect of a quadrivalent meningococcal ACWY glycoconjugate or a

serogroup B meningococcal vaccine on meningococcal carriage: an observer-blind, phase 3 randomised clinical trial. *Lancet.* 2014;384:2123−2131.

112. Sridhar S, Greenwood B, Head C, et al. Global incidence of serogroup B invasive meningococcal disease: a systematic review. *Lancet Infect Dis.* 2015;15:1334−1346.

113. Finne J, Leinonen M, Makela PH. Antigenic similarities between brain components and bacteria causing meningitis. Implications for vaccine development and pathogenesis. *Lancet.* 1983;2:355−357.

114. Jennings HJ, Lugowski C. Immunochemistry of groups A, B, and C meningococcal polysaccharide-tetanus toxoid conjugates. *J Immunol.* 1981;127:1011−1018.

115. Kelly C, Arnold R, Galloway Y, O'Hallahan J. A prospective study of the effectiveness of the New Zealand meningococcal B vaccine. *Am J Epidemiol.* 2007; 166:817−823.

116. Harrison LH. Vaccines for prevention of group B meningococcal disease: not your father's vaccines. *Vaccine.* 2015;33.

117. Sacchi CT, Whitney AM, Popovic T, et al. Diversity and prevalence of PorA types in *Neisseria meningitidis* serogroup B in the United States, 1992−1998. *J Infect Dis.* 2000;182:1169−1176.

118. Luo Y, Friese OV, Runnels HA, et al. The dual role of lipids of the lipoproteins in Trumenba, a self-adjuvanting vaccine against meningococcal meningitis B disease. *AAPS J.* 2016;18:1562−1575.

119. Tettelin H, Saunders NJ, Heidelberg J, et al. Complete genome sequence of *Neisseria meningitidis* serogroup B strain MC58. *Science.* 2000;287:1809−1815.

120. Pizza M, Scarlato V, Masignani V, et al. Identification of vaccine candidates against serogroup B meningococcus by whole-genome sequencing. *Science.* 2000;287:1816−1820.

121. Beernink PT, Caugant DA, Welsch JA, Koeberling O, Granoff DM. Meningococcal factor H-binding protein variants expressed by epidemic capsular group A, W-135, and X strains from Africa. *J Infect Dis.* 2009;199: 1360−1368.

122. Pajon R, Fergus AM, Koeberling O, Caugant DA, Granoff DM. Meningococcal factor H binding proteins in epidemic strains from Africa: implications for vaccine development. *PLoS Negl Trop Dis.* 2011;5:e1302.

123. Harris SL, Zhu D, Murphy E, et al. Preclinical evidence for the potential of a vivalent fHBP vaccine to prevent *Neisseria meningitidis* Serogroup C disease. *Hum Vaccin.* 2011;7.

124. Wang X, Cohn A, Comanducci M, et al. Prevalence and genetic diversity of candidate vaccine antigens among invasive *Neisseria meningitidis* isolates in the United States. *Vaccine.* 2011;29:4739−4744.

125. Esposito S, Prymula R, Zuccotti GV, et al. A phase 2 randomized controlled trial of a multicomponent meningococcal serogroup B vaccine, 4CMenB, in infants (II). *Hum Vaccin Immunother.* 2014;10:2005−2014. PMCID: PMC4186018.

126. Gossger N, Snape MD, Yu LM, et al. Immunogenicity and tolerability of recombinant serogroup B meningococcal vaccine administered with or without routine infant vaccinations according to different immunization schedules: a randomized controlled trial. *Jama.* 2012;307:573−582.

127. Vesikari T, Esposito S, Prymula R, et al. Immunogenicity and safety of an investigational multicomponent, recombinant, meningococcal serogroup B vaccine (4CMenB) administered concomitantly with routine infant and child vaccinations: results of two randomised trials. *Lancet.* 2013;381:825−835.

128. Snape MD, Saroey P, John TM, et al. Persistence of bactericidal antibodies following early infant vaccination with a serogroup B meningococcal vaccine and immunogenicity of a preschool booster dose. *CMAJ.* 2013;185: E715−E724. PMCID: 3796620.

129. Santolaya ME, O'Ryan ML, Valenzuela MT, et al. Immunogenicity and tolerability of a multicomponent meningococcal serogroup B (4CMenB) vaccine in healthy adolescents in Chile: a phase 2b/3 randomised, observer-blind, placebo-controlled study. *Lancet.* 2012; 379:617−624.

130. Kimura A, Toneatto D, Kleinschmidt A, Wang H, Dull P. Immunogenicity and safety of a multicomponent meningococcal serogroup B vaccine and a quadrivalent meningococcal CRM197 conjugate vaccine against serogroups A, C, W-135, and Y in adults who are at increased risk for occupational exposure to meningococcal isolates. *Clin Vaccine Immunol.* 2011;18:483−486.

131. Perrett KP, McVernon J, Richmond PC, et al. Immune responses to a recombinant, four-component, meningococcal serogroup B vaccine (4CMenB) in adolescents: a phase III, randomized, multicentre, lot-to-lot consistency study. *Vaccine.* 2015;33:5217−5224.

132. Marshall HS, Richmond PC, Nissen MD, et al. A phase 2 open-label safety and immunogenicity study of a meningococcal B bivalent rLP2086 vaccine in healthy adults. *Vaccine.* 2013;31:1569−1575.

133. Food and Drug Administration. Highlights of Prescribing Information: TRUMENBA (Meningococcal Group B Vaccine). http://www.fda.gov/downloads/ BiologicsBloodVaccines/Vaccines/ApprovedProducts/UCM 421139.pdf.

134. Vesikari T, Ostergaard L, Diez-Domingo J, et al. Meningococcal serogroup B bivalent rLP2086 vaccine elicits broad and robust serum bactericidal responses in healthy adolescents. *J Pediatr Infect Dis Soc.* 2016;5:152−160. PMCID: 5407127.

135. Folaranmi T, Rubin L, Martin SW, Patel M, MacNeil JR. Centers for disease C. Use of serogroup B meningococcal vaccines in persons aged >/=10 Years at increased risk for serogroup B meningococcal disease: recommendations of the advisory committee on immunization practices, 2015. *MMWR Morb Mortal Wkly Rep.* 2015;64:608−612.

136. Muse D, Christensen S, Bhuyan P, et al. A phase 2, randomized, active-controlled, observer-blinded study to assess the immunogenicity, tolerability and safety of bivalent rLP2086, a meningococcal serogroup B vaccine, coadministered with tetanus, diphtheria and acellular pertussis vaccine and serogroup A, C, Y and W-135

meningococcal conjugate vaccine in healthy US adolescents. *Pediatr Infect Dis J.* 2016;35:673−682.

137. Vesikari T, Wysocki J, Beeslaar J, et al. Immunogenicity, safety, and tolerability of bivalent rLP2086 meningococcal group B vaccine administered concomitantly with diphtheria, tetanus, and acellular pertussis and inactivated poliomyelitis vaccines to healthy adolescents. *J Pediatr Infect Dis Soc.* 2016;5:180−187. PMCID: 5407129.

138. Senders S, Bhuyan P, Jiang Q, et al. Immunogenicity, tolerability and safety in adolescents of bivalent rLP2086, a meningococcal serogroup B vaccine, coadministered with quadrivalent human papilloma virus vaccine. *Pediatr Infect Dis J.* 2016;35:548−554.

139. Santolaya ME, O'Ryan M, Valenzuela MT, et al. Persistence of antibodies in adolescents 18-24 months after immunization with one, two, or three doses of 4CMenB meningococcal serogroup B vaccine. *Hum Vaccin Immunother.* 2013;9:2304−2310. PMCID: 3981837.

140. Lujan E, Winter K, Rovaris J, Liu Q, Granoff DM. Serum bactericidal antibody responses of students immunized with a meningococcal serogroup B vaccine in response to an outbreak on a university campus. *Clin Infect Dis.* 2017.

141. McQuaid F, Snape MD, John TM, et al. Persistence of specific bactericidal antibodies at 5 years of age after vaccination against serogroup B meningococcus in infancy and at 40 months. *CMAJ.* 2015;187:E215−E223. PMCID: PMC4401613.

142. Patton ME, Stephens D, Moore K, MacNeil JR. Updated recommendations for use of MenB-FHbp serogroup B meningococcal vaccine - advisory committee on immunization practices, 2016. *MMWR Morb Mortal Wkly Rep.* 2017;66:509−513.

143. Lujan E, Partridge E, Giuntini S, Ram S, Granoff DM. Breadth and duration of meningococcal serum bactericidal activity in health care workers and microbiologists immunized with the MenB-FHbp vaccine. *Clin Vaccine Immunol.* 2017;24. PMCID: 5583465.

144. De Wals P. Group QMDaVSaE. Results of a mass immunization campagin with 4-components serogroup B meningococcal vaccine (4CMenB) in Quebec Canada. In: *10th Annual Meningitis Research Foundation Meningitis Symposium. Bristol UK.* 2015.

145. De Wals P, Deceuninck G, Lefebvre B, et al. Impact of an immunization campaign to control an increased incidence of serogroup B meningococcal disease in one region of Quebec, Canada. *Clin Infect Dis.* 2017;64: 1263−1267.

146. Parikh SR, Andrews NJ, Beebeejaun K, et al. Effectiveness and impact of a reduced infant schedule of 4CMenB vaccine against group B meningococcal disease in England: a national observational cohort study. *Lancet.* 2016;388: 2775−2782.

147. Wilkins AL, Snape MD. Emerging clinical experience with vaccines against group B meningococcal disease. *Vaccine.* 2017.

148. Block SL, Szenborn L, Daly W, et al. A comparative evaluation of two investigational meningococcal ABCWY vaccine formulations: results of a phase 2 randomized, controlled trial. *Vaccine.* 2015;33:2500−2510.

149. Murdoch H, Wallace L, Bishop J, Robertson C, Claire Cameron J. Risk of hospitalisation with fever following MenB vaccination: self-controlled case series analysis. *Arch Dis Child.* 2017;102:894−898.

150. Nainani V, Galal U, Buttery J, Snape MD. An increase in accident and emergency presentations for adverse events following immunisation after introduction of the group B meningococcal vaccine: an observational study. *Arch Dis Child.* 2017.

151. Kapur S, Bourke T, Maney JA, Moriarty P. Emergency department attendance following 4-component meningococcal B vaccination in infants. *Arch Dis Child.* 2017; 102:899−902.

152. Martinon-Torres F, Gimenez-Sanchez F, Bernaola-Iturbe E, Diez-Domingo J, Jiang Q, Perez JL. A randomized, phase 1/2 trial of the safety, tolerability, and immunogenicity of bivalent rLP2086 meningococcal B vaccine in healthy infants. *Vaccine.* 2014;32: 5206−5211.

153. Food and Drug Administration. Summary Basis for Regulatory Action: Trumenba. http://www.fda.gov/downloads/BiologicsBloodVaccines/Vaccines/ApprovedProducts/UCM424125.pdf.

154. Fiorito TM, Baird GL, Alexander-Scott N, et al. Adverse events following vaccination with bivalent rLP2086 (Trumenba(R)): an observational, longitudinal study during a college outbreak and a systematic review. *Pediatr Infect Dis J.* 2017.

155. Ostergaard L, Lucksinger GH, Absalon J, et al. A phase 3, randomized, active-controlled study to assess the safety and tolerability of meningococcal serogroup B vaccine bivalent rLP2086 in healthy adolescents and young adults. *Vaccine.* 2016;34:1465−1471.

156. Soeters HM, Whaley M, Alexander-Scott N, et al. Meningococcal carriage evaluation in response to a serogroup B meningococcal disease outbreak and mass vaccination campaign at a college-Rhode Island, 2015−2016. *Clin Infect Dis.* 2017;64:1115−1122.

157. MacNeil JR, Rubin L, McNamara L, Briere EC, Clark TA, Cohn AC. Use of MenACWY-CRM vaccine in children aged 2 through 23 months at increased risk for meningococcal disease: recommendations of the Advisory Committee on Immunization Practices, 2013. *MMWR Morb Mortal Wkly Rep.* 2014;63:527−530.

158. MacNeil J, Rubin L, Folaranmi T, Ortega-Sanchez IR, Patel P, Martin SW. Use of serogroup B meningococcal vaccines in adolescents and young adults: recommendations of the Advisory Committee on Immunization Practices, 2015. *MMWR Morb Mortal Wkly Rep.* 2015;64:1171−1176.

159. Advisory Committee on Immunization Practices/Centers for Disease Control and Prevention. Evidence-Based Recommendations—GRADE. https://www.cdc.gov/vaccines/acip/recs/grade/about-grade.html.

160. Bruce MG, Rosenstein NE, Capparella JM, Shutt KA, Perkins BA, Collins M. Risk factors for meningococcal disease in college students. *JAMA.* 2001;286:688−693.

161. Harrison LH, Dwyer DM, Maples CT, Billmann L. Risk of meningococcal infection in college students. *JAMA*. 1999;281:1906—1910.

162. Harrison LH, Pass MA, Mendelsohn AB, et al. Invasive meningococcal disease in adolescents and young adults. *JAMA*. 2001;286:694—699.

163. Harris CM, Wu HM, Li J, et al. Meningococcal disease in patients with HIV infection—a review of cases reported through active surveillance in the United States, 2000—2008. *Open Forum Infect Dis*. 2016.

164. Cohen C, Singh E, Wu HM, et al. Increased incidence of meningococcal disease in HIV-infected individuals associated with higher case-fatality ratios in South Africa. *Aids*. 2010;24:1351—1360.

165. Centers for é Control and Prevention, Infant meningococcal vaccination. Advisory Committee on Immunization Practices (ACIP) recommendations and rationale. *MMWR Morb Mortal Wkly Rep*. 2013;62:52—54.

166. Centers for Disease Control and Prevention. Syncope after vaccination—United States, January 2005—July 2007. *MMWR Morb Mortal Wkly Rep*. 2008;57:457—460.

167. Centers for Disease Control and Prevention. General recommendations on immunization — recommendations of the Advisory Committee on Immunization Practices (ACIP). *MMWR Recomm Rep*. 2011;60:1—64.

168. Centers for Disease Control and Prevention. Guidance for the Evaluation and Public Health Management of Suspected Outbreaks of Meningococcal Disease. (In preparation).

169. Walker TY, Elam-Evans LD, Singleton JA, et al. National, regional, state, and selected local area vaccination coverage among adolescents aged 13—17 Years - United States, 2016. *MMWR Morb Mortal Wkly Rep*. 2017;66: 874—882.

170. National vaccination coverage among adolescents aged 13—17 years—United States, 2006. *MMWR Morb Mortal Wkly Rep*. 2007;56:885—888.

171. Granoff DM, Giuntini S, Gowans FA, Lujan E, Sharkey K, Beernink PT. Enhanced protective antibody to a mutant meningococcal factor H-binding protein with low-factor H binding. *JCI Insight*. 2016;1:e88907. PMCID: 5033880.

CHAPTER 8

Vaccine Immunology: What Do Clinicians Need to Know?

DANIEL M. ALTMANN, PHD

INTRODUCTION

The rationale for immunization is easily articulated and widely understood: When an individual needs defense from attack, whether from infection—bacterial, viral, fungal, parasitic—or from a tumor, there is a need to generate rapid, specific, and potent immunity to do so. However, maturation of an effective immune response is a relatively slow process, so that in the case of a highly pathogenic attacker the battle may have been lost long before this can occur. The aim of a vaccine is thus to potentiate specific immunity that is sufficiently rapid and effective to prevent or ameliorate clinical disease.

Consideration of the benefits of vaccines and the mechanistic requirements of a specifically protective vaccine necessitates a brief refresher on the pertinent components of an effective immune response covered in the following sections.

INDUCING A PROTECTIVE IMMUNE RESPONSE—A TERMINOLOGY REFRESHER

Innate Immunity, Adaptive Immunity, and Memory

The function of the immune system is response to attack. This can be considered an enormously multifaceted network of organs, lymph nodes, cells, and molecules. Immunology makes a distinction between two interconnected limbs of the immune response, innate and adaptive immunity. The term "innate immunity" refers to immune mechanisms that are rapid, sometimes virtually immediate, but lack either antigen specificity or memory. To elicit an immune response, any unwanted invader, whether a tumor, a bacterium, or a virus-infected cell, must be recognized as foreign/dangerous. The initial phase of immunity during which recognition occurs and the first response ensues is through recognition by pattern recognition receptors of the innate

immune response. Thus this is a response that has some degree of specificity—the body has recognized that this cell expresses the molecular patterns of bacterial cells rather than human cells—but it lacks actual antigen specificity, for example, any knowledge of whether this is *Streptococcus pneumoniae*, *Staphylococcus aureus*, or *Streptococcus pyogenes*. The response also lacks memory. That is, the pattern recognition–driven, innate response to the bacterium is essentially of the same character and magnitude, time after time. This is in contrast to specific, adaptive immunity, whereby, as a consequence of having met and responded to a specific bug previously, the B and T lymphocytes of the immune system have memory, are increased in number, and are primed to mount an enhanced and more effective response.

The multilayered steps in innate immune defenses can perhaps best be pictured by imagining the obstacles faced by a pathogenic bacterium inhaled into the human lung. First, there are the physical barriers of respiratory cilia and lysozyme-containing mucous. Then there are antimicrobials, surfactants, defensins, and mannose-binding lectins. Once microbially conserved structures of the bacterium, the so-called pathogen-associated molecular patterns (PAMPs), are recognized by innate receptors on host cells including neutrophils, epithelial cells, macrophages, and dendritic cells, a very rapid innate immune response can kick into action. The innate receptors triggering this array of responses include the toll-like receptors (TLRs) and the nucleotide-binding oligomerization domain (NOD)–like receptors, termed NOD-like receptors. The consequences of this activation can be diverse, depending on the pathogen and context, including activation of mannose-binding lectin, innate cytokines, and interferons, neutrophil chemotaxis, activation and neutrophil extracellular trap formation, phagocytosis, release of reactive oxygen species, and activation of natural killer cells and innate lymphoid cells.

Vaccinations. https://doi.org/10.1016/B978-0-323-55435-0.00008-2

Vaccines are not designed primarily to activate this limb of the immune response, so what is its significance to a consideration of vaccine immunity? The first point to make is that in most healthy individuals, this is an overwhelmingly efficient process, with most pathogens repelled. Second, this activation of innate immunity, which lies at the origins of all pathogen recognition, is intricately linked to activation of successful and appropriate, protective antibody and T cell immunity. Thus the aim of any successful vaccine strategy is to find ways of mimicking the correct, stimulatory components of these innate switches. Sometimes this may be by use of attenuated or apathogenic variants that nevertheless carry all the usual innate activation signals. Other times this is the role of a really stimulatory but safe adjuvant.

Once the cells and pathways of the innate immune response have been alerted to the presence of a pathogenic invader, the adaptive immune response becomes activated. "Adaptive immunity" refers to the response of B and T lymphocytes. By contrast to innate immunity, the key feature of adaptive immunity is that it depends on highly antigen-specific receptors, antibodies in the case of B lymphocytes and the T cell receptor in the case of T lymphocytes. In terms of an effective response to infection, this adaptive arm of the immune response has the disadvantage that developing a response de novo is slow and may take a few weeks to really take off. Maturation of B lymphocyte immunity encompasses an initial lag to produce a detectable, specific antibody response, then the production of relatively low-affinity IgM antibodies, class switching to appropriate immunoglobulin (Ig) subclasses, and then progressive affinity maturation by somatic hypermutation (SHM) to produce an enduring, high-affinity, specific, antibody response, with a subset of cells enduring as a long-term, B cell memory pool. This may take several weeks from the initial entry of a newly encountered antigen. For T lymphocyte immunity as well, the initial antigen encounter is qualitatively and quantitatively different to subsequent encounters. Microbial antigens must be perceived and taken up by dendritic cells, migrating to the follicles of lymph nodes or secondary lymphoid organs, to engage with T lymphocytes that carry a specific T lymphocyte receptor for this antigen, giving rise to germinal centers. Depending on the signals and cytokines that the T lymphocyte has received from the dendritic cell, it will then differentiate into a cell with an appropriate, context-appropriate, antimicrobial effector program.

Priming by vaccination generates a highly antigen-specific, context-appropriate, memory response. The term "memory" in this context carries with it a number of implications. For the antibody-producing B cell pool, engagement with T follicular helper cells within the germinal centers of primary and secondary lymphoid organs generates a pool of antigen-specific B cells that are at enhanced frequency, have undergone SHM to achieve affinity maturation, and class switched to the appropriate antibody subclass. Although the T cell receptor operates by engaging antigenic peptides at moderate affinities and does not undergo any affinity maturation, proliferation of the initial precursor pool means that the frequency of cells specific for this antigen will be greater at any subsequent encounter. Similar to the B lymphocyte pool, responding T lymphocytes from the initial encounter will live on as a long-term, memory population.

Note that T lymphocytes and B lymphocytes act in concert to elicit an effective adaptive response to a vaccine or natural infection—thus the old concept of a requirement for T cell "help." The exception to this is the polysaccharide capsule vaccines that are T cell independent but can only stimulate a B cell response that is IgM, low affinity and lacking in memory. Conjugate vaccines address this issue by linking a B cell–stimulating polysaccharide antigen to a T cell–stimulating protein antigen to supply help, which induces Ig class switch and SHM.

For a vaccine encompassing antigens recognized by both B and T cells, as is the case for all microbes, the notion is that the microbial antigen is processed by antigen-presenting cells such as a dendritic cell that consequently matures and migrates to a lymphoid follicle. This is a specialized structure within lymph nodes and lymphoid organs where B cells can make intimate contact with T follicular helper cells to initiate a response. Antigen processing by the mature dendritic cell results in the presentation of short, proteolytically cleaved fragments within the peptide-binding groove of a human leukocyte antigen (HLA) molecule at the cell surface. This peptide/HLA complex is recognized by the specific T cell receptor of a passing T lymphocyte, leading to cellular activation and cytokine release. The receptor of the B lymphocyte may or may not be specific for the identical antigen within this microbial pathogen. Because T lymphocyte receptors recognize small, processed peptide fragments and B lymphocyte receptors generally recognize conformational, tertiary protein structures, the two receptor types will in any case not necessarily recognize the same stretch of antigens.

Thus the central precept underpinning the immunology of effective vaccinology is that, with respect to the adaptive immune response to specific antigen, secondary immune responses are highly enhanced, both qualitatively and quantitatively, relative to primary encounter. This gives a decisive advantage to the host in the arms race against the pathogen.

DIFFERENT MODES OF PROTECTIVE IMMUNITY—IMMUNE EFFECTOR PHENOTYPES

For much of the early history of vaccinology, from the 10th century in China and from Jenner and Pasteur onwards, elucidation of a nonpathogenic isolate capable of conferring protective immunity to pathogenic exposure was empirical in nature rather than the output of detailed molecular characterization. This approach endured through many highly successful, relatively modern vaccines, including polio and yellow fever virus. In many cases the key "correlate of protection" (CoP) is the titer of antibody capable of neutralizing the input pathogen: Those vaccines most capable of inducing a large amount of antibody that could bind at high affinity and neutralize an incoming virus or bacterium before they could spread and cause systemic damage are considered the most efficacious. Neutralization could encompass bacteriostasis and opsonization for phagocytosis. For much of vaccinology, neutralizing titer as CoP remains a truism. The proof-of-concept evidence for this has come from human or experimental infection examples in which simple passive transfer of the neutralizing antibody is sufficient to reiterate the full protective effect of the original vaccine, without subsequent involvement of immunized cells. Indeed, some highly effective vaccines induce potent antibody-mediated protection in a manner that is largely independent of T lymphocyte immunity. These are vaccines such as the pneumococcal and meningococcal polysaccharide capsule vaccines; they rely on the fact that B lymphocytes seem able to respond to the repeated, multivalent sugar structures, without help from T lymphocytes.[1] However, as the molecular immunology of diverse infections has been characterized in even more detail, it has become clear that it may be optimal for most microbial protein antigens to stimulate different components of the adaptive immune response for maximal protection in different contexts. This is readily appreciated when one considers that different immune effector mechanisms may be needed to slough a nematode from the gut, to eliminate *Aspergillus* fungal spores from the bronchi, or to kill a virus-infected cell in the brain.

Over the past several decades there have been improving details for understanding the functionally distinct immune subsets into which T lymphocytes may be subdivided. This started when it was

appreciated that T cells could be broadly subdivided into those that primarily lyse targets such as virus-infected cells—CD8 cytotoxic T cells—and cells that made batteries of soluble cytokines to facilitate functionality of other cells, especially immunoglobulin class switching of B lymphocytes—CD4 T helper cells. Each of these is now subdivided by effector function and cytokine profile into several subsets (Table 8.1). Why should this matter to vaccinology? The answer comes back to context appropriateness of response: For example, powerful, IgE-driven, eosinophilic, allergic-type responses may be highly desirable for expelling gut parasites and thus desirable in an antiparasite vaccine but highly undesirable for lung pathogens when

TABLE 8.1
Key Features of T Lymphocyte Subsets in the Adaptive Immune Response

T Cell Subset	Markers	Hallmark Cytokines	Infection/ Vaccine Relevance
Th1	CD4, CXCR3, and CCR5	Interferon γ	Intracellular bacteria; viral infection
Th2	CD4, CRTH2, CCR3, and CCR4	Interleukin 4, 5, and 13	Parasitic infection; B cell class switching to IgG1 and IgE
Th9	CD4 and CCR6	Interleukin 9	Proposed role in tumor immunity
Th17	CD4, CCR4, and CCR6	Interleukin 17	Extracellular bacteria; fungi
Tfh	CXCR5	Interleukin 6, 10, and 21	B cell help; B cell memory formation
Treg	CCR6, CD39, CD25-hi, and FoxP3	Interleukin 10 and TGF-β	Regulation of responses to prevent immune pathology
Tc1	CD8, CD183, and CD195	Interferon γ	Viral infections; tumors
Tc17	CD8, CCR5, and CCR6	Interleukin 17	Fungi

Information in this table represents a composite overview of information gathered from analysis of responses both in human patients and in mouse experimental models.

one considers the damage that can be done to the delicate lung mucosal surface by such responses. On the other hand, vaccines capable of inducing the CD4 cells that make the cytokine, interleukin 17 (IL-17), may be highly desirable to prevent mycobacterial infections, but rather ineffective for parasitic disease.[2] While CD8 cells have been defined on the basis of their primary function of cytolysis of targets, they can also be stratified on the basis of their programs for cytokine secretion.

To summarize, it is clear that the adaptive immune response encompasses a highly diverse arsenal of effector mechanisms, from antibody subclasses and their associated functions to T lymphocyte cytokines and cytotoxicity, these exquisitely evolved for their suitability of response to the selection pressure of invading pathogens. There is growing appreciation that vaccines need to be similarly attuned to the particular flavor of protective immunity that needs to be elicited. Although the field of vaccinology has innumerable victories to celebrate for their impact on public health, several seemingly intractably faltering projects, including vaccines for HIV, TB, and malaria, attest to this knowledge gap in how to well achieve fully protective immunity.

DIFFERENT TYPES OF VACCINES

Vaccines are of many types, carrying distinct intrinsic advantages and disadvantages in terms efficacy, immunogenicity, longevity of protection between boosts, appropriateness of response, ease of production, cost of production, and safety.

The overarching distinction in vaccine preparations is between live attenuated vaccines and inactivated/inactive viruses. The term "live attenuated vaccine" encompasses all those whereby repeated passage or mutation results in a protective but nonpathogenic variant. Vaccines of this type include vaccinia, measles, mumps, rubella (MMR), yellow fever, rubella, and bacillus calmette–guérin (BCG). The advantages of these vaccines are that the intact, live microbes replicate normally in the human host and give out the appropriate innate immunity activation cues through PAMP expression to guide the proper protective response. Furthermore, this means that a single dose is generally sufficient. However, these vaccines are more demanding to produce, license, monitor, store, and transport than inactivated virus and may be more likely to be associated with adverse events. As live viruses have a potential risk for reversion to pathogenicity, some are contraindicated in immunosuppressed or pregnant recipients.

Under the heading of inactivated or inactive vaccines falls a wide array of different types of formulations.

This includes heat- or formalin-inactivated vaccines, microbial subunits, toxins, proteins, polysaccharides, and filtrates. It also includes products made by recombinant DNA technology, including recombinant proteins, DNA vaccines, and epitope string vaccines. Within this latter group come the many examples in which genes for microbial antigens or groups of antigens have been cloned into a benign carrier virus such as an adenovirus or vaccinia virus.[3] DNA vaccines and epitope string vaccines appear promising in a research setting, but have not yet had a major impact clinically. Part of the rationale for vaccinating with specific components of the microorganism is the very much lower risk of any adverse events. This very diverse group of vaccines are variably associated with a host of pros and cons depending on the specific case. Common features are that they are less immunogenic than live attenuated vaccines and tend to require two or multiple doses and, in many cases, the use of an adjuvant. Although simple inactivation by heat or by formalin fixation may seem the most simple, conservative approach to try and mimic the immunogenicity of the live pathogen, associated alterations in immunogenicity can have unforeseen consequences. Oft-cited historical examples are formaldehyde-inactivated respiratory syncytial virus (RSV) and measles vaccines: In these cases, the formaldehyde treatment modified the chemical structure of viral antigens, so skewing the effector phenotype of the T cell response to an inappropriate, pathogenic Th2 profile.[4]

Vaccine Immunogens—Antigen Discovery

Vaccines that are widely in use today range from the BCG vaccine for tuberculosis, essentially an attenuated variant carrying the vast majority of the antigens encoded in the genome of the mycobacterium, some 4000 different antigens, to the anthrax vaccine, which contains only one antigen of *Bacillus anthracis*. For any vaccination strategy that is to use some subunit preparation rather a whole microbe, there is the question of which antigens to include so as to maximize protection? This issue of antigen discovery for protective vaccines has been a demanding one. It might be imagined that one could simply look in the serum of people who have recovered from a particular infection and determine whether there is particularly strong antibody (or T cell) response to a given antigen or set of antigens. The limitation of this approach is that many components of the microbial genome may indeed be highly immunogenic, but not everything that is immunogenic is necessarily protective. How to screen to find the most immunogenic and protective component of a complex microbial genome? A number of approaches have been applied, many of these variations on the theme of "reverse vaccinology" as initially proposed by Rappuoli et al.[5,6] The approach was first applied successfully to translation of the MenB (*Neisseria meningitidis*) vaccine and has since been applied in a wide range of other infections. The term describes a pipeline approach, starting with the full genome sequences, filtering on those gene products predicted to have properties of visibility to the host immune system (for example, bacterial cell wall or secreted antigens), and then using high-throughput functional screens such as ability to elicit neutralizing antibodies after injection of each recombinant protein into mice. A related strategy has been the use of "antigen arrays."[7] This involves robotically coating glass slides with several hundred recombinant proteins from a microbial sequence and then using these to screen for common patterns of immune recognition, for example, using antiserum panels from patients who have recovered from the infection in question.

Although it may appear intuitively appealing that the entire antigenic repertoire of the whole microbe must surely elicit a stronger, protective response than some selected subset of purified antigens, experience has shown that this is not necessarily always the case, note, for example, the experience with vaccination against zoster in which the single glycoprotein E vaccine (Shingrix) appears to outperform live attenuated virus.

In general, contemporary, high-throughput approaches to screening for B cell and T cell immunodominant antigens mean that, as has been the case for Zika and Ebola virus infections, it is often possible to move very rapidly from microbial sequencing to antigen discovery and then directly to synthesis of recombinant vaccines for trial.[8,9]

ADJUVANTS

With an ever-increasing number of vaccine candidates being based on inactive protein or polysaccharide immunogen preparations, much of the success of vaccine trials depends on the use of safe but efficacious adjuvants. It will be clear from the previous discussion that the aim of an ideal adjuvant would be to substitute, as faithfully as possible, for the innate danger signals that allow the innate immune system to activate potent and appropriately protective components of the adaptive immune response. The ideal adjuvant needs to bring subunit vaccines on a par with live vaccines in terms of immunogenicity, protection, and efficacy after one or a few doses. Despite immense progress in basic research into innate danger signals, translation of this knowledge into licensed adjuvants for clinical use has

been relatively slow. Many historical studies of experimental mouse immunology have depended on the very strong adjuvant effect of complete Freund's adjuvant—a mineral oil emulsion containing a high dose of heat-killed *Mycobacterium tuberculosis*, a formulation that would be unacceptable for human use. It has been challenging to develop clinical adjuvants with similar potency. Clinical adjuvant development has been largely into vaccine delivery vehicles (including the old notion of generating an "antigen depot" for slow dispersal and uptake) and into immunostimulants, particularly through activation of pattern recognition receptors.[10,11]

Within the category of delivery vehicles is "Alum" (aluminum-potassium sulfate), used in vaccines including those against HPV, HepB, and pertussis. Also in this group is Squalene (MF59) and oil-in-water emulsion (AS03), used in pandemic and seasonal influenza vaccines. Liposomes are used for antigen delivery of HepA vaccine. Saponin-based adjuvants are in use for veterinary vaccines and in trial for various human vaccinology applications.

A large number of immunostimulatory adjuvants are currently in trial for human vaccine use. GSK used the term "Adjuvant Systems" to describe combination adjuvants, of which three are currently in use in licensed vaccines: AS01, AS03, and AS04.[12] AS04, an example of a so-called "combination" adjuvant comprising a mixture of Alum and monophosphoryl lipid A (MPL), is a derivative of bacterial lipopolysaccharide which is the prototypic ligand for the TLR-4 pattern recognition receptor—a key driver of Th1 antimicrobial T cell responses. It is used in some HPV and HepB formulations. The herpes zoster (shingles) candidate vaccine, a recombinant vaccine, comprising VZV glycoprotein E, is adjuvanted using AS01. This was also the adjuvant for the malaria vaccine phase III RTS,S trials. AS01 is a combination of the immunostimulants QS-21 and MPL with liposomes.

Assessing Vaccines—CoPs

Since 2001, Plotkin et al. have argued for vaccinology to develop the methodologies and terminology that would establish validated, measurable vaccine efficacy surrogates for clinical disease endpoints.[13,14] This would facilitate vaccine dosing, evaluation and licensure, and fuel iterative cycles of vaccine development through improved understanding of protective mechanisms. Validated CoPs have been highlighted as a key bottleneck in vaccine development. Investigators, producers, regulators, and policymakers developing new vaccine programmes attach central importance to

CoPs in trial evaluation. CoPs were often traditionally based on antibody titers deduced to offer a correlate of in vivo protection. Ability of an immunization regimen to attain the required absolute value could have profound impact on trial evaluation, "stop-go" decisions. However, for many pathogens that impose a high disease burden, we lack pertinent mechanistic insights and thus validated relevant assays. Many vaccines currently in development may depend variably on innate immunity, antibodies of different functions and specificities, and T cell subsets. Relevant approaches to validation of CoPs may thus include T cell analysis, transcriptomics/systems biology, animal models and human challenge studies, mathematical modeling, and in vitro neutralization/bactericidal models.

CoP approaches can thus be highly context specific, lacking "one-size-fits-all" approaches across pathogens or even across cohorts. There can be geographical or population differences between antibody levels required for protection, as with pneumococcal disease, influenza, or BCG vaccination, in which protective responses differ with age. For some ongoing vaccine trials such as Ebola and Zika, there is a need for rapid evaluation and licensure, yet only sparse knowledge of the specific, protective, correlates. In other vaccine trials such as RTS,S for malaria or RV144 for HIV, there is evidence of partial protection with the need to delineate the associated CoP, leading to iterative improvements.[15] In some cases, as with Group B meningococcal vaccines, licensure was based on the correlate itself rather than on efficacy trials. However, as vaccines are developed more rapidly to address healthcare crises with emerging infectious diseases, we often have little starting information on immune pathways or specific CoP.

Pollard proposed the starting point that a CoP is "a biomarker that is statistically associated with protection." Beyond this, there may be relative and absolute correlates and cocorrelates, that is, multiple pathways involved in protection.[16] A further refinement was the distinction between a mechanistic CoP, indicating an immune parameter—mediating protection, and a nonmechanisitic CoP. In many cases the ability to define a pertinent CoP may require detailed knowledge of the pathophysiology/immunology of the specific disease: Which are the implicated protective antigens? What is the clinical spectrum of response to exposure and, thus, which protective endpoint is relevant? Is there an issue of cross-reactive baseline immunity to related microbial species? Is there baseline, asymptomatic exposure to the pathogen in the trial population? What is the functionally pertinent immune assessment: IFN γ—secreting T cell frequency? Frequency of positive T or B cells for immunodominant epitopes? Transcriptomic biosignatures from nonhuman primate models, human challenge models, or from asymptomatic versus symptomatic natural exposure? Neutralizing or bactericidal antibodies? What about monitoring multivalent vaccines? Are the largest responses the best—what about immunopathogenic responses and immune potentiation and the effect of antibody-dependent enhancement of disease that has been of concern in Dengue vaccine trials? Are there different CoP answers with age or ethnicity?

The toolbox for vaccine research is changing rapidly in an age of large-scale "systems biology." CoP research can now encompass vast, diverse, bioinformatic datasets, including transcriptomics (that is, the RNA profile of patients' responding cells), flow cytometry, T cell and antibody analyses, and experimental protection data.[17] Even analysis of patient antibodies has been expanded to integrate computational analysis across multiple assay systems of effector function—so-called "systems serology."[18] This highlights a need in this field to train and nurture those graduates with the numeracy and computer literacy to work with this new type and scale of integrated data.

FUTURE DIRECTIONS IN THE IMMUNOLOGY OF VACCINES—CONCLUDING REMARKS

Recent decades have witnessed an explosion of knowledge across immunology, microbiology, systems biology, and bioinformatics. In many respects this offers enormous hope for prospects of new and much-needed vaccines. Vaccine candidates can be rationally and rapidly produced and comprehensively evaluated. On the other hand, despite enormous successes in areas such as pathogen whole genome sequencing, innate immunity, antigen discovery, and fundamental T cell immunology, this has not yet been translated into quick wins for currently intractable infection challenges including HIV, TB, and malaria.

REFERENCES

1. Defrance T, Taillardet M, Genestier L. T cell-independent B cell memory. *Curr Opin Immunol*. 2011;23(3):330—336.
2. Ottenhoff TH. New pathways of protective and pathological host defense to mycobacteria. *Trends Microbiol*. 2012; 20(9):419—428.
3. Ewer KJ, Lambe T, Rollier CS, Spencer AJ, Hill AV, Dorrell L. Viral vectors as vaccine platforms: from immunogenicity to impact. *Curr Opin Immunol*. 2016;41: 47—54.

4. Moghaddam A, Olszewska W, Wang B, et al. A potential molecular mechanism for hypersensitivity caused by formalin-inactivated vaccines. *Nat Med*. 2016;12(8): 905−907.

5. Rappuoli R, Bottomley MJ, D'Oro U, Finco O, De Gregorio E. Reverse vaccinology 2.0: human immunology instructs vaccine antigen design. *J Exp Med*. 2016;213(4): 469−481.

6. Rappuoli R, Covacci A. Reverse vaccinology and genomics. *Science*. 2003;302(5645):602.

7. Crompton PD, Kayala MA, Traore B, et al. A prospective analysis of the Ab response to *Plasmodium falciparum* before and after a malaria season by protein microarray. *Proc Natl Acad Sci U S A*. 2010;107(15):6958−6963.

8. Zhou Y, Sullivan NJ. Immunology and evolvement of the adenovirus prime, MVA boost Ebola virus vaccine. *Curr Opin Immunol*. 2015;35:131−136.

9. Pierson TC, Graham BS. Zika virus: immunity and vaccine development. *Cell*. 2016;167(3):625−631.

10. Matzinger P. Tolerance, danger, and the extended family. *Annu Rev Immunol*. 1994;12:991−1045.

11. Pradeu T, Cooper EL. The danger theory: 20 years later. *Front Immunol*. 2012;3:287.

12. Garcon N, Di Pasquale A. From discovery to licensure, the Adjuvant System story. *Hum Vaccines Immunother*. 2017; 13:19−33.

13. Plotkin SA. Complex correlates of protection after vaccination. *Clin Infect Dis*. 2013;56(10):1458−1465.

14. Plotkin SA, Gilbert PB. Nomenclature for immune correlates of protection after vaccination. *Clin Infect Dis*. 2012; 54(11):1615−1617.

15. White MT, Verity R, Griffin JT, et al. Immunogenicity of the RTS,S/AS01 malaria vaccine and implications for duration of vaccine efficacy: secondary analysis of data from a phase 3 randomised controlled trial. *Lancet Infect Dis*. 2015; 15(12):1450−1458.

16. Carter MJ, Blomke CJ, Pollard AJ. Immunological correlates of vaccine-mediated protection. In: Bloom BR, Lambert P-H, eds. *The Vaccine Book*. Amsterdam; Boston: Elsevier; 2017:122 [chapter 7].

17. Furman D, Davis MM. New approaches to understanding the immune response to vaccination and infection. *Vaccine*. 2015;33(40):5271−5281.

18. Arnold KB, Chung AW. Prospects from systems serology research. *Immunology*. 2018;153(3):279−289. https:// doi.org/10.1111/imm.12861.

CHAPTER 9

Vaccine Use in Immunocompromised Adults: Challenges and Solutions

JENNIFER A. WHITAKER, MD, MS • KENNETH VALLES, BS • PRITISH K. TOSH, MD • GREGORY A. POLAND, MD, FIDSA, MACP, FRCP (LONDON)

INTRODUCTION

The term "immunocompromised" represents a broad spectrum, relating to primary immunodeficiencies, secondary acquired medical conditions that alter immune competence, the effects of advanced aging, and immunosuppressive treatments. New biologic agents continue to be added to the immunosuppressive armamentarium on a nearly daily basis. It is challenging to predict the impact of these agents, immunocompromising medical conditions, and their interactions on vaccine response. Furthermore, correlates of protection have not been defined for many vaccines, adding another layer to the complexity of predicting vaccine response and safety in this heterogeneous group. In this chapter we will discuss these challenges and provide potential solutions.

The spectrum of immunocompromise that will be addressed in this chapter includes altered immune states due to primary and secondary immunodeficiencies, HIV, chronic inflammatory diseases treated with immunosuppressive agents, functional or anatomic asplenia, malignancy, chemotherapy, and hematologic stem cell transplant and solid organ transplant (SOT). Vaccination during the relatively immunocompromised state of pregnancy will also be reviewed. The effects of aging and immunosenescence on vaccine responses and special considerations for vaccines in older adults will be addressed in the chapter "Vaccines for the Elderly: How, When, Why?"

GENERAL PRINCIPLES

The general principles of vaccine use in this patient population include consideration of vaccine type, level of immunosuppression, medical comorbidities, safety, and timing of vaccination. It is vital to understand the categories of vaccines (live and inactivated, toxoid, adjuvanted) to appropriately use them in this patient population. One must also account for degrees of immunosuppression and medical comorbidities when using vaccines in this population. Finally the optimal timing of vaccination for safety (in the cases of live vaccines) and to maximize the likelihood of developing protective immunity (immunogenicity) should be evaluated. After reviewing these general principles, we will then review details of vaccine use in this population by specific vaccine type.

LIVE ATTENUATED VACCINES

Vaccines are classified into two categories: inactivated and live attenuated. Live attenuated vaccines are created by attenuating or "weakening" live viruses or bacteria to produce a vaccine strain that still demonstrates limited replication and yet is able to induce immune responses but does not lead to disease. However, in severely immunocompromised patients, live attenuated vaccines have been reported to cause disease. A more in depth discussion of these instances will occur under each live vaccine section. The live attenuated vaccines that are available in the United States are listed in Table 9.1.[1] Live vaccines that are routinely used in the adult civilian population will be discussed under each vaccine type. Live vaccines are not recommended for persons with high-level immunosuppression (Table 9.2)[2] or during pregnancy because of the possibility that they could cause harm. When a live attenuated vaccine does cause disease, it is generally a milder form of disease than would occur with the same pathogen, had it not been in the attenuated vaccine form. The disease or infection caused by the vaccine strain is generally referred in such a case as an

---

TABLE 9.1
Live Attenuated Vaccines Available in the United States

Vaccine	Trade Name; Manufacturer	Abbreviation	Route	Approved Ages
LIVE VIRAL VACCINES				
Adenovirus	Adenovirus Type 4 and Type 7; Barr Laboratories Inc		Oral	Only for use in military personnel aged 17−50 years
Herpes zoster (shingles)	Zostavax	HZV	SC	≥50 years
Influenza	FluMist	LAIV4	Intranasal	2−49 years; not currently recommended by ACIP
Measles, mumps, rubella	M-M-R II; Merck	MMR	SC	Minimum age = 12 months
Measles, mumps, rubella, varicella	ProQuad; Merck	MMRV	SC	1−12 years
Rotavirus	Rota Teq; Merck	RV5	Oral	3 dose series through 8 months
Rotavirus	Rotarix; GlaxoSmithKline	RV1	Oral	2 dose series through 8 months
Varicella	Varivax; Merck	VAR	SC	Minimum age = 12 months
Vaccinia (smallpox)	ACAM2000; Sanofi		Percutaneous	All ages
Yellow fever	YF-Vax; Sanofi	YF	SC	Minimum age = 9 months
Yellow fever	Stamaril		SC	Alternative vaccine that is available at approved sites during YF-Vax shortage Minimum age = 9 months
Live attenuated influenza vaccine	FluMist; MedImmune FluMist Quadrivalent; AstraZeneca	LAIV	Intranasal	Ages 2−49 years Will be recommended during the 2018−19 influenza season
LIVE BACTERIAL VACCINES				
Cholera	Vaxchora; PaxVax		Oral	18−64 years
Typhoid	Vivotif; PaxVax	Ty21a	Oral	Minimum age = 6 years

ACIP, advisory committee on immunization practices; *SC*, subcutaneous.

---

adverse reaction or serious adverse event depending on severity.[1] Live vaccines have posed specific challenges and barriers for severely immunosuppressed patients. As one example, up until recently the only vaccine approved for the prevention of herpes zoster has been a live, attenuated varicella zoster virus (VZV) vaccine. The development of a newly Food and Drug Administration (FDA)−approved non-live recombinant adjuvanted subunit herpes zoster vaccine offers a potential solution for many persons who have previously been ineligible for zoster vaccination.

THE SPECTRUM OF IMMUNOCOMPROMISED HOSTS

The spectrum of immunocompromised hosts is highly complex. In the context of this chapter this spectrum will be simplified and in some instances further categorized into levels of "low-level immunosuppression" and "high-level immunosuppression" in the same manner that has been described by the 2013 Infectious Disease Society of America (IDSA) Clinical Practice Guidelines for Vaccination of the Immunocompromised Host (Table 9.2).[2] The category of "high-level

TABLE 9.2
Classification of Immunosuppression[2]

LOW-LEVEL IMMUNOSUPPRESSION
HIV-infected adults with CD4 T-lymphocyte counts of 200–499 cells/mm^3
Systemic corticosteroid therapy that is less than what is listed for high-level immunosuppression (which is prednisone 20 mg/day orally for $\geq$ 14 days or equivalent dosing of other systemic corticosteroid therapy)
Methotrexate $\leq$0.4 mg/kg per week, azathioprine $\leq$3 mg/kg per day, or 6-mercaptopurine $\leq$1.5 mg/kg per day
HIGH-LEVEL IMMUNOSUPPRESSION
HIV infection with CD4 T-lymphocyte count <200
Prednisone oral therapy 20 mg/day for $\geq$ 14 days (or equivalent dosing of other systemic corticosteroid therapy)
Biologic immune modulators, including tumor necrosis factor-α inhibitors or rituximab
Receiving cancer chemotherapy
$\leq$2 months from solid organ transplantation
Combined primary immunodeficiency disorder

immunosuppression" represents the same conditions that are listed in the US Centers for Disease Control and Prevention (CDC) Advisory Committee on Immunization Practices (ACIP) "Recommended Immunization Schedule for Adults Aged 19 Years or Older, United States, 2017" under the umbrella of "severe immunosuppression."[3] The categorization of immunosuppression into these levels is an oversimplification, but some framework is needed for vaccine decision-making and administration. This categorization does not take into account many disease states that may lead to immunosuppression even in their untreated states, such as untreated hematologic malignancies.

VACCINATION TIMING

It is always preferable for vaccination to occur before the initiation of immunosuppression to maximize vaccine response and avoid safety concerns with live vaccines in cases of immunosuppression. If possible, it is recommended that inactivated vaccines be administered $\geq$14 days before immunosuppression.[3] IDSA guidelines recommend that live vaccines be administered $\geq$4 weeks before initiation of immunosuppression. It is recommended that they be completely avoided within 14 days of starting immunosuppression.[3] There are different considerations for timing of vaccination depending on the underlying medical comorbidity and anticipated duration of immunosuppression. These will be addressed by disease type in the following section.

SPECIFIC IMMUNOSUPPRESSIVE CONDITIONS AND THERAPIES
HIV Infection
Persons living with HIV are at increased risk of infection and severity of disease from vaccine-preventable diseases. All persons living with HIV should be vaccinated against influenza annually, pneumococcus, meningococcus, tetanus-diphtheria-acellular pertussis (Tdap), and hepatitis B (HB), regardless of other specific risk factors (Table 9.3).[4] The US guidelines do not recommend routine vaccination against *Haemophilus influenza* type b (Hib) infection in adults and adolescents with HIV infection.[3] Persons living with HIV have been found to be at increased risk for invasive pneumococcal and meningococcal disease. For this reason, HIV infection itself is an indication for adults to receive the 13-valent pneumococcal conjugate vaccine (PCV13), followed by boosting with the 23-valent pneumococcal polysaccharide vaccine (PPSV23), the conjugate quadrivalent meningococcal vaccine, and the HB vaccine. HB vaccination is recommended for all persons with HIV because of its similar mode of acquisition as HIV infection and because patients with HIV/HB coinfection have higher morbidity and mortality. Other vaccinations should be administered to persons with HIV infection if there are specific indications or if the patient lacks immunity (Table 9.3). Hepatitis A vaccine is recommended for the following persons living with HIV who have additional risk factors such as men who have sex with men, travel in countries with endemic hepatitis A, chronic liver disease, need for clotting factor concentrates, and those who inject illicit drugs.

TABLE 9.3
Recommended Vaccine Schedule for Adults With HIV Infection, United States, 2017

Vaccine	Indications	CD4 Requirement	Comments
Influenza	Annual immunization for all persons	None; vaccinate with each influenza season	Live attenuated nasal immunization is contraindicated
Pneumococcal PCV13 and PPSV23	All persons	None; start immunization at entry to care	
Meningococcal MCV4	All persons	None; start immunization at entry to care	2-dose primary series, 2-month interval, revaccinate every 5 years
Tdap	One dose if never vaccinated with Tdap as adolescent or adult; during each pregnancy at 27–36 weeks	None	Boost with Td every 10 years
Hepatitis B	All persons who are not immune (anti-HBs negative, includes those who have isolated anti-HBc positivity)	None	Hemodialysis dose formulation and other vaccine strategies may be used to optimize seroprotection
Hepatitis A	If risk factors for infection or liver disease (chronic liver disease, receive clotting factor concentrates, men who have sex with men, inject illicit drugs, and travel in countries with endemic hepatitis A)		2-dose series of single-antigen vaccine or 3 dose series of combined hepatitis A/hepatitis B vaccine
HPV	Same guidelines as for all adults and adolescents through the age of 26 years	None	2-dose series may be used if series is started at the age $\leq$ 14 years 3-dose series is recommended for those starting series $\geq$ 15 years
MMR	Those without evidence of immunity to MMR. Immunity = born before 1957, documentation of receipt of MMR, or laboratory evidence of immunity or disease.	CD4 $\geq$ 200 cells/μL	
Varicella	Those with no evidence of immunity to varicella. Immunity = documented receipt of 2 doses of VAR, born in the United States before 1980, diagnosis of varicella or zoster by a healthcare provider or laboratory evidence of immunity	CD4 $\geq$ 200 cells/μL	
Zoster (live)	Recommended for immunocompetent adults $\geq$ 60 years; FDA-approved for adults $\geq$ 50 years	Contraindicated if CD4 < 200 cells/μL	
Zoster (nonlive, recombinant subunit vaccine)	Recommended for immunocompetent adults $\geq$ 50 years		

anti-HBs, hepatitis B surface antibody titer; anti-HBc, hepatitis B core antibody; FDA, Food and Drug Administration; MCV4, meningococcal conjugate quadrivalent vaccine; MMR, measles-mumps-rubella; PCV13, 13-valent pneumococcal conjugate vaccine; PPSV23, 23-valent pneumococcal polysaccharide vaccine; Tdap, tetanus-diphtheria-acellular pertussis vaccine; Td, tetanus-diphtheria vaccine.

In general, live vaccines are contraindicated in patients with a CD4 cell count <200 cells/μL. Those who have a CD4 cell count ≥200 cells/μL and who do not have evidence of immunity to measles, mumps, and rubella or varicella (Table 9.3) should receive a two-dose series of the measles-mumps-rubella (MMR) vaccine.[2] No specific guidance is given by ACIP regarding the live zoster vaccination for patients with HIV infection. The live zoster vaccine is contraindicated in those with CD4 cell count <200 cells/μL; however, the ACIP has recommended the preferred use of the inactivated adjuvanted herpes zoster subunit vaccine for all immunocompetent adults aged ≥50 years.[5] This vaccine has been found to be safe and immunogenic in persons living with HIV, including those with CD4 count <200 cells/μL.[6]

Vaccine immunogenicity for HIV-infected patients tends to be better in patients who have achieved virologic suppression on antiretroviral therapy before the time of vaccination[7–11] and have higher CD4 T-cell counts.[8,11–16] In studies that evaluated both the effects of HIV virologic suppression and CD4 count, virologic suppression was a better predictor of vaccine immunogenicity than CD4 count at the time of vaccination.[7,8,10] However, in the cases of *Streptococcus pneumoniae* and influenza, the risk posed by these pathogens is significant enough that vaccination should not be delayed until viral suppression or immune reconstitution has been achieved.[4,17] Influenza vaccines have been demonstrated to be effective in preventing symptomatic influenza infection among persons living with HIV.[8,18] PCV13 should be administered on entry into care at time of HIV diagnosis, regardless of CD4 count or virologic suppression. The PPSV23 may be delayed until virologic suppression has been achieved or until virologic suppression and CD4 count is > 200 cells/μL is achieved. It is important providers recognize that some individuals may never reach a CD4 count >200/μL, and these persons will still need PPSV23. We are still awaiting data on the efficacy of the PCV13/PPSV23 prime boost strategy in the prevention of invasive pneumococcal vaccine among adults living with HIV.[19] Specific vaccine strategies including high-dose vaccine (for influenza and HB vaccine), adjuvanted vaccines, and vaccine timing for optimizing immunogenicity will be discussed in under individual vaccine types.

Autoimmune Inflammatory Rheumatic Diseases and Immunosuppressive Therapy

Patients with autoimmune inflammatory rheumatic disease (AIRD) are at increased risk of incidence and severity of infection due to their underlying conditions and their complications, immunosuppressive and immunomodulatory drug use, and increased frequency of hospitalizations and surgeries. Influenza, pneumococcal, herpes zoster and human papillomavirus (HPV) infections occur more frequently in patients with AIRD than those without these conditions.[20–24] Many studies have investigated and demonstrated the safety of inactivated vaccines in this patient population.[20,25–29]

Vaccine status should be addressed at the time of diagnosis of an AIRD and at each visit. If possible, vaccines should be administered two or more weeks before initiation of immunosuppressive therapy. If immunosuppressive therapy has already been started, vaccines should be given at the time of lowest level of immunosuppressive therapy and disease activity. Persons with AIRD should receive PCV13 vaccination, followed by a dose of PPSV23 at a minimum of 8 weeks later. They should receive another booster dose of PPSV23 5 years later if they were immunized before the age of 65 years and the subsequent dose 5 years later would be due before the age 65 years.[3] Other vaccines should be administered according to age and specific indications. Live vaccines are contraindicated in patients receiving tumor necrosis factor (TNF)-α inhibitors or corticosteroids at a dose of ≥20 mg/day prednisone or equivalent for >2 weeks.[2,3,29] The timing of administration of live vaccines in this patient population with respect to safety is a subject that has not been entirely elucidated. In general, experts recommend that patients should be off high-level immunosuppression for at least 4 weeks before administration of a live vaccine.[2,30] Some have advocated waiting five half-lives after the administration of biological agents and waiting a minimum of 6 months after rituximab before administration of a live vaccine.[30] IDSA guidelines recommend waiting ≥4 weeks after administration of a live vaccine before initiating high-level immunosuppression. The European League Against Rheumatism recommends waiting 2–4 weeks after live vaccine administration before initiating high-level immunosuppression.[26]

In the case of herpes zoster the zoster subunit vaccine containing recombinant glycoprotein E in combination with a novel adjuvant (AS01$_B$) recombinant zoster (shingles) vaccine (RZV) offers a much needed vaccine solution for these patients. ACIP has preferentially recommended this vaccine for healthy adults aged ≥50 years.[5] The immunogenicity and effectiveness of RZV in patients with AIRD needs to be further evaluated. Because this is a subunit vaccine that does not contain live virus, this vaccine avoids the risks posed to this patient population by live virus vaccines. The ACIP recommends the preferential use of this vaccine in all patients on low-dose immunosuppressives but has not made a definitive recommendation yet for patients on mid- to high-dose immunosuppressive therapy.[5]

Vaccine immunogenicity in this patient population varies across the spectrum of disease type, type of immunosuppressive therapy, and vaccine type. Disease-modifying antirheumatic drugs or TNF-α inhibitors have not diminished humoral immune responses to inactivated influenza vaccine (IIV) in numerous studies.[27,31–34] TNF-α inhibitors alone have also not been shown to not affect the efficacy of pneumococcal vaccination.[20] Tocilizumab, a humanized monoclonal antibody against the interleukin-6 receptor, has not been shown to decrease the humoral immune response to influenza vaccine[35] or for pneumococcal vaccine.[36] In contrast, rituximab, a chimeric monoclonal antibody against the CD20 protein, has been shown to markedly decrease humoral immune responses to influenza vaccine, particularly within 8 weeks after its administration,[37–39] as well as humoral responses to the conjugate pneumococcal[40] and polysaccharide pneumococcal vaccines.[41] Abatacept, a fusion protein that selectively blocks the interaction of CD80/CD86 receptors with CD28, thereby inhibiting T-cell proliferation and B-cell immunological response, has also been shown to diminish humoral responses to influenza vaccine.[42]

Malignancy and Chemotherapy

Patients with solid tumor and hematologic malignancies, except those receiving intensive chemotherapy (such as induction or consolidation therapy for acute leukemia) or those receiving anti–B-cell antibodies, should be vaccinated with annual influenza vaccination.[2] Pneumococcal immunization (both conjugate and polysaccharide pneumococcal vaccines) should be administered if feasible to patients with newly diagnosed malignancy as outlined under the section "Pneumococcal Vaccines." In some cases, such as acute leukemia, it may not be beneficial to administer immunizations at the time of diagnosis. The IDSA Clinical Practice Guidelines for Vaccination of the Immunocompromised Host suggest that inactivated vaccines administered during cancer chemotherapy not be counted as valid doses, unless there has been evidence of seroprotection documented by laboratory assay. Furthermore, those guidelines also recommend waiting until 3 months after completion of chemotherapy to administer inactivated vaccines to maximize vaccine immunogenicity.[2] Live vaccines are contraindicated during

chemotherapy and for 3 months after the completion of chemotherapy. When anti–B-cell antibodies are administered, it is recommended to wait a minimum 6 months before administering either inactivated vaccines (due to decreased likelihood of immunogenicity) or live vaccines (for safety consideration).[2] These recommendations differ in the case of patients who have had hematologic malignancies and hematopoietic stem cell transplant (HSCT) recipients, in which a longer period of time is recommended before giving living vaccines. (see below)

HSCT Recipients

The duration of high-level immunosuppression after HSCT depends on the type of transplant (autologous vs. allogenic), myeloablative conditioning and immunosuppressive regimens used, graft source and degree of match, and complications after HSCT, such as graft versus host disease (GVHD). Posttransplant immune recovery begins with neutrophil engraftment. Lymphocyte engraftment varies depending on the factors noted previously. In most patients, after HSCT, pretransplant antigen-specific immunity is lost, and the general dogma is that post-HSCT recipients should be viewed as "never vaccinated" patients, irrespective of pre-HSCT donor or recipient immunity.[2] Vaccination practices in the HSCT recipient population have varied widely over the years. Through a collaborative effort between US, Canadian, and the European Blood and Marrow Transplantation Society, in addition to IDSA, and the CDC, guidelines for preventing infectious complications after HSCT were published in 2009.[43] Previous recommendations had recommended waiting until 12 months after transplant to initiate vaccination. However, it was recognized that patients generally can mount protective responses to certain vaccines earlier than 1 year after HSCT. The 2009 guidelines and newer IDSA guidelines for vaccination in the immunocompromised host recommend starting immunization at variable times after HSCT (Table 9.4). Conjugate vaccines appear to be the most immunogenic in general, and this appears to hold true for this patient population. Studies of the 7-valent PCV (PCV7) demonstrated similar antibody responses whether the vaccine was administered at 3 or 9 months after HSCT.[44]

Live vaccines (MMR, varicella), however, should not be administered until ≥ 24 months after HSCT and only if GVHD is not present and the patient is not on significant immunosuppression (Table 9.4). In general, live zoster vaccine has not been recommended (this vaccine contains 14 times the live virus dose as varicella vaccine). With the FDA approval of the new inactivated

TABLE 9.4
Recommended Vaccines for Adult Recipients of HSCTs

	Earliest Time of Initiation after HSCT	Doses	Comments
INACTIVATED VACCINES			
Influenza	4–6 months	1 dose annually	May be started as early as 3 months after HSCT in setting of influenza outbreak
PCV13	3 months	3 doses	
PPSV23	12 months	1 dose	If patient has GVHD, then fourth dose of PCV13 may be administered in place of PPSV23
MCV4	6 months	2 doses	
Hib	6 months	2 doses	
DTap, Tdap, Td	6 months	3 doses	Various strategies using DTap and Tdap/Td combinations are discussed in text
IPV	6 months	3 doses	
HPV	6 months	2 doses (based on updated HPV guidelines)	Only for those aged 11–26 years
Hepatitis B	6 months	3 doses	May consider giving high-dose (hemodialysis dose) vaccine; check anti-HBs at 1 month after vaccination
LIVE ATTENUATED VACCINES—DO NOT ADMINISTER TO PATIENTS WITH ACTIVE GVHD OR ONGOING IMMUNOSUPPRESSION			
MMR	24 months	2 doses	Delay until 8–11 months after the last IVIG
Varicella	24 months	2 doses	Delay until 8–11 months after the last IVIG
Zoster (live)	Not recommended		

DTaP, diphtheria (full dose), tetanus, acellular pertussis vaccine; *GVHD*, graft versus host disease; *Hib*, Haemophilus influenza vaccine; *HPV*, human papillomavirus vaccine; *HSCTs*, hematopoietic stem cell transplants; *IPV*, inactivated polio vaccine; *IVIG*, intravenous immunoglobulin; *MCV4*, meningococcal conjugate quadrivalent (ACWY) vaccine; *MMR*, measles-mumps-rubella vaccine; *PCV13*, 13-valent pneumococcal conjugate vaccine; *PPSV23*, 23-valent polysaccharide pneumococcal vaccine; *Tdap*, tetanus, diphtheria (reduced dose), acellular pertussis vaccine; *Td*, tetanus, diphtheria (reduced dose) vaccine.

subunit zoster vaccine, zoster immunization practices in this patient population have now changed. This vaccine has been studied and found to be safe and immunogenic in autologous HSCT recipients.[45]

There has been little research performed on subsequent booster immunizations in this patient population. Booster vaccines are recommended based on general recommendations for booster vaccines for healthy adults (tetanus) and other immunosuppressed patients (pneumococcal and meningococcal vaccines). For patients less than the age of 65 years who are immunosuppressed, the ACIP recommends one single revaccination with PPSV23 ≥ 5 years after the first dose. Some European public health organizations recommend repeat vaccination with PPSV23 every 5 years. ACIP recommends booster vaccines with meningococcal conjugate

vaccine containing serotypes A, C, Y, and W135 (meningococcal conjugate quadrivalent vaccine [MCV4]) every 5 years. These patients also need to have booster vaccination with tetanus vaccine every 10 years.

SOT Recipients
Before transplant
Potential SOT candidates should be vaccinated as early as possible in the course of their end-stage organ disease in accordance with ACIP guidelines based on disease-specific indications.[2,3,46] The pretransplant evaluation is a good time to review immunization status and initiate immunizations. SOT candidates are more likely to develop vaccine-induced immunity before transplant than after transplant.[46,47] Current guidelines recommend standard-dose injectable, inactivated influenza,

PCV13/PPSV23, Tdap, hepatitis A, HB, and HPV vaccines for all SOT candidates who have not been previously vaccinated, who lack serologic evidence of immunity (for hepatitis A and B), and who are in the appropriate age range (for HPV).[46] Postvaccination hepatitis B surface antibody titer (anti-HBs) should be checked 1−2 months after HB vaccination. If a protective anti-HBs titer is not present, a second three-dose series should be administered. Patients with end-stage renal disease (ESRD) should receive the hemodialysis dose of HB vaccine. HPV vaccines should be administered for both males and females in the appropriate age groups.[3]

In general, live vaccines are contraindicated after transplant when the patient is on maintenance immunosuppression. The American Society for Transplantation (AST) recommends that antibody levels for measles, mumps, and rubella and varicella be obtained before transplant and the candidate be immunized with MMR vaccine and varicella vaccine if any of the respective antibody levels are negative.[46] Both MMR and varicella require a two-dose vaccine series that is administered 4 weeks apart. MMR and varicella vaccines should only be administered if it is anticipated that there will be a period of 4 weeks after vaccination before the anticipated time of transplantation. With the availability of the new recombinant zoster subunit vaccine, this will change shingles prevention immunization practices in this population.

After transplant

Vaccinations are usually withheld in the first 2 months after transplant as this is a time of more intense immunosuppression that may affect vaccine response. SOT recipients should receive yearly seasonal influenza vaccination. Current guidelines by IDSA and the ATS recommend standard-dose influenza vaccine for SOT recipients starting a minimum of 2−3 months after transplant, with the option for administration as early as 1 month after transplant in the event of an outbreak.[2,46] At this time there has been no recommendation for SOT recipients to receive high-dose or adjuvanted influenza vaccines, or booster doses—although either is appropriate for those patients aged 65 years and older. The use of additional influenza vaccine strategies to increase vaccine immunogenicity and effectiveness is an area that warrants additional study. A pilot study demonstrated safety and increased influenza vaccine humoral response after receipt of the MF59-adjuvanted influenza vaccine in kidney transplant recipients.[48] A randomized controlled trial (RCT) among pediatric SOT recipients demonstrated significantly

higher rates of seroconversion for H3N2, but not seroprotection, among children vaccinated with high-dose trivalent influenza vaccine (TIV) compared with standard-dose trivalent vaccine.[49] A phase III trial evaluating the efficacy and safety of a single dose of seasonal TIV compared with two doses of vaccine for prevention of influenza in SOT recipients found that a booster dose 5 weeks after initial vaccination induced increased antibody responses, with the booster arm having higher rates of seroconversion for all three vaccine influenza stains compared with the single-dose arm.[50] AST notes that if a patient is vaccinated very early after transplant, revaccination 3−6 months after transplant could be considered if it is still within the seasonal time period for influenza.[46] From a safety point of view it is reassuring to note that large studies have failed to demonstrate evidence for influenza immunizations triggering allograft rejection.[51−55]

Other inactivated vaccines (hepatitis A and B, HPV if indicated by age, PCV13, PPSV23, Tdap) are recommended to be started 2−6 months after transplantation if the transplant recipient did not complete the series before transplant or remains seronegative despite prior immunization. When given after transplant, the hemodialysis dose of HB vaccine may help improve vaccine response, as compared with the standard-dose HB vaccine. However, this is an area that still needs to be studied and demonstrated that the higher antigen dose actually results in high rates of seroprotection. Another vaccine strategy that warrants additional study in the SOT transplant population is a newly FDA-approved adjuvanted HB vaccine Heplisav-B (Dynavax). The adjuvant in Heplisav-B is a synthetic cytosine phosphoguanine oligonucleotide (CpG 1018). The other FDA-approved HB vaccines (Engerix-B, GSK; Recombivax HB, Merck; and Twinrix, GSK) use aluminum hydroxide as an adjuvant. In clinical trials of healthy adults[56−58] and adults with diabetes,[58] two doses of Heplisav-B have been shown to be more immunogenic than three doses of Engerix-B.

Pregnancy

Immunologic and physiologic changes during pregnancy may increase a woman's susceptibility to infection. This is particularly true in the case of influenza infection. Ideally, women should be fully vaccinated before pregnancy, and vaccination status should be addressed during prenatal visits. When considering whether a woman should be vaccinated during pregnancy, one should consider whether the benefits of vaccination to both the mother and fetus outweigh the potential risks of vaccination. Inactivated vaccines

TABLE 9.5
Vaccines Recommended for Adults With Functional or Anatomic Asplenia

Vaccine	Primary Vaccine Series	Repeat Vaccination
Pneumococcal	**No prior pneumococcal vaccine:** PCV13 × 1 dose, followed by PPSV23 × 1 dose ≥8 weeks later **Previous PPSV23 receipt:** PCV13 × 1 dose ≥1 year after the last PPSV23 dose **Previous PCV13 receipt:** PPSV23 × 1 dose ≥8 weeks after the last PCV13 dose	• PPSV23 × 1 dose 5 years after the last dose of PPSV23 • Repeat 1 final dose of PPSV23 after age 65 years (as long as it has been at least 5 years since the last PPSV23 dose)
MCV4	2 doses given 8 weeks apart	Repeat MCV4 every 5 years
Meningococcal B	2 doses of MenB-4C given 4 weeks apart or 3 doses of MenB-FHbp at 0, 2, and 6 months	No recommendation at this time
Haemophilus influenzae B	1 dose in those not previously vaccinated	None

MCV4, meningococcal conjugate quadrivalent (ACWY) vaccine; *MenB-4C*, Bexsero, GlaxoSmithKline Biologicals, Inc.; *MenB-FHbp*, Trumenba, Pfizer, Inc.; *PCV13*, 13-valent pneumococcal conjugate vaccine; *PPSV23*, 23-valent polysaccharide pneumococcal vaccine.

are safe for pregnant women.[59] Influenza poses a risk of significant morbidity to the mother and fetus; therefore IIV is recommended for women during pregnancy. One study has reported an association between IIV and spontaneous abortion in a post hoc analysis.[60] However, this study had numerous weaknesses in the study design, and multiple other well-designed studies have not demonstrated this association.[61–63]

Tdap administration during the third trimester has been used as part of a "cocooning" strategy to provide passive maternal antibody transfer to the fetus and protection until the child can begin pertussis vaccination at the age of 2 months.[64] Because pertussis immunity wanes relatively quickly with time, the Tdap vaccine should be administered during each pregnancy.[3] Live vaccines may pose a potential risk to the developing fetus and are not recommended during pregnancy. In general, vaccine responses in women during pregnancy seem to be similar to those of women who are not pregnant.[65]

Splenectomy and functional asplenia
Persons with functional or anatomic asplenia are at particular risk for infection with the encapsulated bacteria that are also vaccine preventable: *S. pneumoniae*, *Neisseria meningitidis*, and Hib.[66] When the splenectomy is planned, vaccination should be administered > 2 weeks before the surgery. In cases where this is not possible, vaccination has generally been

recommended at least 2 weeks after the surgery. Where there is concern that a patient may not follow up later for vaccination, it would be reasonable to go ahead and initiate the vaccine series when the patient is stable postoperatively. The recommended vaccines are in Table 9.5. It is important to note that meningococcal B vaccines are included in this recommendation.[67]

Primary immunodeficiencies
Many primary immunodeficiencies are diagnosed in childhood. These will not be reviewed in detail here. Patients with combined immunodeficiencies (both B- and T-cell immunodeficiencies) or T-cell immunodeficiencies (with CD3 T-cell lymphocyte count <500 cells/mm[3], Wiskott-Aldrich syndrome, or X-linked lymphoproliferative disease and familial disorders that predispose them to hemophagocytic lymphohistiocytosis) should be considered to have high-level immunosuppression (Table 9.2) and should not be given live vaccines. Inactivated vaccines may be given as part of the initial assessment of the immunodeficiency, before treatment with immunoglobulin therapy.[2]

Adults aged ≥19 years with primary complement deficiencies should receive the same vaccines against encapsulated organisms as outlined previously for patients with splenectomy. They should also be up to date with other routine vaccines that are recommended based on their other medical indications. Patients with phagocytic cell deficiencies should receive all inactivated vaccines based on the CDC ACIP schedule. Those with chronic granulomatous disease may receive live viral vaccines. Those with leukocyte adhesion deficiency, defects of cytotoxic granule release, other undefined phagocyte defects, or innate immunity defects should not receive live viral vaccines.[2] Inactivated vaccines other than influenza vaccine are not routinely given to persons with major antibody deficiencies when they are being treated with immunoglobulin therapy. Live vaccines should not be administered to these patients.[2]

VACCINES FOR HOUSEHOLD CONTACTS OF IMMUNOSUPPRESSED PERSONS AND HEALTHCARE WORKERS WHO WORK WITH IMMUNOSUPPRESSED PERSONS

Healthcare providers (HCPs), family members, and close contacts of immunosuppressed persons should be fully immunized. Providers caring for immunosuppressed patients should serve as a "double check" to ensure that close contacts of their immunosuppressed patients are fully immunized. Annual influenza vaccination is very important. In the past when a live attenuated influenza vaccine (LAIV) was offered in the United States, it was recommended that health care workers (HCWs) and close contacts of highly immunosuppressed patients receive the IIV and not the LAIV, if possible. This was because viral shedding with LAIV had been reported for up to 11 days after administration of this vaccine, even though transmission leading to disease has not been documented.[68-71] LAIV is currently not being offered in the United States because of vaccine low effectiveness; however, some vaccination programs are still using LAIV as part of their influenza immunization programs, and ACIP has voted to recommend LAIV for the 2018–19 influenza season.[72] If LAIV has been administered to a close contact of a person within 2 months of HSCT, a person with chronic GVHD, or severe combined immunodeficiency, then contact between the vaccinated person and immunosuppressed person should be avoided for 7 days after vaccination.[2] Other live vaccines administered to close contacts of immunosuppressed persons have not been found to place the immunosuppressed person at risk (Table 9.1), with the exception of smallpox vaccine (generally only administered to select members of the military) and oral polio vaccines (which are no longer available in the United States).[2,46] All live vaccines, with the exception of smallpox and oral polio vaccines, may be administered to HCPs and close contacts of

immunosuppressed persons. In the case of rotavirus vaccine being administered to an infant, it is recommended that persons with high-level immunosuppression avoid handling diapers of the infants for 4 weeks after vaccination.[2] It has been demonstrated that children may have viral shedding for up to 28 days after rotavirus vaccination.[73] It is also recommended that pets be fully immunized. There is no concern for transmission of infection due to pets receiving live vaccines.[46]

INACTIVATED VACCINES
Influenza Vaccines

In the United States and several other countries, annual IIVs are recommended for all adults, regardless of immunosuppression. Influenza causes significant morbidity and mortality among immunosuppressed persons. For example, influenza-related mortality of 30% at 60 days in HSCT recipients has been reported in a multicenter study.[74] Numerous strategies have been proposed as solutions to the problem of suboptimal influenza vaccine efficacy and effectiveness in immunocompromised adults. These potential vaccine solutions include increased antigen dose (high-dose) vaccines, adjuvanted vaccines, intradermal administration, and administration of booster doses during the influenza season. We will only briefly discuss strategies to increase influenza vaccine efficacy in older adults here as this topic is discussed in detail in the chapters "Vaccines for the Elderly: How, When, Why?" and "Influenza Vaccines—Are They Efficacious or Not?"

LAIV has not been recommended by ACIP for prevention of influenza during the 2016–17 and 2017–18 influenza seasons[75,76] because of studies demonstrating low vaccine effectiveness against influenza A(H1N1)pdm09 viruses during the 2013–14 and 2016–17 influenza seasons in the United States. During the 2017–18 influenza season, IIVs are available as both TIV (two strains of influenza A and one strain of influenza B) and quadrivalent influenza vaccine (QIV; two strains of influenza A and two strains of influenza B) formulations in the United States. The trivalent and quadrivalent vaccines are available in standard dose (15 μg of each hemagglutinin per 0.5 mL dose) and high dose (60 μg of each hemagglutinin antigen per 0.5 mL dose). The quadrivalent vaccine is available in standard dose alone. Recombinant influenza vaccines (RIVs) produced using egg-free cell-based culture technology are also available in trivalent and quadrivalent formulations with 45 μg of each hemagglutinin antigen per 0.5 mL dose. Finally an approved

MF-59 adjuvanted TIV is available and FDA approved for adults ≥65 years.[75]

ACIP has recommended adults aged ≥65 years receive any standard/high dose, trivalent/quadrivalent, or adjuvanted/non-adjuvanted IIV or RIV without specifying any preference for a specific vaccine formulation.[75] Studies have demonstrated that older adults have decreased antibody responses to standard-dose influenza vaccines compared with younger adults.[77,78] Studies of influenza vaccine immunogenicity do not necessarily correlate to vaccine efficacy (how the vaccine protects against disease in a controlled trial setting) or vaccine effectiveness (how a vaccine protects against disease in an observational setting). A hemagglutination inhibition (HAI) assay titer ≥ 1:40 has generally been associated with 50% clinical protection from infection. However, this association was determined in young healthy adults,[79] and data are lacking on this correlation with protection in older adults or immunocompromised persons. Studies among older adults have demonstrated varying vaccine efficacy for standard-dose IIV depending on strain type and match. A metaanalysis of individual patient data for 5210 participants reported vaccine strain match–adjusted vaccine effectiveness (defined as relative reduction in risk of laboratory-confirmed influenza in vaccinated patients compared with unvaccinated patients) among community-dwelling older adults during influenza epidemic seasons of 44% (95% confidence interval [CI] 22%–63%) and vaccine strain mismatched–adjusted vaccine effectiveness of 20% (95% CI 3%–33%).[80] This systematic review reported that seasonal influenza vaccine was not effective during nonepidemic influenza seasons among community-dwelling older adults.[80] Few studies have evaluated TIV influenza vaccine efficacy or effectiveness among immunosuppressed groups.[81] A few studies have demonstrated TIV efficacy in reducing symptomatic influenza infection among persons living with HIV,[8,18] SOT recipients,[51,82,83] and HSCT recipients.[84] Most studies in immunosuppressed adult populations have only assessed influenza vaccine immunogenicity.[81,85,86] Therefore our understanding of suboptimal influenza vaccine efficacy in many of these heterogenous immunosuppressed patient populations is not clear and warrants further evaluation.

High-dose IIVs

High-dose influenza vaccine has been proposed as a potential solution to suboptimal influenza vaccine effectiveness for both older adults and other immunocompromised adult populations. Immunogenicity studies of the high-dose TIV in older adults demonstrated that the high-dose TIV led to higher HAI titers for influenza A viruses than the standard-dose vaccine.[87,88] An RCT comparing efficacy of the high-dose TIV versus standard-dose TIV among 31,989 persons ≥65 years during the 2011–12 and 2012–13 influenza seasons did note superior vaccine efficacy for high-dose TIV.[89] This study reported a 24.2% (95% CI 9.7%–36.5%) greater relative vaccine efficacy for high-dose TIV compared with standard-dose TIV in preventing culture and/or reverse transcriptase–polymerase chain reaction (RT-PCR)–confirmed influenza caused by any influenza viral types/subtypes with protocol-defined influenza-like illness (ILI).[89]

There are few studies evaluating the immunogenicity of the high-dose TIV among immunocompromised adults and no studies evaluating its efficacy in any of these populations. Among 195 adults living with HIV (with 10% having a CD4 <200 cells/μL), an RCT compared the immunogenicity of high-dose TIV versus standard-dose TIV. Higher seroprotection rates were seen in the high-dose group for influenza A (H1N1) (96% vs. 87%; P = .029) and influenza B (91% vs. 80%; P = .030).[90] Another RCT of standard-dose TIV versus high-dose TIV among adult HSCT patients (median time after transplantation 8 months) demonstrated that the group receiving the high-dose vaccine had a higher postvaccine geometric mean titer (GMT) for one influenza strain (H3N2) and higher percentage of seroprotective rates (81% vs. 36%; P = .004) in the high-dose group. No significant differences were found for seroprotection or seroconversion for the influenza A/H1N1 or influenza B strains.[91] A study of adult oncology patients aged 18–64 years randomized to TIV high-dose versus standard-dose showed HAI GMTs were higher with the high-dose vaccine for influenza A/H3N2 and B strains, and seroconversion rates were higher with the high-dose vaccine for all three strains.[92] Larger studies evaluating the efficacy and effectiveness of high-dose influenza vaccines are needed in many immunocompromised groups (HIV, HSCT, SOT, AIRD) to know if this vaccine strategy might be a solution for various groups within the heterogenous population of immunocompromised adults.

Adjuvanted IIVs

Two oil-in-water adjuvants (AS03 and MF59) have been used in combination with influenza vaccines to boost their immunogenicity. The MF59-adjuvanted influenza vaccine has been FDA approved for those aged ≥65 years. AS03 adjuvanted influenza vaccines have been used widely in Europe and other parts of the world, particularly in combination with H1N1 vaccines. In studies comparing the immunogenicity of MF59-adjuvanted TIV to standard-dose TIV, the adjuvanted QIV met noninferiority for the three vaccine viruses for seroconversion rates and GMT ratios in adults aged $\geq$65 years.[93] One study evaluated the immunogenicity of MF59-adjuvanted H1N1 vaccine among persons living with HIV, but it did not have a comparison group receiving standard-dose, nonadjuvanted vaccine.[94] Additional studies have evaluated the AS03 adjuvanted H1N1 vaccine in HSCT recipients[95] and persons with AIRD.[96] Neither of these studies compared adjuvanted vaccine with nonadjuvanted vaccine. No studies have evaluated the efficacy or effectiveness of adjuvanted vaccines in preventing influenza infection among immunocompromised adults. More research is needed to determine if adjuvanted influenza vaccines offer a solution for influenza prevention in immunocompromised persons.

Intradermal Vaccine

Intradermal administration of vaccines has been suggested as a solution to improve vaccine immunogenicity. Intradermal administration results in antigen presentation by dendritic cells in the skin, which may improve the antigen presentation process. In healthy adults, intradermal vaccines have allowed for lower doses of vaccine antigens than in intramuscular vaccines with similar immunogenicity outcomes.[97] A metaanalysis of RCTs comparing the immunogenicity and safety of intradermal influenza vaccines with intramuscular vaccines in immunocompromised patients (including SOT recipients, persons with cancer and HIV, those treated with TNF-α inhibitors, and HSCT patients) demonstrated that intradermal vaccines were safe and showed similar vaccine immunogenicity as intramuscular vaccines, with lower doses of antigen being used in intradermal vaccines.[98] However, a solution for immunocompromised patient in terms of influenza prevention would not merely match the immunogenicity of intramuscular influenza vaccines, but rather would result in increased vaccine immunogenicity. One RCT among lung transplant recipients did compare immunogenicity outcomes in SOT recipients receiving standard-dose intramuscular TIV versus high-dose intradermal TIV. This study did not report any higher immunogenicity outcomes for the intradermal vaccine.[99] Based on immunogenicity data from this study, intradermal influenza vaccination is unlikely to be the solution for influenza vaccine prevention in the SOT population, although it appears to be a safe and acceptable alternative to intramuscular vaccine. A solution for influenza prevention in immunocompromised adults

would also result in increased influenza vaccine efficacy and effectiveness, which have yet to be studied with intradermal influenza vaccines in many subgroups of this diverse population. A QIV (Fluzone Intradermal Quadrivalent; Sanofi Pasteur) is currently an FDA-approved vaccine and listed as an option for influenza vaccine by ACIP for the 2017–18 influenza season.[75] ACIP has not preferentially recommended one influenza vaccine formulation over another for persons in whom each influenza vaccine is licensed. Fluzone Intradermal Quadrivalent influenza vaccine is recommended for adults aged 18–64 years.[75]

Recombinant Influenza Vaccines

There are two FDA-approved RIVs available in the United States with indications for adults $\geq$18 years: Flublok (RIV3) and Flublok Quadrivalent (RIV4). These vaccines are not produced in eggs and are egg free. Unlike the other influenza vaccines that have been discussed, these vaccines contain only hemagglutinin antigens (not hemagglutinin and neuraminidase antigens). An RCT involving >9000 adults aged $\geq$50 years comparing Flublok Quadrivalent (45 μg of each hemagglutinin antigen per strain) with the SD QIV IIV (15 μg of each hemagglutinin antigen per strain) was conducted during the 2014–15 influenza season to compare the relative vaccine efficacy of these vaccines against RT-PCR–confirmed, protocol-defined ILI. This study was powered to show noninferiority of the relative vaccine efficacy of RIV4. Based on prespecified criteria for the primary noninferiority analysis, RIV4 was found to be noninferior to QIV.[100] The authors reported an exploratory superiority analysis of RIV over QIV. They noted that among the modified per-protocol population the probability of ILI was 30% lower with RIV4 than with QIV (hazard ratio 0.69; 95% CI, 0.53–0.90; P = .006).[101] RCTs comparing HD TIV or QIV with Flublok TIV or QIV have not been conducted. Further study of Flublok TIV and QIV in older adults and other immunocompromised populations is needed.

Booster Doses

The use of more than one influenza vaccine (or booster doses) in a single influenza season has been studied in several immunocompromised groups as a way to improve vaccine immunogenicity and waning immunity. Booster influenza vaccines have been studied in patients with end-stage renal disease,[102] SOT recipients,[50,103] and HSCT recipients.[104] In these studies, with the exception of the TRANSGRIPE 1–2 RCT,[50] influenza booster doses did not lead to sufficient improvement in influenza vaccine immunogenicity to lead to endorsement of the booster dose strategy in these populations. TRANSGRIPE 1−2 was a randomized controlled multicenter trial where 499 patients were stratified by the study site, organ type, and time since transplantation and randomized to receive one dose or two doses (booster group) of the influenza vaccine 5 weeks apart. Seroconversion rates were higher in the booster group compared with single-dose vaccine group for the per-protocol population for all three influenza strains (54% vs. 38% for H1N1; 48% vs. 32% for H3N2; and 91% vs. 43% for influenza B; $P < .05$ for all vaccine strains). Seroprotection rates at 10 weeks were also higher in the booster group for all vaccine strains ($P < .05$). It is also important to note that seroconversion rates did not meet significance in the modified intention-to-treat population. Interestingly the clinical efficacy against microbiologically confirmed cases of influenza (99.2% vs. 98.8%) was similar for both groups.[50] Therefore one wonders whether this practice is justified on the basis of improved immunogenicity but no increased efficacy? The current AST guidelines on vaccination in SOT recipients recommend one standard dose of influenza vaccine for SOT recipients. Some experts have suggested that if influenza vaccine was given earlier than 2 months after transplantation, at a time of higher immunosuppression and when vaccination may have been less effective, then consideration may be given to administering a second dose of vaccine later in the influenza season.[47] The TRANSGRIPE 1−2 study was not powered to provide a basis for this recommendation of booster doses in the immediate transplant period as only 16% of the participants were <6 months since the time of transplantation.[50] At this time, influenza booster doses seem unlikely to solve the problem of poorer vaccine immunogenicity in immunocompromised persons.

PNEUMOCOCCAL VACCINES

There are more than 90 serotypes of S. pneumoniae, several of which have the propensity to cause invasive disease.[105] A PPSV23 was licensed in 1983 and contains 25 μg of purified capsular polysaccharide antigen for each of 23 different serotypes of pneumococcus. Immunity generated by polysaccharides is largely T-cell independent.[106] This is problematic in children younger than the age of 2 years who are largely unable to mount a T-cell−independent immune response and in older adults and immunocompromised hosts whose antibody response is less robust and wanes more quickly than that seen in younger, healthy adults.[106] A PCV7, licensed in

2000, was created by conjugating 2.2 μg of the capsular polysaccharide of each serotype of pneumococcus to 34 μg of diphtheria toxin.[105] This created pneumococcal antigens capable of generating T-cell−dependent immune responses that are more immunogenic and long-lasting than T-cell−independent responses. Furthermore, conjugate vaccines are able to generate mucosal immunity and prevent nasopharyngeal carriage of pneumococcus.[107] The 7-valent conjugate vaccine was first recommended as part of routine vaccination for children.[105] A PCV13 was licensed in 2010 for use in children and adults.[105]

A vaccine series comprises one dose of PCV13 followed by one dose of PPSV23 at least 8 weeks later, and a second dose of PPSV23 at least 5 years later is recommended for immunocompromised adults including those with sickle cell disease, asplenia, HIV, solid organ malignancies, hematologic malignancies, SOT, chronic high-dose corticosteroid use, or any other congenital or acquired immunodeficiency that puts someone at increased risk of complications from pneumococcal disease.[105] After HSCT, patients should receive three monthly PCV13 doses starting 3−6 months after transplantation followed by a dose of PPSV23 12 months after transplantation if there is no evidence of GVHD or a fourth dose of PCV13 if there is evidence of GVHD.[2] The data supporting this strategy are very limited, and further study is needed to determine the optimal vaccination strategy for pneumococcal vaccine (and other vaccines) in this population.

TETANUS, DIPHTHERIA, PERTUSSIS VACCINES

Tdap and tetanus-diphtheria (Td) vaccines are indicated for all adults aged ≥ 19 years who have not received a dose according to the ACIP guidelines.[3] Tdap vaccination of pregnant women is discussed in the earlier section on pregnancy. HSCT recipients will need to complete a three dose series of a Td-containing vaccine beginning as early as 6 months after transplantation (Table 9.4).[2] The 2013 IDSA Clinical Practice Guidelines for Vaccination of the Immunocompromised Host recommend that for HSCT recipients aged ≥7 years (including adults), three doses of diphtheria (full dose)-tetanus-acellular pertussis (DTaP) vaccine be considered (weak recommendation with low-quality evidence).[2] The authors note that alternative strategies might include a dose of Tdap followed by either two doses of diphtheria-tetanus or Td vaccine. There is little evidence to support which regimen is most immunogenic in this patient population. DTaP contains higher doses of diphtheria toxoid and pertussis antigens than then Tdap vaccine, so theoretically it may be more immunogenic in this patient population. The trade-off is that DTaP is usually more reactogenic than Tdap. Further study is needed to determine if three doses of DTaP are indeed more immunogenic in persons after HSCT.

MENINGOCOCCAL VACCINES

Meningococcal vaccines are discussed in detail in the chapter "Practical use of meningococcal vaccines." The discussion here will be limited to vaccine use in immunocompromised adults. Conjugate meningococcal vaccines are preferred in every indication for meningococcal vaccination over polysaccharide vaccines because they are more immunogenic. In the United States there are two available meningococcal conjugate vaccines containing serotypes A, C, Y, and W135 conjugated to diphtheria toxin (MCV4). The quadrivalent polysaccharide meningococcal vaccine that had previously been available in the United States was discontinued in 2017. There are two serogroup B conjugate (MenB) vaccines available in the United States. As discussed in the respective medical condition sections in the first half of this chapter, adults living with HIV, persons with functional or anatomic asplenia, persons with complement deficiencies (C3, C5−C9, properdin, factor H, and factor D), and HSCT recipients should be immunized with two doses of MCV4 with at least 8 weeks between doses. In addition to these indications, persons treated with eculizumab (a monoclonal antibody terminal complement inhibitor used to treat paroxysmal nocturnal hemoglobinuria and complement-mediated hemolytic uremic syndrome) must be vaccinated with MCV4 and MenB because of extremely high risks of meningococcal infection with this medication.[108] Other immunocompromised adults who should receive MenB vaccination are those with functional or anatomic asplenia, the complement deficiencies noted previously, and those treated with eculizumab. Booster doses of MCV4 should be administered every 5 years. At the current time there has been no guidance from ACIP on booster doses of MenB.

HIB VACCINES

Medical conditions and medications resulting in immunosuppression are risk factors for Hib disease. Hib vaccine was first licensed in the United States in 1985. An improved conjugate Hib vaccine was licensed in the United States in December 1987. The widespread vaccination of children with the Hib vaccine has led to "herd immunity" and reduced exposure to this organism in adults—as well as near elimination of Hib disease in the United States.[109] Conditions that place patients at particularly high risk include the following: hemoglobinopathies, complement deficiency, antibody deficiencies, functional and anatomic asplenia, and HSCT recipients.[109] HSCT recipients are recommended to be immunized with three doses of Hib at 6−12 months after transplantation.[2,109] The ACIP guidelines and 2013 IDSA Clinical Practice Guidelines for Vaccination of the Immunocompromised Host report that one dose of Hib vaccine should be administered to previously unvaccinated persons with sickle cell disease aged ≥5 years or asplenia.[2,109] In the case of splenectomy, persons should be vaccinated with Hib if they were not previously vaccinated. Persons with terminal complement component deficiencies should receive Hib vaccine as recommended by the ACIP guidelines (most will have received this during childhood). Hib vaccine is not recommended for persons with malignancy unless they undergo HSCT. There have been no recommendations for use of Hib vaccines in SOT recipients.

Hepatitis B

Vaccine strategies to increase HB vaccine immunogenicity have been the subject of intense research over the years for both immunocompetent adults and immunocompromised adults. Strategies to increase HB vaccine responsiveness have included increased antigen dose (double-dose) administration in immunocompromised persons, intradermal administration, and adjuvanted vaccines. The correlate of protection for HB vaccine efficacy is an anti-HBs concentration of ≥10 mIU/mL measured 1−3 months after completion of the vaccine series. The HB vaccine series leads to a seroconversion rate of 90%−95% in healthy younger adults. Seroconversion rates decline with age to 47% by the sixth decade of life.[110] Seroconversion rates are also affected by immunosuppression. Seroconversion rates vary widely in this heterogeneous patient population. Seroconversion rates of 18%−71% have been reported among persons living with HIV infection who received the standard-dose HB vaccine series.[111] In persons with end-stage renal disease on hemodialysis, the response rate to the standard-dose vaccine series is 50%−60%.[112] Even with the recommended double-dose vaccine along with an extra fourth dose (at 0, 1, 2, and 6 months), the response rate is about 70% in persons on hemodialysis.[113] Seroconversion rates in persons with decompensated cirrhosis are 37%.[114]

High-dose vaccines

High-dose HB vaccines have been shown to result in higher seroprotection (anti-HBs concentration of ≥ 10 mIU/mL) rates among persons with end-stage renal disease/on hemodialysis[115] and persons living with HIV.[111] ACIP and IDSA have recommended that patients with chronic kidney disease and hemodialysis[3,115] receive a high-dose HB vaccine series. IDSA has recommended that persons living with HIV receive a high-dose HB vaccine series. ACIP and IDSA guidelines do not outline a preference of high-dose vaccine for other immunocompromised persons. More data are needed to determine the immunogenicity and efficacy of high-dose HB vaccine series in other immunocompromised populations, such as SOT and HSCT recipients.

Intradermal vaccines

Intradermal administration of HB vaccine has been shown to initially result in higher vaccine immunogenicity than intramuscular administration; however, a metaanalysis of 12 studies demonstrated that the difference was not significant with follow-up over 6−60 months.[116] A few other studies have demonstrated increased rates of seroprotection among hemodialysis patients vaccinated intradermally versus intramuscularly in previous HB vaccine nonresponders.[117,118] It may be that intradermal vaccine administration is a solution for prior vaccine nonresponders but not a vaccine strategy that should be recommended initially for all immunocompromised persons.

Adjuvanted vaccines

Heplisav-B is a recombinant HB vaccine that contains the CpG 1018 adjuvant (Dynavax, proprietary Toll-like receptor 9 adjuvant) that was FDA-approved in 2017.[119] Heplisav-B is approved to be administered as two intramuscular doses 1 month apart. Two doses of Heplisav-B have been shown to be significantly more immunogenic than three standard-doses of Engerix-B (GlaxoSmithKline Biologicals) in adults aged 18−55 years (95% [95% CI 93.9, 96.1] vs. 81.3% [77.8, 84.9]),[56] 40−70 years (90.1% [88.2,91.8] vs. 70.5 [65.5, 75.2]),[57] and among those with type 2 diabetes mellitus (90.0% vs. 65.1%, with a difference of 24.9% [19.3%, 30.7%]).[58] This vaccine will need to be studied in other immunocompromised populations to determine if it is a solution for low seroprotection rates in these populations. A phase four study is being conducted to further evaluate for any signals of adverse effects related to the vaccine.

Fendrix (HB-AS04) is a recombinant HB vaccine with AS04 adjuvant (GlaxoSmithKline). AS04 combines aluminum salt and the Toll-like receptor 4 agonist 3-O-desacyl-4′-monophosphoryl lipid A. Fendrix was approved by the European Medicines Agency in 2005 but has not been FDA approved. Completion of the Fendrix four-dose vaccine series was shown to result in higher GMT anti-HBs titers in predialysis and hemodialysis patients than a standard four-dose series of Engerix-B.[120] However, the percentage of persons who achieved seroprotection against HB virus was not significantly different between the HB-AS04 and Engerix-B vaccine groups at 1 month after completion of the vaccine series. HB-AS04 did result in a greater number of predialysis and hemodialysis patients maintaining seroprotection at 36 months (72.9% vs. 52%, $P = .029$). HB-AS04 has been studied in a nonrandomized controlled manner among renal transplant recipients. In one study of 17 renal transplant recipients who had received at least three vaccines against HB virus and not achieved seroprotection, one dose of HB-AS04 resulted in seroprotection in seven of these persons.[121] Further RCTs are needed to compare the safety and immunogenicity of high-dose HB vaccines and adjuvanted HB vaccines among transplant recipients.

In one brief communication, HB-AS04 was been administered to persons living with HIV who failed to respond to prior HB vaccine series and resulted in a significant number of these persons (95%) achieving seroprotection.[122] The authors of this communication acknowledge that it is possible that there were confounding factors, such as higher CD4 count at time of HB-AS04 administration compared with other HB vaccine series.[122] Nonetheless, it seems worthwhile to study adjuvanted HB vaccines in persons living with HIV in an RCT.[121]

Hepatitis A

Hepatitis A vaccination is recommended for persons traveling or working in countries outside the United States with high or intermediate rates of hepatitis A virus infection, men who have sex with men, illicit drug users, persons working in research with the virus, individuals with chronic liver disease (including all persons with chronic hepatitis B and C infection), and persons with clotting factor disorders.[123] Immunocompromised persons who meet any of these indications should be vaccinated. The hepatitis A vaccines available in the United States are inactivated vaccines and are available as Hepatitis A single-antigen vaccines, as well as in combination with HB vaccine. Live attenuated hepatitis A vaccines are available in some countries outside the

United States. Hepatitis A vaccines, both single-antigen and combination vaccines, are highly immunogenic in healthy adults; therefore postvaccination serologic testing is not recommended. In healthy adults >95% of those vaccinated with hepatitis A vaccines have protective antibody titers at 20 years after follow-up.[124,125] Vaccine immunogenicity may be lower in those with chronic liver disease and immunosuppression. Persons with chronic hepatitis B/C infection or those with other causes of liver disease should be vaccinated before the development of decompensated liver disease because vaccine immunogenicity is better in persons with early-stage liver disease. In patients with HIV infection, vaccine seroconversion (developing a positive hepatitis A antibody titer) varies from 48% to 96%.[126,127] Suppression of HIV replication through antiretroviral therapy is associated with an improved likelihood of vaccine response.[126] In persons living with HIV, US guidelines recommend that the antibody response be assessed 1 month after completion of the series. If seroprotective antibody level has not been achieved, then repeat vaccination is recommended.[4] The question of whether to check total or IgG hepatitis A antibody level before vaccination is less clear. It may be more cost-effective to vaccinate persons rather than check titers. In those who have strong risk factors for having had prior hepatitis A infection, such as living for a prolonged time in country with high rates of hepatitis A infection, hepatitis A antibody screening at baseline may be cost-effective. Hepatitis A vaccines are highly immunogenic, and, in general, seroprotective antibody titers are able to be achieved with repeat vaccination. It does not appear that additional vaccine strategies to increase hepatitis A vaccine immunogenicity or efficacy are needed at this time.

HPV VACCINES

HPV vaccines protect against acquisition of HPV infection, and, thus, subsequent development of the HPV-associated disease. Several different HPV vaccines are available worldwide (bivalent, quadrivalent, and 9-valent). Only the 9-valent HPV vaccine is available in the United States. The US AICP recommends HPV vaccine at the age of 11–12 years for females. HPV vaccine may be administered starting at the age of 9 years. Catch-up vaccination is recommended for females up to the age of 26 years. The ACIP recommends HPV vaccine for males at the age of 11–12 years. The ACIP also notes HPV vaccine may be started in males at the age of 9 years. Catch-up vaccination is recommended for males up to the age of 21 years. ACIP notes permissive use of HPV vaccine for men up to the age of 26 years if these men are immunocompromised or have sex with men.[128] Immunocompromised adolescents and adults should complete the HPV vaccine series. HSCT recipients should receive this vaccine series again after transplant if they meet age criteria.

LIVE VACCINES

MMR Vaccines

MMR was licensed in 1971 and combines three live vaccines directed against measles (first licensed in 1963), mumps (first licensed in 1967), and rubella (first licensed in 1969). The MMR series of 2 doses given at 12–15 months and 4–6 years is part of the routine recommended childhood vaccination series in the United States.[129] Although adults who have received their complete childhood vaccination series or were born before 1957 are likely immune, there are circumstances for which vaccination of an immunocompromised adult may be a consideration, including catch-up vaccination, in the setting of an outbreak, or after HSCT. Because it is a live vaccine with the potential for vaccine-derived disease in immunocompromised hosts, MMR is generally contraindicated in those with low- and high-level immunosuppression.[2] However, newer studies have found that the vaccine may be able to be given safely in certain immunocompromised populations such as patients with HIV infection with a CD4 count greater than 200,[130] after recovery from chemotherapy,[131] and 1–2 years after HSCT without evidence of GVHD.[132] If immunosuppression is planned and a patient does not demonstrate immunity to measles, mumps, or rubella by serology, it is recommended to provide a dose at least 4 weeks before the start of immunosuppression.[2] In the setting of a measles or mumps outbreak resulting in a high-risk exposure of an immunocompromised patient to a known or suspected case, immunoglobulin should be administered instead of MMR vaccine.[1] After HSCT, primary immunity should be reestablished with a 2-dose MMR series starting 24 months after transplant, provided there is no evidence of GVHD or ongoing immunosuppression.[2]

VZV Vaccines

Before vaccination (which was introduced to the routine childhood immunization schedule in the United States with one dose in 1995 and a two-dose schedule in 2007), nearly all people in temperate climates had developed immunity to VZV by adulthood. Primary varicella infection is often a largely mild disease in immunocompetent patients; however, some cases will evolve to severe disease and significant morbidity and mortality can be seen.[133] Severe outcomes are far more common in immunosuppressed individuals, and these patients can develop life-threatening illnesses with disseminated disease and complications.

Evidence of immunity

According to ACIP, evidence of varicella immunity includes one or more of the following criteria: written documentation of immunization; HCP documentation of typical previous varicella disease (atypical cases require laboratory verification or documented epidemiologic link); laboratory evidence of immunity (serology); or a person being born in the United States before 1980. Birth before 1980 is not allowed as evidence for varicella immunity for immunosuppressed individuals, pregnant patients, and healthcare workers. Patients born outside of the United States before 1980 must fulfill one or more of the other criteria.[134]

Varicella vaccine indications for adults

It is strongly recommended that all immunocompetent household members of immunocompromised patients be vaccinated according to the ACIP schedule with varicella and zoster vaccines.[2] Should a household member develop a postvaccination rash from a live varicella vaccine, they should cover the rash and avoid contact and close interactions with any household members who lack evidence of immunity until a period of 24 h or more has passed since the last new lesion developed or all lesions are resolved.[135] The single-antigen VZV vaccine Varivax (Merck) was approved for the prevention of varicella in children aged ≥12 months in 1995, and this is the vaccine that would be used for adult varicella immunization. It contains the Oka strain VZV and has no less than 1350 plaque-forming units (PFUs). At present there are no known efforts to bring an inactivated varicella vaccine to market.

Varicella vaccine immunogenicity and correlates of protection

Vaccine licensing studies have used a measurement of humoral immunity (VZV glycoprotein antigen-based enzyme-linked immunosorbent assay [ELISA]) as a measure of vaccine immunogenicity.[136,137] Varicella vaccine efficacy has been evaluated in healthy children but data are lacking for immunosuppressed patients. For children the postvaccination VZV glycoprotein ELISA antibody response correlates with VZV neutralizing antibody level, VZV-specific T-cell proliferative responses, vaccine efficacy, and long-term protection

against varicella.[134] No varicella vaccine correlates of protection have been studied for adults.[134]

Contraindications to varicella vaccine administration

Contraindications to the varicella vaccine include the following: pregnancy or chance of pregnancy in 4 weeks after administration; previous severe allergic reaction to the vaccine or any of its components; active, untreated tuberculosis; and severe immunosuppression (Table 9.2). HIV-positive patients: Adults and children without evidence of severe immunodeficiency (HIV-infected persons with CD4+T-lymphocytes count >200 cells/μL) are appropriate candidates for varicella vaccination.[4,138] Varicella vaccine is generally deferred in HSCT recipients until 24 months after transplant, provided there is no evidence of GVHD or ongoing immunosuppression.[2]

Zoster Vaccines
Live attenuated vaccine

In the past, ACIP has recommended live attenuated zoster immunization for immunocompetent individuals aged ≥60 years, including those with prior herpes zoster infection.[139] The live attenuated zoster vaccine Zostavax (Merck) is FDA approved for immunocompetent adults at the age of ≥ 50 years. Zostavax is the lyophilized preparation that contains the Oka/Merck strain VZV and no less than 19,400 PFUs per dose, 14 times the potency of the varicella vaccine Varivax (Merck).[140] The live zoster vaccine has been shown to be 70% effective for prevention of herpes zoster in patients between the age of 50 and 59 years; 51% in patients between the age of 60 and 69 years; and 38% in patients older than the age of 70 years.[140,141] The live zoster vaccine was shown to be effective in reducing PHN by 67% in the 60- to 69-year-old cohort and by 67% in the ≥70-year-old cohort.[140] Significant waning immunity was seen with the live zoster vaccine. Vaccinated patients older than the age of 60 years experienced a decrease in vaccine efficacy from 68% in the first year, to only 4% in year eight, and to no protection from shingles by year 10.[142]

Recombinant subunit vaccine

In October 2017 the US FDA approved the inactivated recombinant zoster subunit vaccine containing 50 μg of recombinant VZV glycoprotein E in combination with the liposome-based adjuvant system AS01$_B$ (RZV) (GlaxoSmithKline Biologicals).[143] ACIP has recommended that this vaccine be preferentially administered in a two-dose series to adults aged ≥50 years (the second dose should be given 2–6 months after the first). ACIP has recommended that this vaccine be administered to those who have previously been vaccinated with the live shingles vaccine, provided that 8 weeks has elapsed since live attenuated zoster vaccination.[5] The RZV vaccine is a much needed solution to the decreased effectiveness of the live zoster vaccine seen in older adults. As an inactivated vaccine, it also fills the void of a nonreplicating vaccine incapable of causing infection in adults who are highly immunosuppressed. Efficacy for shingles prevention in patients older than 50 years was shown to be 97% over a 3-year study, and, importantly, no significant difference in efficacy was seen between age groups.[144] Clinical trials involving immunosuppressed patients show that the vaccine was generally well tolerated. The RZV vaccine group did demonstrate more reactogenicity (84%) than the placebo group (38%). No major adverse events were seen; however, up to 17% of participants reported grade 3 adverse events significant enough to limit daily activities for 1–2 days after vaccination.[144] A subsequent study showed that RZV was 90% efficacious in preventing PHN, and no significant discrepancy was seen among the age cohorts.[145] This vaccine has been found to be safe and immunogenic in an autologous HSCT population[45] and among patients with HIV, including those with a CD4 count <200 cells/μL.[6] Multiple studies of the safety and efficacy of this vaccine in other immunosuppressed patient populations are ongoing.

Zoster vaccine correlates of protection

The correlate of protection for HZ has not been completely elucidated. While uncommon, recurrent herpes zoster (HZ) is observed and previous shingles disease does not protect patients from future episodes.[146] Various studies suggest that cell-mediated immunity (CMI) to VZV is needed to protect against herpes zoster and that antibody to VZV does not play a significant role in prevention of herpes zoster.[146–148] When VZV-specific CMI decreases, as it does with aging, medical illnesses, or iatrogenic immunosuppression, the incidence and severity of herpes zoster and its complications rise.[147–150] VZV antibody levels in immunosuppressed persons do not correlate with levels of VZV CMI or with the risk of herpes zoster.[148,151] In one study of the live zoster vaccine, older adults had significantly lower CMI responses to the vaccine compared with younger adults.[152] Immunogenicity studies of the RZV vaccine have evaluated both VZV antibodies, as well as VZV-specific CMI. The RZV vaccine has demonstrated robust VZV-specific humoral and CMI responses.[153–155]

Contraindications to Zoster vaccine administration

The live attenuated herpes zoster vaccine is contraindicated in all significantly immunosuppressed patients regardless of the cause. Specific contraindications include the following: pregnancy or intent to become pregnant in 4 weeks after administration; previous severe allergic reaction to the vaccine or any of its components; active, untreated tuberculosis; and severe immunosuppression (Table 9.2). The only contraindications for RZV are known allergy to any component of the vaccine. For patients who are ineligible for live varicella or zoster vaccines, it is also important to note that acyclovir and valacyclovir prophylaxis are highly effective and safe in severely immunocompromised patients for prevention of varicella zoster.

LIVE TRAVEL VACCINATIONS

Specific considerations for live travel vaccines and immunocompromised persons are discussed in detail in the chapter "Vaccines for Adult Travelers: When and Why?"

CONCLUSIONS

One of the greatest challenges for vaccine use in immunocompromised adults is the lack of data regarding vaccine efficacy (and, in some cases, even immunogenicity and safety) in this heterogeneous population. How can one create a solution until one first understands the problem? Potential vaccine strategies include vaccines with higher antigen doses, adjuvanted vaccines, intradermal administration, and inclusion of booster doses. Conjugate vaccines have been shown to be more immunogenic than polysaccharide vaccines (pneumococcal and meningococcal vaccines). Pneumococcal conjugate vaccines have been the solution for improving vaccine responses in immunocompromised adults (and other populations, such as children). Conjugate meningococcal vaccines have largely replaced the use of polysaccharide vaccines in all populations, not just the immunocompromised. High-dose and adjuvanted vaccines for influenza have been FDA approved and may be solutions for immunocompromised adults, but these require further study and head-to-head comparisons. High-dose HB vaccines have been shown to be superior in patients with chronic kidney disease and in persons living with HIV. One might assume that these high-dose and adjuvanted HB vaccines would be more immunogenic in other immunocompromised populations, but this has yet to be proven. Furthermore, head-to-head comparisons of high-dose HB vaccines and the newly FDA-approved adjuvanted HB vaccine among various immunocompromised populations are needed.

Perhaps one of the greatest success stories of a vaccine solution for immunocompromised adults is that of the RZV vaccine containing the AS01$_B$ adjuvant. This vaccine solution solved the need for a nonlive vaccine that could be administered to immunocompromised persons, who previously had no options for zoster vaccine, despite their high risk for disease. In addition to providing an option for zoster vaccination, it also improved vaccine immunogenicity. One lesson for us to learn is that through finding ways to meet the vaccine challenges for immunocompromised adults, we might discover better vaccine solutions for immunocompetent persons, as well.

REFERENCES

1. Centers for Disease Control and Prevention. Principles of vaccination. In: Hamborsky J, Kroger A, Wolfe S, eds. *Epidemiology and Prevention of Vaccine-preventable Diseases.* 13th ed. Washington, DC: Public Health Foundation; 2015.
2. Rubin LG, Levin MJ, Ljungman P, et al. 2013 IDSA clinical practice guideline for vaccination of the immunocompromised host. *Clin Infect Dis.* 2014;58:309−318.
3. Kim DK, Riley LE, Harriman KH, Hunter P, Bridges CB. Advisory committee on immunization practices recommended immunization schedule for adults aged 19 Years or older—United States, 2017. *MMWR Morb Mortal Wkly Rep.* 2017;66:136−138.
4. Panel on Opportunistic Infections in HIV-Infected Adults and Adolescents. Guidelines for the Prevention and Treatment of Opportunistic Infections in HIV-infected Adults and Adolescents: Recommendations from the Centers for Disease Control and Prevention, the National Institutes of Health, and the HIV Medicine Association of the Infectious Diseases Society of America. Available from: http://aidsinfo.nih.gov/contentfiles/lvguidelines/adult_oi.pdf. Accessed October 7, 2017.
5. Dooling KL, Guo A, Patel M, et al. Recommendations of the advisory committee on immunization practices for use of herpes zoster vaccines. *MMWR Morb Mortal Wkly Rep.* 2018;67:103−108.
6. Berkowitz EM, Moyle G, Stellbrink HJ, et al. Safety and immunogenicity of an adjuvanted herpes zoster subunit candidate vaccine in HIV-infected adults: a phase 1/2a randomized, placebo-controlled study. *J Infect Dis.* 2015;211:1279−1287.
7. Evison J, Farese S, Seitz M, Uehlinger DE, Furrer H, Muhlemann K. Randomized, double-blind comparative trial of subunit and virosomal influenza vaccines for immunocompromised patients. *Clin Infect Dis.* 2009;48:1402−1412.
8. Yamanaka H, Teruya K, Tanaka M, et al. Efficacy and immunologic responses to influenza vaccine in HIV-1-infected patients. *J Acquir Immune Defic Syndr.* 2005;39:167−173.
9. Gonzalez R, Castro P, Garcia F, et al. Effects of highly active antiretroviral therapy on vaccine-induced humoral immunity in HIV-infected adults. *HIV Med.* 2010;11:535−539.
10. Sogaard OS, Schonheyder HC, Bukh AR, et al. Pneumococcal conjugate vaccination in persons with HIV: the effect of highly active antiretroviral therapy. *AIDS.* 2010;24:1315−1322.
11. Siberry GK, Williams PL, Lujan-Zilbermann J, et al. Phase I/II, open-label trial of safety and immunogenicity of meningococcal (groups A, C, Y, and W-135) polysaccharide diphtheria toxoid conjugate vaccine in human immunodeficiency virus-infected adolescents. *Pediatr Infect Dis J.* 2010;29:391−396.
12. Malaspina A, Moir S, Orsega SM, et al. Compromised B cell responses to influenza vaccination in HIV-infected individuals. *J Infect Dis.* 2005;191:1442−1450.
13. Wallace MR, Brandt CJ, Earhart KC, et al. Safety and immunogenicity of an inactivated hepatitis A vaccine among HIV-infected subjects. *Clin Infect Dis.* 2004;39:1207−1213.
14. Kemper CA, Haubrich R, Frank I, et al. Safety and immunogenicity of hepatitis A vaccine in human immunodeficiency virus-infected patients: a double-blind, randomized, placebo-controlled trial. *J Infect Dis.* 2003;187:1327−1331.
15. Rodriguez-Barradas MC, Musher DM, Lahart C, et al. Antibody to capsular polysaccharides of Streptococcus pneumoniae after vaccination of human immunodeficiency virus-infected subjects with 23-valent pneumococcal vaccine. *J Infect Dis.* 1992;165:553−556.
16. Loeliger AE, Rijkers GT, Aerts P, et al. Deficient antipneumococcal polysaccharide responses in HIV-seropositive patients. *FEMS Immunol Med Microbiol.* 1995;12:33−41.
17. Crum-Cianflone NF, Wallace MR. Vaccination in HIV-infected adults. *AIDS Patient Care STDS.* 2014;28:397−410.
18. Tasker SA, Treanor JJ, Paxton WB, Wallace MR. Efficacy of influenza vaccination in HIV-infected persons. A randomized, double-blind, placebo-controlled trial. *Ann Intern Med.* 1999;131:430−433.
19. Feldman C, Anderson R, Rossouw T. HIV-related pneumococcal disease prevention in adults. *Expert Rev Respir Med.* 2017;11:181−199.
20. Westra J, Rondaan C, van Assen S, Bijl M. Vaccination of patients with autoimmune inflammatory rheumatic diseases. *Nat Rev Rheumatol.* 2015;11:135−145.
21. Nichol KL, Wuorenma J, von Sternberg T. Benefits of influenza vaccination for low-, intermediate-, and high-risk senior citizens. *Arch Intern Med.* 1998;158:1769−1776.
22. Wotton CJ, Goldacre MJ. Risk of invasive pneumococcal disease in people admitted to hospital with selected immune-mediated diseases: record linkage cohort analyses. *J Epidemiol Community Health.* 2012;66:1177−1181.

23. Smitten AL, Choi HK, Hochberg MC, et al. The risk of herpes zoster in patients with rheumatoid arthritis in the United States and the United Kingdom. *Arthritis Rheum.* 2007;57:1431–1438.

24. Tam LS, Chan AY, Chan PK, Chang AR, Li EK. Increased prevalence of squamous intraepithelial lesions in systemic lupus erythematosus: association with human papillomavirus infection. *Arthritis Rheum.* 2004;50:3619–3625.

25. Puges M, Biscay P, Barnetche T, et al. Immunogenicity and impact on disease activity of influenza and pneumococcal vaccines in systemic lupus erythematosus: a systematic literature review and meta-analysis. *Rheumatology (Oxford).* 2016;55:1664–1672.

26. Heijstek MW, Ott de Bruin LM, Bijl M, et al. EULAR recommendations for vaccination in paediatric patients with rheumatic diseases. *Ann Rheum Dis.* 2011;70:1704–1712.

27. Del Porto F, Lagana B, Biselli R, et al. Influenza vaccine administration in patients with systemic lupus erythematosus and rheumatoid arthritis. Safety and immunogenicity. *Vaccine.* 2006;24:3217–3223.

28. Borchers AT, Keen CL, Shoenfeld Y, Silva Jr J, Gershwin ME. Vaccines, viruses, and voodoo. *J Investig Allergol Clin Immunol.* 2002;12:155–168.

29. Singh JA, Saag KG, Bridges Jr SL, et al. 2015 American College of Rheumatology guideline for the treatment of rheumatoid arthritis. *Arthritis Care Res Hob.* 2016;68:1–25.

30. Tanriover MD, Akar S, Turkcapar N, Karadag O, Ertenli I, Kiraz S. Vaccination recommendations for adult patients with rheumatic diseases. *Eur J Rheumatol.* 2016;3:29–35.

31. Chalmers A, Scheifele D, Patterson C, et al. Immunization of patients with rheumatoid arthritis against influenza: a study of vaccine safety and immunogenicity. *J Rheumatol.* 1994;21:1203–1206.

32. Fomin I, Caspi D, Levy V, et al. Vaccination against influenza in rheumatoid arthritis: the effect of disease modifying drugs, including TNF alpha blockers. *Ann Rheum Dis.* 2006;65:191–194.

33. Gelinck LB, van der Bijl AE, Beyer WE, et al. The effect of anti-tumour necrosis factor alpha treatment on the antibody response to influenza vaccination. *Ann Rheum Dis.* 2008;67:713–716.

34. Kubota T, Nii T, Nanki T, et al. Anti-tumor necrosis factor therapy does not diminish the immune response to influenza vaccine in Japanese patients with rheumatoid arthritis. *Mod Rheumatol.* 2007;17:531–533.

35. Mori S, Ueki Y, Hirakata N, Oribe M, Hidaka T, Oishi K. Impact of tocilizumab therapy on antibody response to influenza vaccine in patients with rheumatoid arthritis. *Ann Rheum Dis.* 2012;71:2006–2010.

36. Mori S, Ueki Y, Akeda Y, et al. Pneumococcal polysaccharide vaccination in rheumatoid arthritis patients receiving tocilizumab therapy. *Ann Rheum Dis.* 2013;72:1362–1366.

37. van Assen S, Holvast A, Benne CA, et al. Humoral responses after influenza vaccination are severely reduced in patients with rheumatoid arthritis treated with rituximab. *Arthritis Rheum.* 2010;62:75–81.

38. Gelinck LB, Teng YK, Rimmelzwaan GF, van den Bemt BJ, Kroon FP, van Laar JM. Poor serological responses upon influenza vaccination in patients with rheumatoid arthritis treated with rituximab. *Ann Rheum Dis.* 2007;66:1402–1403.

39. Oren S, Mandelboim M, Braun-Moscovici Y, et al. Vaccination against influenza in patients with rheumatoid arthritis: the effect of rituximab on the humoral response. *Ann Rheum Dis.* 2008;67:937–941.

40. Kapetanovic MC. Further evidence for influenza and pneumococcal vaccination in patients treated with disease modifying antirheumatic drugs and anti-tumor necrosis factor agents. *J Rheumatol.* 2014;41:626–628.

41. Bingham 3rd CO, Looney RJ, Deodhar A, et al. Immunization responses in rheumatoid arthritis patients treated with rituximab: results from a controlled clinical trial. *Arthritis Rheum.* 2010;62:64–74.

42. Ribeiro AC, Laurindo IM, Guedes LK, et al. Abatacept and reduced immune response to pandemic 2009 influenza A/H1N1 vaccination in patients with rheumatoid arthritis. *Arthritis Care Res Hob.* 2013;65:476–480.

43. Tomblyn M, Chiller T, Einsele H, et al. Guidelines for preventing infectious complications among hematopoietic cell transplantation recipients: a global perspective. *Biol Blood Marrow Transpl.* 2009;15:1143–1238.

44. Cordonnier C, Labopin M, Chesnel V, et al. Randomized study of early versus late immunization with pneumococcal conjugate vaccine after allogeneic stem cell transplantation. *Clin Infect Dis.* 2009;48:1392–1401.

45. Stadtmauer EA, Sullivan KM, Marty FM, et al. A phase 1/2 study of an adjuvanted varicella-zoster virus subunit vaccine in autologous hematopoietic cell transplant recipients. *Blood.* 2014;124:2921–2929.

46. Danziger-Isakov L, Kumar D. Practice ASTIDCo. Vaccination in solid organ transplantation. *Am J Transpl.* 2013;13(suppl 4):311–317.

47. Chong PP, Avery RK. A comprehensive review of immunization practices in solid organ transplant and hematopoietic stem cell transplant recipients. *Clin Ther.* 2017;39:1581–1598.

48. Kumar D, Campbell P, Hoschler K, et al. Randomized controlled trial of adjuvanted versus nonadjuvanted influenza vaccine in kidney transplant recipients. *Transplantation.* 2016;100:662–669.

49. GiaQuinta S, Michaels MG, McCullers JA, et al. Randomized, double-blind comparison of standard-dose vs. high-dose trivalent inactivated influenza vaccine in pediatric solid organ transplant patients. *Pediatr Transpl.* 2015;19:219–228.

50. Cordero E, Roca-Oporto C, Bulnes-Ramos A, et al. Two doses of inactivated influenza vaccine improve immune response in solid organ transplant recipients: results of TRANSGRIPE 1-2, a randomized controlled clinical trial. *Clin Infect Dis.* 2017;64:829–838.

51. Hurst FP, Lee JJ, Jindal RM, Agodoa LY, Abbott KC. Outcomes associated with influenza vaccination in the first year after kidney transplantation. *Clin J Am Soc Nephrol.* 2011;6:1192–1197.

52. Avery RK. Influenza vaccines in the setting of solid-organ transplantation: are they safe? *Curr Opin Infect Dis.* 2012; 25:464–468.

53. White-Williams C, Brown R, Kirklin J, et al. Improving clinical practice: should we give influenza vaccinations to heart transplant patients? *J Heart Lung Transpl.* 2006; 25:320–323.

54. Cohet C, Haguinet F, Dos Santos G, et al. Effect of the adjuvanted (AS03) A/H1N1 2009 pandemic influenza vaccine on the risk of rejection in solid organ transplant recipients in England: a self-controlled case series. *BMJ Open.* 2016;6:e009264.

55. Perez-Romero P, Bulnes-Ramos A, Torre-Cisneros J, et al. Influenza vaccination during the first 6 months after solid organ transplantation is efficacious and safe. *Clin Microbiol Infect.* 2015;21(1040):e11–e18.

56. Halperin SA, Ward B, Cooper C, et al. Comparison of safety and immunogenicity of two doses of investigational hepatitis B virus surface antigen co-administered with an immunostimulatory phosphorothioate oligodeoxyribonucleotide and three doses of a licensed hepatitis B vaccine in healthy adults 18-55 years of age. *Vaccine.* 2012;30:2556–2563.

57. Heyward WL, Kyle M, Blumenau J, et al. Immunogenicity and safety of an investigational hepatitis B vaccine with a Toll-like receptor 9 agonist adjuvant (HBsAg-1018) compared to a licensed hepatitis B vaccine in healthy adults 40-70 years of age. *Vaccine.* 2013;31:5300–5305.

58. Jackson S, Lentino J, Kopp J, et al. Immunogenicity of a two-dose investigational hepatitis B vaccine, HBsAg-1018, using a toll-like receptor 9 agonist adjuvant compared with a licensed hepatitis B vaccine in adults. *Vaccine.* 2018;36:668–674.

59. Marshall H, McMillan M, Andrews RM, Macartney K, Edwards K. Vaccines in pregnancy: the dual benefit for pregnant women and infants. *Hum Vaccin Immunother.* 2016;12:848–856.

60. Donahue JG, Kieke BA, King JP, et al. Association of spontaneous abortion with receipt of inactivated influenza vaccine containing H1N1pdm09 in 2010-11 and 2011-12. *Vaccine.* 2017;35:5314–5322.

61. Chambers CD, Johnson DL, Xu R, et al. Safety of the 2010-11, 2011-12, 2012-13, and 2013-14 seasonal influenza vaccines in pregnancy: birth defects, spontaneous abortion, preterm delivery, and small for gestational age infants, a study from the cohort arm of VAMPSS. *Vaccine.* 2016;34:4443–4449.

62. Chambers CD, Johnson D, Xu R, et al. Risks and safety of pandemic H1N1 influenza vaccine in pregnancy: birth defects, spontaneous abortion, preterm delivery, and small for gestational age infants. *Vaccine.* 2013;31: 5026–5032.

63. Chambers CD, Xu R, Mitchell AA. Commentary on: "Association of spontaneous abortion with receipt of inactivated influenza vaccine containing H1N1pdm09 in 2010-11 and 2011-12". *Vaccine.* 2017;35:5323–5324.

64. Committee on Obstetric Practice I. Emerging infections expert work G. Committee Opinion No. 718: update on immunization and pregnancy: tetanus, diphtheria, and pertussis vaccination. *Obstet Gynecol.* 2017;130:e153–e157.

65. Tsatsaris V, Capitant C, Schmitz T, et al. Maternal immune response and neonatal seroprotection from a single dose of a monovalent nonadjuvanted 2009 influenza A(H1N1) vaccine: a single-group trial. *Ann Intern Med.* 2011;155:733–741.

66. Kuchar E, Miskiewicz K, Karlikowska M. A review of guidance on immunization in persons with defective or deficient splenic function. *Br J Haematol.* 2015;171: 683–694.

67. Folaranmi T, Rubin L, Martin SW, Patel M, MacNeil JR. Centers for disease C. Use of serogroup B meningococcal vaccines in persons aged ≥10 years at increased risk for serogroup B meningococcal disease: recommendations of the advisory committee on immunization practices, 2015. *MMWR Morb Mortal Wkly Rep.* 2015;64:608–612.

68. Levin MJ, Song LY, Fenton T, et al. Shedding of live vaccine virus, comparative safety, and influenza-specific antibody responses after administration of live attenuated and inactivated trivalent influenza vaccines to HIV-infected children. *Vaccine.* 2008;26:4210–4217.

69. Block SL, Yogev R, Hayden FG, Ambrose CS, Zeng W, Walker RE. Shedding and immunogenicity of live attenuated influenza vaccine virus in subjects 5-49 years of age. *Vaccine.* 2008;26:4940–4946.

70. Mallory RM, Yi T, Ambrose CS. Shedding of Ann Arbor strain live attenuated influenza vaccine virus in children 6-59 months of age. *Vaccine.* 2011;29:4322–4327.

71. Boikos C, Joseph L, Martineau C, et al. Influenza virus detection following administration of live-attenuated intranasal influenza vaccine in children with cystic fibrosis and their healthy siblings. *Open Forum Infect Dis.* 2016;3:ofw187.

72. Pebody R, McMenamin J, Nohynek H. Live attenuated influenza vaccine (LAIV): recent effectiveness results from the USA and implications for LAIV programmes elsewhere. *Arch Dis Child.* 2018;103(1):101–105.

73. Hsieh YC, Wu FT, Hsiung CA, Wu HS, Chang KY, Huang YC. Comparison of virus shedding after lived attenuated and pentavalent reassortant rotavirus vaccine. *Vaccine.* 2014;32:1199–1204.

74. Reid G, Huprikar S, Patel G, et al. A multicenter evaluation of pandemic influenza A/H1N1 in hematopoietic stem cell transplant recipients. *Transpl Infect Dis.* 2013; 15:487–492.

75. Grohskopf LA, Sokolow LZ, Broder KR, et al. Prevention and control of seasonal influenza with vaccines: recommendations of the advisory committee on immunization practices—United States, 2017-18 influenza season. *MMWR Recomm Rep.* 2017;66:1–20.

76. Grohskopf LA, Sokolow LZ, Broder KR, et al. Prevention and control of seasonal influenza with vaccines. *MMWR Recomm Rep.* 2016;65:1–54.

77. Reber AJ, Chirkova T, Kim JH, et al. Immunosenescence and challenges of vaccination against influenza in the aging population. *Aging Dis.* 2012;3:68–90.

78. Goodwin K, Viboud C, Simonsen L. Antibody response to influenza vaccination in the elderly: a quantitative review. *Vaccine.* 2006;24:1159–1169.

79. Potter CW, Oxford JS. Determinants of immunity to influenza infection in man. *Br Med Bull.* 1979;35:69–75.

80. Darvishian M, van den Heuvel ER, Bissielo A, et al. Effectiveness of seasonal influenza vaccination in community-dwelling elderly people: an individual participant data meta-analysis of test-negative design case-control studies. *Lancet Respir Med.* 2017;5:200–211.

81. Zbinden D, Manuel O. Influenza vaccination in immunocompromised patients: efficacy and safety. *Immunotherapy.* 2014;6:131–139.

82. Schuurmans MM, Tini GM, Dalar L, Fretz G, Benden C, Boehler A. Pandemic 2009 H1N1 influenza virus vaccination in lung transplant recipients: coverage, safety and clinical effectiveness in the Zurich cohort. *J Heart Lung Transpl.* 2011;30:685–690.

83. Scharpe J, Evenepoel P, Maes B, et al. Influenza vaccination is efficacious and safe in renal transplant recipients. *Am J Transpl.* 2008;8:332–337.

84. Machado CM, Cardoso MR, da Rocha IF, Boas LS, Dulley FL, Pannuti CS. The benefit of influenza vaccination after bone marrow transplantation. *Bone Marrow Transpl.* 2005;36:897–900.

85. Beck CR, McKenzie BC, Hashim AB, Harris RC, University of Nottingham I, the ImmunoCompromised Study G, et al. Influenza vaccination for immunocompromised patients: systematic review and meta-analysis by etiology. *J Infect Dis.* 2012;206:1250–1259.

86. Bitterman R, Eliakim-Raz N, Vinograd I, Zalmanovici Trestioreanu A, Leibovici L, Paul M. Influenza vaccines in immunosuppressed adults with cancer. *Cochrane Database Syst Rev.* 2018;2:CD008983.

87. Falsey AR, Treanor JJ, Tornieporth N, Capellan J, Gorse GJ. Randomized, double-blind controlled phase 3 trial comparing the immunogenicity of high-dose and standard-dose influenza vaccine in adults 65 years of age and older. *J Infect Dis.* 2009;200:172–180.

88. Summary Basis for Regulatory Action. *Fluzone High-dose. U.S. Department of Health and Human Services.* Food and Drug Administration; December 23, 2009.

89. DiazGranados CA, Dunning AJ, Kimmel M, et al. Efficacy of high-dose versus standard-dose influenza vaccine in older adults. *N Engl J Med.* 2014;371:635–645.

90. McKittrick N, Frank I, Jacobson JM, et al. Improved immunogenicity with high-dose seasonal influenza vaccine in HIV-infected persons: a single-center, parallel, randomized trial. *Ann Intern Med.* 2013;158:19–26.

91. Halasa NB, Savani BN, Asokan I, et al. Randomized double-blind study of the safety and immunogenicity of standard-dose trivalent inactivated influenza vaccine versus high-dose trivalent inactivated influenza vaccine in adult hematopoietic stem cell transplantation patients. *Biol Blood Marrow Transpl.* 2016;22:528–535.

92. Jamshed S, Walsh EE, Dimitroff LJ, Santelli JS, Falsey AR. Improved immunogenicity of high-dose influenza vaccine compared to standard-dose influenza vaccine in adult oncology patients younger than 65 years receiving chemotherapy: a pilot randomized clinical trial. *Vaccine.* 2016;34:630–635.

93. *Fluad [Package Insert].* Holly Springs, NC: Seqirus; 2017.

94. Fabbiani M, Di Giambenedetto S, Sali M, et al. Immune response to influenza A (H1N1)v monovalent MF59-adjuvanted vaccine in HIV-infected patients. *Vaccine.* 2011;29:2836–2839.

95. Mohty B, Bel M, Vukicevic M, et al. Graft-versus-host disease is the major determinant of humoral responses to the AS03-adjuvanted influenza A/09/H1N1 vaccine in allogeneic hematopoietic stem cell transplant recipients. *Haematologica.* 2011;96:896–904.

96. Gabay C, Bel M, Combescure C, et al. Impact of synthetic and biologic disease-modifying antirheumatic drugs on antibody responses to the AS03-adjuvanted pandemic influenza vaccine: a prospective, open-label, parallel-cohort, single-center study. *Arthritis Rheum.* 2011;63:1486–1496.

97. Hung IFN, Yuen KY. Immunogenicity, safety and tolerability of intradermal influenza vaccines. *Hum Vaccin Immunother.* 2017:1–6.

98. Pileggi C, Lotito F, Bianco A, Nobile CG, Pavia M. Immunogenicity and safety of intradermal influenza vaccine in immunocompromised patients: a meta-analysis of randomized controlled trials. *BMC Infect Dis.* 2015; 15:427.

99. Baluch A, Humar A, Eurich D, et al. Randomized controlled trial of high-dose intradermal versus standard-dose intramuscular influenza vaccine in organ transplant recipients. *Am J Transpl.* 2013;13:1026–1033.

100. Izikson R, Leffell DJ, Bock SA, et al. Randomized comparison of the safety of Flublok((R)) versus licensed inactivated influenza vaccine in healthy, medically stable adults ≥50 years of age. *Vaccine.* 2015;33: 6622–6628.

101. Dunkle LM, Izikson R, Patriarca P, et al. Efficacy of recombinant influenza vaccine in adults 50 years of age or older. *N Engl J Med.* 2017;376:2427–2436.

102. Liao Z, Xu X, Liang Y, Xiong Y, Chen R, Ni J. Effect of a booster dose of influenza vaccine in patients with hemodialysis, peritoneal dialysis and renal transplant recipients: a systematic literature review and meta-analysis. *Hum Vaccin Immunother.* 2016;12:2909–2915.

103. Blumberg EA, Albano C, Pruett T, et al. The immunogenicity of influenza virus vaccine in solid organ transplant recipients. *Clin Infect Dis.* 1996;22:295–302.

104. Engelhard D, Nagler A, Hardan I, et al. Antibody response to a two-dose regimen of influenza vaccine in allogeneic T cell-depleted and autologous BMT recipients. *Bone Marrow Transpl.* 1993;11:1–5.

105. Pneumococcal Vaccination: Information for Healthcare Professionals; Available from: https://www.cdc.gov/vaccines/vpd/pneumo/hcp/index.html; Accessed February 2, 2018.

106. Daniels CC, Rogers PD, Shelton CM. A review of pneumococcal vaccines: current polysaccharide vaccine recommendations and future protein antigens. *J Pediatr Pharmacol Ther*. 2016;21:27–35.

107. van Deursen AMM, van Houten MA, Webber C, et al. The impact of the 13-valent pneumococcal conjugate vaccine on pneumococcal carriage in the community acquired Pneumonia immunization trial in adults (CAPiTA) study. *Clin Infect Dis*. 2018;67(1):42–49.

108. Benamu E, Montoya JG. Infections associated with the use of eculizumab: recommendations for prevention and prophylaxis. *Curr Opin Infect Dis*. 2016;29:319–329.

109. Briere EC, Rubin L, Moro PL, et al. Prevention and control of haemophilus influenzae type b disease: recommendations of the advisory committee on immunization practices (ACIP). *MMWR Recomm Rep*. 2014;63:1–14.

110. Poland GA. Hepatitis B immunization in health care workers. Dealing with vaccine nonresponse. *Am J Prev Med*. 1998;15:73–77.

111. Whitaker JA, Rouphael NG, Edupuganti S, Lai L, Mulligan MJ. Strategies to increase responsiveness to hepatitis B vaccination in adults with HIV-1. *Lancet Infect Dis*. 2012;12:966–976.

112. Propst T, Propst A, Lhotta K, Vogel W, Konig P. Reinforced intradermal hepatitis B vaccination in hemodialysis patients is superior in antibody response to intramuscular or subcutaneous vaccination. *Am J Kidney Dis*. 1998;32:1041–1045.

113. Eleftheriadis T, Pissas G, Antoniadi G, Liakopoulos V, Stefanidis I. Factors affecting effectiveness of vaccination against hepatitis B virus in hemodialysis patients. *World J Gastroenterol*. 2014;20:12018–12025.

114. Horlander JC, Boyle N, Manam R, et al. Vaccination against hepatitis B in patients with chronic liver disease awaiting liver transplantation. *Am J Med Sci*. 1999;318:304–307.

115. Centers for Disease Control and Prevention. *Guidelines for Vaccinating Kidney Dialysis Patients and Patients with Chronic Kidney Disease*. July 2015.

116. Fabrizi F, Dixit V, Magnini M, Elli A, Martin P. Meta-analysis: intradermal vs. intramuscular vaccination against hepatitis B virus in patients with chronic kidney disease. *Aliment Pharmacol Ther*. 2006;24:497–506.

117. Fabrizi F, Andrulli S, Bacchini G, Corti M, Locatelli F. Intradermal versus intramuscular hepatitis B re-vaccination in non-responsive chronic dialysis patients: a prospective randomized study with cost-effectiveness evaluation. *Nephrol Dial Transpl*. 1997;12:1204–1211.

118. Yousaf F, Gandham S, Galler M, Spinowitz B, Charytan C. Systematic review of the efficacy and safety of intradermal versus intramuscular hepatitis B vaccination in end-stage renal disease population unresponsive to primary vaccination series. *Ren Fail*. 2015;37:1080–1088.

119. Barry M, Cooper C. Review of hepatitis B surface antigen-1018 ISS adjuvant-containing vaccine safety and efficacy. *Expert Opin Biol Ther*. 2007;7:1731–1737.

120. Tong NK, Beran J, Kee SA, et al. Immunogenicity and safety of an adjuvanted hepatitis B vaccine in pre-hemodialysis and hemodialysis patients. *Kidney Int*. 2005;68:2298–2303.

121. Lindemann M, Zaslavskaya M, Fiedler M, et al. Humoral and cellular responses to a single dose of Fendrix in renal transplant recipients with non-response to previous hepatitis B vaccination. *Scand J Immunol*. 2017;85:51–57.

122. de Silva TI, Green ST, Cole J, Stone BJ, Dockrell DH, Vedio AB. Successful use of Fendrix in HIV-infected non-responders to standard hepatitis B vaccines. *J Infect*. 2014;68:397–399.

123. Advisory Committee on Immunization P, Fiore AE, Wasley A, Bell BP. Prevention of hepatitis A through active or passive immunization: recommendations of the advisory committee on immunization practices (ACIP). *MMWR Recomm Rep*. 2006;55:1–23.

124. Hens N, Habteab Ghebretinsae A, Hardt K, Van Damme P, Van Herck K. Model based estimates of long-term persistence of inactivated hepatitis A vaccine-induced antibodies in adults. *Vaccine*. 2014;32:1507–1513.

125. Theeten H, Van Herck K, Van Der Meeren O, Crasta P, Van Damme P, Hens N. Long-term antibody persistence after vaccination with a 2-dose Havrix (inactivated hepatitis A vaccine): 20 years of observed data, and long-term model-based predictions. *Vaccine*. 2015;33:5723–5727.

126. Overton ET, Nurutdinova D, Sungkanuparph S, Seyfried W, Groger RK, Powderly WG. Predictors of immunity after hepatitis A vaccination in HIV-infected persons. *J Viral Hepat*. 2007;14:189–193.

127. Launay O, Grabar S, Gordien E, et al. Immunological efficacy of a three-dose schedule of hepatitis A vaccine in HIV-infected adults: HEPAVAC study. *J Acquir Immune Defic Syndr*. 2008;49:272–275.

128. Petrosky E, Bocchini Jr JA, Hariri S, et al. Use of 9-valent human papillomavirus (HPV) vaccine: updated HPV vaccination recommendations of the advisory committee on immunization practices. *MMWR Morb Mortal Wkly Rep*. 2015;64:300–304.

129. Measles Mumps, and Rubella (MMR): Vaccination Information for Healthcare Professionals; Available from: https://www.cdc.gov/vaccines/vpd/mmr/hcp/index.html; Accessed February 2, 2018.

130. Scott P, Moss WJ, Gilani Z, Low N. Measles vaccination in HIV-infected children: systematic review and meta-analysis of safety and immunogenicity. *J Infect Dis*. 2011;204(suppl 1):S164–S178.

131. Koochakzadeh L, Khosravi MH, Pourakbari B, Hosseinverdi S, Aghamohammadi A, Rezaei N. Assessment of immune response following immunization with DTP/Td and MMR vaccines in children treated for acute lymphoblastic leukemia. *Pediatr Hematol Oncol*. 2014;31:656–663.

132. Machado CM, de Souza VA, Sumita LM, da Rocha IF, Dulley FL, Pannuti CS. Early measles vaccination in bone marrow transplant recipients. *Bone Marrow Transpl.* 2005;35:787–791.

133. Gershon AA, Breuer J, Cohen JI, et al. Varicella zoster virus infection. *Nat Rev Dis Primers.* 2015;1:15016.

134. Marin M, Guris D, Chaves SS, et al. Prevention of varicella: recommendations of the advisory committee on immunization practices (ACIP). *MMWR Recomm Rep.* 2007;56:1–40.

135. Advisory Committee on Immunization P. Centers for disease C, prevention. Immunization of health-care personnel: recommendations of the advisory committee on immunization practices (ACIP). *MMWR Recomm Rep.* 2011;60:1–45.

136. Kuter BJ, Ngai A, Patterson CM, et al. Safety, tolerability, and immunogenicity of two regimens of Oka/Merck varicella vaccine (Varivax) in healthy adolescents and adults. Oka/Merck Varicella Vaccine Study Group. *Vaccine.* 1995;13:967–972.

137. Ngai AL, Staehle BO, Kuter BJ, et al. Safety and immunogenicity of one vs. two injections of Oka/Merck varicella vaccine in healthy children. *Pediatr Infect Dis J.* 1996;15:49–54.

138. Crum-Cianflone NF, Sullivan E. Vaccinations for the HIV-infected adult: a review of the current recommendations, Part II. *Infect Dis Ther.* 2017;6:333–361.

139. Harpaz R, Ortega-Sanchez IR, Seward JF, Advisory Committee on Immunization Practices Centers for Disease C, Prevention. Prevention of herpes zoster: recommendations of the advisory committee on immunization practices (ACIP). *MMWR Recomm Rep.* 2008;57:1–30;quiz CE2–4.

140. Oxman MN, Levin MJ, Johnson GR, et al. A vaccine to prevent herpes zoster and postherpetic neuralgia in older adults. *N Engl J Med.* 2005;352:2271–2284.

141. Schmader KE, Levin MJ, Gnann Jr JW, et al. Efficacy, safety, and tolerability of herpes zoster vaccine in persons aged 50-59 years. *Clin Infect Dis.* 2012;54:922–928.

142. Tseng HF, Harpaz R, Luo Y, et al. Declining effectiveness of herpes zoster vaccine in adults aged ≥60 years. *J Infect Dis.* 2016;213:1872–1875.

143. Food and Drug Administration. "SHINGRIX." Avaialbe from: https://www.fda.gov/biologicsbloodvaccines/vaccines/approvedproducts/ucm581491.htm; Accessed August 20, 2018.

144. Lal H, Cunningham AL, Godeaux O, et al. Efficacy of an adjuvanted herpes zoster subunit vaccine in older adults. *N Engl J Med.* 2015;372:2087–2096.

145. Cunningham AL, Lal H, Kovac M, et al. Efficacy of the herpes zoster subunit vaccine in adults 70 years of age or older. *N Engl J Med.* 2016;375:1019–1032.

146. Weinberg A, Zhang JH, Oxman MN, et al. Varicella-zoster virus-specific immune responses to herpes zoster in elderly participants in a trial of a clinically effective zoster vaccine. *J Infect Dis.* 2009;200:1068–1077.

147. Oxman MN, Gershon AA, Poland GA. Zoster vaccine recommendations: the importance of using a clinically valid correlate of protection. *Vaccine.* 2011;29:3625–3627.

148. Oxman MN. Zoster vaccine: current status and future prospects. *Clin Infect Dis.* 2010;51:197–213.

149. Hayward A, Levin M, Wolf W, Angelova G, Gilden D. Varicella-zoster virus-specific immunity after herpes zoster. *J Infect Dis.* 1991;163:873–875.

150. Hayward AR, Herberger M. Lymphocyte responses to varicella zoster virus in the elderly. *J Clin Immunol.* 1987;7:174–178.

151. Hata A, Asanuma H, Rinki M, et al. Use of an inactivated varicella vaccine in recipients of hematopoietic-cell transplants. *N Engl J Med.* 2002;347:26–34.

152. Weinberg A, Canniff J, Rouphael N, et al. Varicella-zoster virus-specific cellular immune responses to the live attenuated zoster vaccine in young and older adults. *J Immunol.* 2017;199:604–612.

153. Chlibek R, Smetana J, Pauksens K, et al. Safety and immunogenicity of three different formulations of an adjuvanted varicella-zoster virus subunit candidate vaccine in older adults: a phase II, randomized, controlled study. *Vaccine.* 2014;32:1745–1753.

154. Leroux-Roels I, Leroux-Roels G, Clement F, et al. A phase 1/2 clinical trial evaluating safety and immunogenicity of a varicella zoster glycoprotein e subunit vaccine candidate in young and older adults. *J Infect Dis.* 2012;206:1280–1290.

155. Cunningham AL, Heineman T. Vaccine profile of herpes zoster (HZ/su) subunit vaccine. *Expert Rev Vaccines.* 2017;16:1–10.

CHAPTER 10

Vaccines for Adult Travelers: When and Why?

MARIA D. MILENO, MD • COLLEEN LAU, MBBS (UWA), MPH&TM (JCU), PHD (UQ), FRACGP, FFTM (ACTM), FACTM • JOHN R. LONKS, MD • JOSEPH M. GARLAND, MD • MARTHA C. SANCHEZ, MD • GERARD J. NAU, MD, PHD • JEROME M. LARKIN, MD

VACCINES FOR ADULT TRAVELERS: WHEN AND WHY?

The value of a pretravel consultation extends well beyond the provision of immunizations that are mandatory for entry into countries with required immunizations. Travel can be a pivotal health experience in the life of an individual traveler. Often it is a touchpoint for assessment of an individual's wellness and ability to embark—clearly it is not "just shots." Travel continues to grow substantially—increasing numbers of individuals of all ages with diverse baseline medical wellness or underlying immune compromise are traveling to remote places for business, pleasure as well as planned and unexpected distant family visits to congregate with their loved ones, and sometimes even to bury them. For occupational purposes or just fun, travelers may plan trips with unexpected high risk for malaria or with need for yellow fever vaccine which may itself pose risk in older individuals. Often, expert conversation and guidance can encourage and impact further preparation and prophylaxis. Other infectious exposures may vary based on the travel itinerary, likely activity while traveling, underlying health, and prior immunizations. The pretravel consultation is an optimal time to ensure that routine immunizations are up to date particularly if infectious risks may increase during travel, e.g., diphtheria, measles, and varicella. As well, practical preemptive dosing of tetanus boosters helps to avoid need for the traveler to seek healthcare to obtain a tetanus booster at the time of an injury. Tdap includes protection against pertussis that has spread in small epidemics throughout the US even among adults. Influenza is the most common vaccine-preventable, travel-related disease, and transmission in the tropics is year-round rather than seasonal. An evaluation of cardiac fitness and general mobility is often

important for elderly travelers. Immune responses may wane—indeed elderly people are not all the same! Concise and complete educational guidance should help individuals understand the need to attempt to bolster immunity to *Streptococcus pneumoniae*, hepatitis B, and herpes zoster. Here we summarize the approach to vaccinating adult travelers using the most current guidelines. Routine vaccinations for all adult travelers can be found through the Centers for Disease Control.[1,2]

HEPATITIS A VACCINE

Hepatitis A virus is a nonenveloped positive strand RNA virus, member of the Picornavirus family that is mainly transmitted through fecal-oral routes and exposure to contaminated food and water sources. It commonly causes a self-limited inflammatory response in the liver which is associated with nonspecific symptoms and signs including fatigue, nausea, vomiting, or low-grade fever, but in rare cases it may progress to fulminant hepatitis and liver failure.[1] It affects about 1.5 million people worldwide per year, and it is one of the most common vaccine-preventable infectious diseases in travelers.[2] Ideally individuals should plan to receive the hepatitis A vaccine at least 1 month in advance of travel. In practice, last-minute vaccination is given, and there is good evidence that hepatitis A vaccine is protective soon after it is given.[3] The individual's immune response rises in response to acute encounters with hepatitis A virus during travel. This highly immunogenic vaccine is thought to provide lifelong protection once the primary course has been completed.[4]

There are two licensed Hepatitis A antigen vaccines available in the United States for individuals aged 12 months and above, HAVRIX (manufactured by

Vaccinations. https://doi.org/10.1016/B978-0-323-55435-0.00010-0

GlaxoSmithKline) and VAQTA (manufactured by Merck & Co., Inc.). The schedule for HAVRIX is at 0 and 6–12 months and for VAQTA at 0 and 6–18 months. Vaccine is recommended for travelers to countries with intermediate-to-high prevalence for Hepatitis A.

Protective antibody levels are detected in 54%–62% of healthy adults at 14 days and >94% 1 month after vaccination.

A combined inactivated hepatitis A and hepatitis B vaccine (Twinrix, GlaxoSmithKline) is available for those aged 18 years and above to be given in a three-dose series at 0, 1, and 6 months or an accelerated schedule at 0, 7, and 21–30 days with a booster at 12 months.

Adverse effects: Pain at the injection site (56%–67%) and headache (14%–16%) are the most common vaccine side effects reported in adults.

Contraindications: Hepatitis A vaccine should not be administered to those with a history of severe allergic reaction such as anaphylaxis to any component of the vaccine.

Pregnancy: The risk to the fetus when the vaccine is given during pregnancy has not been determined; because the vaccine is inactivated, it is suspected to be low.[5] If the risk of hepatitis A at destination is moderate to high, this outweighs the risk of giving hepatitis A vaccine.

Safety: The vaccine may be given to immunocompromised patient because it is inactivated.

Hepatitis A immunoglobulin: GamaSTAN S/D is available in the United States for temporary protection against hepatitis A infection, with recommended dosing of 0.1 mL/kg for up to 1 month of planned travel duration and 0.2 mL/kg for up to 2 months.[6] It may be given in conjunction with the Hepatitis A vaccine for those traveling in less than 2 weeks, and it should be given at the same time at separate anatomic sites. It is rarely needed given the high immunogenicity of the Hepatitis A vaccine but is considered for use in older adult, immunocompromised persons, and those with chronic liver disease or other chronic medical conditions.[7] Travelers may receive the Hepatitis A immunoglobulin alone if they are aged <12 months, are allergic to a component of the vaccine, or choose not to receive the vaccine.

For postexposure prophylaxis, immunoglobulin must be given within 2 weeks of exposure.[6]

HEPATITIS B VACCINE

Hepatitis B is a DNA virus in the Hepadnavirus family which is an important cause of chronic liver disease worldwide that may lead to liver cirrhosis and hepatocellular carcinoma. The forms of transmission in travelers are through unprotected sexual contact and parenteral or mucosal exposure to infected blood and body fluids. The liver is the main site of infection causing asymptomatic and symptomatic disease. The primary infection is usually self-limited in immunocompetent adults causing chronic infection in about 5%, but it may be as high as 30%–90% in children aged <5 years.[1,2]

The pretravel consultation is an ideal time to offer hepatitis B vaccine to adults who have escaped the pediatrician for its administration. Persons born in 1992 and beyond have had this vaccine as part of their pediatric schedule. Travelers to areas of intermediate and high endemicity are at risk of acquiring infection, particularly healthcare workers, disaster relief personnel, recipients of medical care, and those engaging in sexual activity, intravenous drug use, and tattooing.

Two single-antigen vaccines against Hepatitis B are available in the United States, Recombivax HB (Merck & Co., Inc., Whitehouse Station, New Jersey) and Engerix-B (GlaxoSmithKline Biologicals, Rixensart, Belgium). Either should be administered at 0, 1, and 6 months, but alternate schedules of 0, 2, and 4 months or 0, 1, and 4 months will provide similar immunological responses. Thirty to fifty percent of healthy adults will have protective antibody levels after the first dose, 75% after the second dose, and 90% after the third dose.

An accelerated schedule may be given on days 0, 7, and 21, followed by a booster at 12 months.[3]

The Hepatitis B vaccine, after the completed vaccination series, provides protection for about 20 years and possibly lifelong.

It may make it easier for travelers to complete a protective series against hepatitis B infection now that the Food and Drug Administration (FDA) has approved Heplisav-B (hepatitis B vaccine, recombinant [adjuvanted]; Dynavax)—a two-dose series spaced 1 month apart—for the prevention of infection caused by all known subtypes of hepatitis B virus for use in adults aged 18 years and above.[5] A combined inactivated hepatitis A and hepatitis B vaccine (Twinrix, GlaxoSmithKline) is available for those aged 18 years and above to be given at 0, 1, and 6 months or in an accelerated schedule at 0, 7, and 21–30 days with a booster dose at 12 months.

Adverse events: Most common reported side effects are pain at the injection site in >10%. Other reactions such as low-grade fever, myalgia, and headaches are rare (<1%).

Contraindications: Hepatitis B vaccine should not be administered to those with a history of severe allergic reaction, such as anaphylaxis to yeast or any other component of the vaccine.

Safety: The vaccine may be given to immunocompromised patients because it is inactivated.

Pregnancy: The vaccine contains a noninfectious Hepatitis B surface antigen, and there is no known risk to the developing fetus.

Postexposure prophylaxis: Hepatitis B immunoglobulin may be administered in case of conjunction of the hepatitis B vaccines in patients after high risk exposure with infected blood or body fluids within 24 h of exposure.[4]

TYPHOID VACCINE

Travelers to destinations beyond North America, Western Europe, Australia and New Zealand, and high-income countries in Asia e.g., Hong Kong, Japan, and Singapore are at risk for typhoid fever, the clinical disease caused by *Salmonella enterica* serovar Typhi (*S. enterica* serovar *Typhi*). A similar disease is also caused by the related organisms *S. enterica* serovar Paratyphi types A, B, and C. Collectively causing enteric fevers, the disease is transmitted by fecal-oral transmission of the bacteria. Ingestion results in local replication within the intestine followed by systemic spread during which blood cultures can be positive in 60%–80% of patients.[1] Clinically the disease is characterized by insidious onset of fatigue and fever, along with malaise, headache, and anorexia.[2]

S. enterica serovar *Typhi* and *S. paratyphi* are globally distributed but principally found in developing countries.[1,3] The highest prevalence is found in southern and southeast Asia, especially in children: The incidence can be as high as 30 cases per 1000 per year.[3] Together, these infections account for approximately 1% of all enteric fever–related deaths globally.[3]

Ongoing progression and geographic expansion of antibiotic resistance has complicated the management of typhoid fever. Mortality rates approach 26% if treated without effective antimicrobials, but resistance has compromised standard therapy with trimethoprim-sulfamethoxazole, ampicillin, and even the fluoroquinolones.[3] Reports of *S. enterica* serovar *Typhi* strains with extended-spectrum B-lactamases are also increasing.[3] Owing to these concerns, azithromycin has become the recommended antibiotic for treatment of severe traveler's diarrhea.

Prevention is the preferred strategy for protecting travelers from typhoid fever. In addition to scrupulous water and food precautions, two vaccines are approved to prevent this disease. Vaccination is recommended for all travelers who may encounter *S. enterica* serovar *Typhi*, especially those with prolonged exposure to possibly contaminated food and drink.[2] Conversely, routine typhoid vaccination is not recommended for nontraveling residents of the United States. Vaccination is recommended, however, for household members of carriers of *S. enterica* serovar *Typhi* or laboratory workers at risk of exposure.

One typhoid vaccine is Ty21a, an oral vaccine comprised of a live, attenuated derivative of *S. enterica* serovar *Typhi* strain Ty21. In the United States this is available as a four-dose blister pack that must be refrigerated until taken. The administration is complex, requiring that one capsule is taken by mouth 1 h before a meal every other day until completion of all the doses.[2,4] This vaccine is licensed for use in individuals aged 6 years. Clinical trials evaluating a three-dose regimen of Ty21a were performed in endemic countries. These trials demonstrated that protection is approximately 60%.[2,4] It is recommended that the four-dose regimen be repeated every 5 years if there is a risk of reexposure. Because it is a live vaccine, it is contraindicated in immunocompromised individuals and pregnant mothers.[2] It should also be avoided in individuals with an acute febrile illness or gastroenteritis.[2] In addition, antibiotics may compromise the efficacy of Ty21a. Therefore the regimen should begin at least 3 days after the last dose of an antibiotic and finish at least 3 days before initiating antibiotic therapy.

The alternative for typhoid prevention is an inactivated parenteral vaccine containing the Vi capsular polysaccharide of the bacteria. This product is administered as a single intramuscular injection of the polysaccharide. It has the advantage of approved use for individuals older than 2 years, although efficacy in the 2- to 4-year-old group is uncertain.[2] Depending on the study, efficacy of this vaccine is 60%–80%, and readministration is recommended every 2 years.[2,4] There are fewer precautions with this formulation, although its activity and safety are undefined for immunocompromised patients or during pregnancy.[2]

There is great interest in improving typhoid vaccination because the efficacy of the existing vaccines is less than 100% and it can be overcome by a high inoculum of *S. enterica* serovar *Typhi*.[2] Moreover, neither of the vaccines is recommended for children younger than 2 years, principally because data are lacking. A new generation of vaccines, however, is being developed. These are conjugate vaccines in which the Vi polysaccharide is linked to an immunogenic protein, such as tetanus toxoid, diphtheria toxoid, or a recombinant exoprotein from *Pseudomonas aeruginosa*.[3] Early trials suggest these vaccines are at least as effective as the existing vaccines and have activity in infants younger than 2 years.[3,4] Combined hepatitis A/typhoid vaccine is available in Australia.

YELLOW FEVER VACCINE

Pathogen and transmission: Yellow fever is a mosquito-borne viral disease. It occurs in many African and South American countries. A list of countries is available in the online version of the *CDC Health Information for International Travel* book.[1] The mosquito vector, *Aedes* species, that carries the yellow fever virus does not live at high altitudes. For some countries there is marked regional variation in the risk of acquiring yellow fever with high risk for acquisition at low altitudes and no risk at high altitudes.

Epidemiology: Worldwide there are about 200,000 cases with about 30,000 deaths each year. An exact number of cases and deaths is not known because most cases occur in areas of the world which are largely rural where there is a lack of ability to make an exact diagnosis, as well there is inadequate surveillance and reporting available.

Clinical disease: Most cases of yellow fever are asymptomatic; however, symptomatic disease can be very severe, and often fatal. The incubation period for yellow fever virus infection is approximately 3–6 days. Systemic symptoms include fever, headache, photophobia, myalgia, arthralgia, anorexia, abdominal pain, vomiting, jaundice, hemorrhagic complications, and multisystem organ failure. Some patients show leukopenia during the first week of illness and leukocytosis during the second week of illness. Bleeding dyscrasia can occur with elevated prothrombin and partial thromboplastin levels and decreased platelet counts. For those with severe yellow fever, the mortality rate is approximately 25%–50%.

There is no specific treatment for yellow fever virus infections, and management is totally with supportive care.

Risk for travelers: From 1970 to 2015 there were 10 cases of yellow fever reported in unvaccinated travelers from the United States and Europe; five traveled to West Africa and five to South America. Eight of these 10 travelers died.[2] Lack of data on human disease in a specific area does not mean that there is no risk for the acquisition of yellow fever in that area because reporting mechanisms may be poor. It is estimated that for a 2-week stay, the risk of acquiring yellow fever in West Africa is 50 cases per 100,000 population with approximately 10 deaths, whereas travelers to South America are estimated to experience five cases per 100,000 population with one death.

Prevention: Use of repellants (N,N-diethyl-m-toluamide or N,N-diethyl-3 methyl-benzamide [DEET] or picaridin) on skin and insecticide (permethrin) on clothing as well as minimizing exposure to mosquitos can reduce the risk of acquisition. Additionally, there is an effective yellow fever vaccine.

Vaccine: The Yellow Fever Vaccine (YF-VAX), a live attenuated vaccine, is given as a single dose in an authorized, licensed center. The vaccine once reconstituted must be used within 1 h or discarded. Vaccination should be documented on the International Certificate of Vaccination or Prophylaxis (ICVP) commonly referred to as the "yellow card." The certificate of vaccination is valid beginning 10 days after the date of vaccination. Hence vaccination must occur at least 10 days before entering a country that requires yellow fever vaccination. The CDC and WHO now recognize that yellow fever vaccine is needed only once in a lifetime. The vaccine is only available at authorized yellow fever vaccination centers. A list of authorized yellow fever vaccination centers in the U.S. can be found at the CDC website.[3] However, YF-VAX is not currently available; it is expected to be available sometime in the late 2018. Through an Expanded Access Investigational New Drug process, an alternative live attenuated yellow fever vaccine, Stamaril, is currently available at some designated clinics.[4]

Efficacy: There have been no human studies carried out to determine the correlates of protection from the vaccine. The efficacy of the vaccine is not known; however, there are observational data that show that human protection does occur. Eighty to hundred percent of vaccine recipients develop neutralizing antibodies 10 days after vaccination. There have been reports of five cases in which yellow fever occurred in a vaccine recipient; however, it is unknown whether they were vaccinated properly and/or the vaccine was handled appropriately.

Long-term duration of immunity is documented at high titer in 80% of healthy individuals after 40 years.[5] Neutralizing antibodies decrease more quickly in persons with HIV, and revaccination may be considered in 10 years.

The yellow fever vaccine is a live vaccine but can be given at the same time as other live virus vaccines, such as measles, mumps, rebella (MMR), varicella vaccine, and zoster vaccine or separated from their administration by 30 days. The concomitant use of yellow fever vaccine with oral typhoid vaccine is acceptable.

Adverse side effects: Headache, fever, myalgia, malaise, and chills have been reported in approximately 11%–33% of vaccine recipients. Symptoms tend to be mild. Yellow fever vaccine–associated neurologic disease (YEL-AND)—a serious but rarely fatal adverse complication—which includes meningoencephalitis, acute disseminated encephalomyelitis, bulbar palsy, and Guillain-Barre syndrome. It is estimated that 0.4–0.8 cases of YEL-AND occur per 100,000 doses distributed. Higher rates occur in those aged ≥60 years, 1.6 cases per 100,000 for those aged 60–69 years, and about 1.1–2.3 cases per 100,000 in those aged ≥70 years.[6] Yellow fever vaccine–associated viscerotropic disease (YEL-AVD) is another serious complication. This syndrome mimics naturally acquired yellow fever disease with a mortality rate of about 65%. Patients usually develop nonspecific symptoms of headache, nausea, vomiting, diarrhea, malaise, and myalgia within 1 week of vaccination, which can progress to more severe disease. Estimated risk of developing yellow fever–associated viscerotropic disease is 0.3–0.4 cases per 100,000 doses distributed. This rate is higher among those older than 60 years; 1.0–1.1 cases per 100,000 for those aged 60–69 years and 2.3–3.2 cases per 100,000 for those aged ≥70 years.[6] Two specific risk factors for the development of YEL-AVD are older age and history of thymus disease or thymectomy.

Pregnancy: There are no data available to show whether pregnant women are at increased risk of developing yellow fever. Outbreak data do not suggest an increased risk of more severe disease. Vaccination during pregnancy has not been studied in a large prospective trial. In pregnancy, yellow fever vaccine should be given only if clearly needed, and risk of disease at the destination outweighs potential unknown risks of this live virus vaccine. Furthermore, seroconversion after vaccination is lower among pregnant women (38.6%) than among nonpregnant women (81.5%); thus serologic testing to determine seroconversion should be considered.

Use of the yellow fever vaccine: Laboratory workers have potential for exposure to yellow fever or the yellow fever vaccine, and travelers to yellow fever–endemic areas are candidates for vaccination.

Vaccination of travelers: Some countries require yellow fever vaccination for entry. Vaccine entry requirements are established by countries to prevent the importation and transmission of the yellow fever virus. Travelers must comply with these requirements. Some countries require vaccination of travelers arriving from all countries, whereas some countries require vaccination only for travelers arriving from a country with risk of yellow fever transmission, even if only in transit. Yellow fever vaccine is recommended for those travelers who are at risk of acquiring yellow fever depending on their specific destination, time of year, outbreak exposures, and uncertain travel plans to risk areas. The CDC and WHO now recognize that only one dose of yellow fever vaccine is needed in a lifetime.

Because the yellow fever vaccine is a live vaccine and can cause serious side effects, the risk/benefit ratio for vaccination needs to be seriously considered before a patient is vaccinated. Travelers entering a country that requires the yellow fever vaccine and have not received it can be quarantined for up to 6 days. A medical provider may issue a waiver of yellow fever vaccination for certain travelers who are judged to have a contraindication to receiving the yellow fever vaccine. The medical contraindication needs to be filled out and shown on the ICVP card. The medical provider should inform the traveler that they are at increased risk of developing yellow fever infection because they have not been vaccinated. The destination country may or may not accept the medical waiver.

> **Contraindications to Yellow Fever Vaccine**
>
> - Hypersensitivity to any of the components of the vaccine.
> - Hypersensitivity to eggs or egg products (allergies to feathers is not a contraindication to the vaccine; in general, anybody who can eat eggs or egg products may be vaccinated).
> - Infants <6 months of age.
> - Women who are breastfeeding infants.
> - Those with thymus removal or disorders associated with abnormal immune function such as a thymoma or myasthenia gravis
> - AIDS/HIV, including those with CD4 counts less than 200
> - Those with a known immunodeficiency.
> - Those taking immunosuppressive or immunomodulatory therapy.

Precautions: Yellow fever vaccine can be safely given to infants at 9 months of age and generally should not be given to infants younger than 6 months.

HIV infection: Data about the immune response to the vaccine are scarce but show consistent immunogenicity in HIV-positive people with CD4 counts >200 cells/mm^3. We carefully consider giving the vaccine if at risk, on a case-by-case basis. Asymptomatic HIV-infected individuals with moderate immune suppression (CD4 200–499/mm^3) should be able to receive the vaccine.

Older individuals: The overall rate of serious adverse side effects for those aged 60 years and above is approximately 8.3 per 100,000 doses compared to 4.7 events per 100,000 doses for younger recipients. If travel to an endemic area is unavoidable for a person aged ≥60 years, then the risk/benefit ratio of vaccination needs to be considered.

MENINGOCOCCAL VACCINE

Infection with *Neisseria meningitidis* is of concern to travelers to certain parts of the globe, particularly the so-called "meningitis belt" across Sub-Saharan Africa, which stretches across the continent from Senegal, Gambia, Guinea-Bissau, and Guinea in the west to Sudan, South Sudan, Eritrea, Ethiopia, and northwest Kenya in the east. It also includes parts of the nations of Mauritania, Mali, Burkina Faso, Côte d'Ivoire, Ghana, Togo, Benin, Nigeria, Niger, Cameroon, Chad, Central African Republic, Democratic Republic of Congo, and Uganda. There is also a concern for meningococcal exposure in the countries of Mozambique and Namibia, which, although not in the "meningitis belt," do have outbreaks of the disease with a frequency to be of concern to travelers. Meningococcal vaccination is recommended to all travelers to these countries. Several nearby countries, and areas within the aforementioned countries not within the belt itself are also considered "at risk," and travelers with expected prolonged contact with the local population and all healthcare workers are recommended to receive vaccination (see map).[1,2] In addition, travelers to Mecca, Saudi Arabia, for the annual Hajj and Umrah pilgrimages have, since 2002, following a series of outbreaks, been required to provide proof of meningococcal vaccination for entry into Saudi Arabia. Since its implementation, there have been no further outbreaks. Finally, there are rare outbreaks in other parts of the world prompting temporary recommendations for travel vaccination to those locations.[3]

N. meningitidis infections in humans can cause a range of clinical presentations, from asymptomatic carriage to severe life-threatening clinical meningitis. When it presents with clinical disease, *N. meningitidis* presents with meningitis in more than 50% of cases. Person-to-person transmission of bacteria occurs through close personal contact with respiratory secretions or saliva of infected persons. There are six major serogroups associated with human disease: A, B, C, X, Y, and W-135. Serogroup A is the most common serogroup found in the meningitis belt, although other serogroups are also present. *N. meningitidis* is found worldwide, with some regional serogroup variation, and at any given time 5%–10% of the population

may be carriers of the organism. Invasive disease is rare in nonepidemic areas, occurring at a rate of 0.5–10 cases per 100,000, but in the epidemic region of the meningitis belt, infections can occur in up to 1000 cases per 100,000, particularly during the dry season from December through June. Rates in Hajj pilgrims are also elevated and estimated to be around 25 per 100,000.[5] Despite these elevated rates in the local populations, the incidence of meningococcal disease in travelers is much lower than that of most other vaccine-preventable diseases; however, because of its high morbidity and mortality, meningococcal disease remains an important consideration in travelers.

Available vaccines: A number of vaccines directed against meningococcal infections are available in the U.S. and other countries for travelers. As most disease in the meningitis belt is caused by serotypes A, C, and W-135, the quadrivalent vaccination against A, C, Y, and W-135 is recommended for all travelers going to this region. Although protein-based vaccines against serotype B exist (in the U.S., MenB-4C [Bexsero] and MenB-FHbp [Trumenba]), they are not recommended for travelers as most serotype B disease occurs in isolated outbreaks within the U.S. and Western Europe and travelers are not considered at risk for this disease when traveling. Several monovalent and bivalent vaccines are also available around the world, but are not routinely recommended for travelers, and are targeted toward outbreaks.

Both conjugate and polysaccharide quadrivalent vaccines against serotypes A, C, Y, and W-135 have been developed, but the manufacturers of the most prevalent quadrivalent polysaccharide vaccine (MPSV4, or Menomune) have discontinued production, and this vaccine is no longer available as of August 2017. Although polysaccharide vaccines do still exist in some countries, recommendations for travelers have largely shifted to conjugate vaccines. In the U.S., only conjugate vaccines are available. Conjugate vaccines carry the advantage of eliciting immunologic memory (generally with recommended revaccination only every 5 years in adults), a reduction in nasopharyngeal carriage, and hence interruption of transmission and establishment of population protection.[4] Polysaccharide vaccines, in contrast, although well tolerated and protective in 85%–100% of vaccines, are comparatively short-lived and demonstrate hyporesponsiveness with repeated vaccination, particularly to serogroup C, and are less effective at preventing nasopharyngeal carriage.[5]

Currently in the U.S., two conjugate quadrivalent vaccines are available: MenACWY-D (Menactra) and MenACWY-CRM (Menveo). In other countries, including

Australia, Canada, and the U.K., ACWY-TT (Nimenrix) is also available. These vaccines are approved for adults through the age of 55 years, although most authorities advise off-label usage in individuals older than 55 years as, with the withdrawal of MPSV4, there is now no approved vaccine for this age group.

With quadrivalent conjugate vaccination, protective antibody levels against all four serogroups develop within 10–14 days after vaccination, and protection of 90%–95% is estimated. The duration of protection is shorter in children younger than 5 years but generally considered to be 5 years in adults. Most guidelines recommend that travelers who have frequent travel to epidemic regions be revaccinated every 5 years, although Saudi Arabia requires vaccination within 3 years for the Hajj.[3,5]

Considerations: Meningococcal vaccines have been found safe to administer with all other vaccines. Studies on the conjugate quadrivalent vaccine MenACWY-D (Menactra) with the pneumococcal conjugate vaccine PCV13 (Prevnar) did show a reduction in subsequent pneumococcal antibody levels, although they were still considered within the protective range. However, given this finding, the US CDC has recommended considering waiting at least 4 weeks after administration of PCV13 before administering the MenACWY-D vaccine in children. This effect was not seen with MenACWY-CRM. No other interactions have been reported for coadministration of vaccines (CDC).

Contraindications and adverse events: The meningococcal conjugate vaccines have demonstrated an excellent safety profile over millions of doses administered worldwide. Adverse reactions are rare and generally mild, most commonly as injection-site erythema and tenderness. Postvaccination headache, fever, and dizziness are also reported. A small number of cases of Guillain-Barre syndrome have been reported, but US and Canadian data do not suggest any elevation in risk.[4] These vaccines have not been studied extensively during pregnancy, although the Vaccine Adverse Event Reporting System in the U.S. has identified no major safety concerns to the mother or fetus, and pregnancy or breastfeeding is not considered an exclusion criterion for vaccination.[4]

Immunosuppression is also not considered a contraindication to vaccination. Rather, all individuals with a history of splenectomy, HIV, or complement deficiency should receive the meningococcal vaccination regardless of travel plans, based on current US guidelines (CDC).[6]

Additional prophylaxis strategies: Prophylactic antibiotic use is recommended in individuals with close contact to patients with known invasive meningococcal disease, including household members and any individuals exposed to the patient's oral secretions within the preceding 7 days. A number of antibiotics are appropriate for postexposure prophylaxis, including ciprofloxacin 500 mg once, ceftriaxone 250 mg IM once, rifampin 600 mg orally twice daily for 2 days, or azithromycin 500 mg orally once. As some regional resistance patterns exist, the geographic area of acquisition may favor one regimen over another. In addition, antibiotic allergies, drug/drug interactions with other medications taken by the patient, other conditions (such as pregnancy), and side effect profiles should be considered in choosing a prophylactic regimen. In general, however, prophylactic antibiotics for meningococcus exposure should not be prescribed for travelers unless they have had a known exposure to oral secretions from an individual with invasive disease.

CHOLERA VACCINE

Cholera is a serious and potentially fatal diarrheal illness caused by infection with the gram-negative bacterium *Vibrio cholera* and is characterized by the sudden onset of severe watery diarrhea—defined as greater than 3 L of output per 24 h—which may lead to rapid life-threatening dehydration.[1]

Vaxchora, lyophilized CBD 103-HGR, is a single-dose live attenuated oral cholera vaccine that was approved by the FDA in 2016 for the prevention of cholera caused by the 01 serogroup of *V. cholerae*—the most common circulating strain to consider for adults traveling to cholera-infected areas.[2] It is the only cholera vaccine licensed for use in the United States. Personal protection measures include following safe food and water precautions and proper sanitation and personal hygiene. These are the primary strategies to prevent cholera. Live oral cholera vaccine has good efficacy: It is estimated to reduce severe diarrheal symptoms at a rate of 90% protective 10 days after vaccination and 80% protective 3 months after vaccination. The vaccine is effective in inducing a vibriocidal antibody response which is the best available correlate of protection against cholera infection. No serious vaccine-related adverse events were reported.

The vaccine is used for travel to areas of active cholera transmission defined as a state, province, or other administrative subdivision within a country with endemic or epidemic cholera caused by toxigenic cholera O1 and includes areas with cholera activity within the last year which are prone to recurrence of cholera epidemics. It does not include areas where only rare, imported, or sporadic cases have been reported and is not routinely recommended for travelers who are not visiting active endemic areas. Clearly, relief workers going to aid cholera victims are advised to take it. Others who are visiting active areas for significant stays should receive it as well.

Considerations: Cholera vaccine should not be given to patients who have received oral or parenteral antibiotics in the preceding 14 days because antibiotics might have activity against the vaccine strain. How long an individual needs to be off of antibiotics before receiving the vaccine is unknown: Duration relates to the antimicrobial activity and half-life of the antimicrobial agent or agents. Duration of fewer than 14 days between stopping antibiotics and giving the cholera vaccine may be acceptable for certain clinical settings if travel cannot be avoided before 14 days have elapsed after stopping antibiotics.

Contraindications

Allergy: Cholera vaccine should not be administered to those with a history of severe allergic reaction such as anaphylaxis to any component of this vaccine or any cholera vaccine.[3]

Age: Data exist only for individuals who are aged between 18 and 65 years.

Pregnancy: No data exist. The vaccine is not absorbed systemically. Maternal exposure to the vaccine is not expected to result in exposure of the fetus or breast-fed infant to the vaccine; however, the vaccine strain may be shed in stool for greater than 7 days after vaccination and theoretically could be transmitted to the infant during vaginal delivery.

Compromised hosts: No data exist on the use of vaccine in compromised hosts. A study of HIV-positive individuals in Mali found vibriocidal antibody conversion was slightly lower among HIV-positive than in HIV-negative participants. No difference in adverse events is found.

Shedding and transmission: The bacterial strain in this oral live attenuated vaccine can be shed in stool and potentially be transmitted to close contacts. Vaccine strain from a previously available formulation was cultured from stool in more than 11% of vaccinated persons 7 days after they were vaccinated with that product. None of the stool cultures of household contacts of persons vaccinated with the currently available product had the vaccine strain isolated. Less than 1% had it isolated from stool cultured 5 days after vaccination with the previously available product.

However, late transmission was not pursued and could have been missed. This may be the case and would explain that 3.7% of family contacts of vaccine recipients seroconverted at 9 or 28 days after vaccination.

Outside the US the following cholera vaccines are available:

Dukoral is a killed whole-cell oral vaccine that also provides limited protection against infection with enterotoxigenic *E. coli* as well as cholera and has been in use both in Canada and many other countries for more than 10 years.

Shanchol and **Euvichol** are other killed whole-cell oral vaccines that have received prequalification and are being stockpiled along with Dukoral by the WHO for emergency use.

Dosing of Vaxchora[3]

Vaxchora is given as a single oral dose at least 10 days before travel. Duration of protection lasts 3 months, and there is no recommendation for boosters at this time. Eating and drinking should be avoided for 1 h before and after vaccine administration. It should not be administered within 2 weeks of antibiotic administration. It should be given at least 10 days before antimalarial prophylaxis with chloroquine. Administration is performed in the clinic to be sure of the timing of the product reconstitution, with the buffer component reconstituted before the mix with the active vaccine component, and to confirm ingestion within 15 min of reconstitution. Reconstitution should be completed within 15 min of removal from the freezer. Empty the buffer component packet into 100 mL of cold or room temperature purified bottled water—effervescence occurs—and stir until dissolved. Then empty the active component into the cup of buffer solution. Stir for 30 s until the active component disperses into a cloudy suspension. The recipient may then drink the entire cup at once within 15 min of reconstitution. Remaining residue may be discarded.[4]

Adverse reactions: The oral vaccine for cholera is well tolerated. Diarrhea occurred in 3.9% of study recipients. Other infrequently reported adverse effects included fatigue, headache, and abdominal pain.

JAPANESE ENCEPHALITIS VACCINE

Japanese encephalitis (JE) is caused by a *Flavivirus* closely related to West Nile virus and is transmitted predominantly by *Culex* mosquitoes that feed from dusk to dawn. The JE virus is maintained in nature by mosquitoes and animal hosts, mainly pigs and water birds. Infection risk is therefore highest in rural farming areas but is also present in urban and periurban areas in Asia.

JE is endemic in most of Asia and parts of the western Pacific region and is one of the most common causes of encephalitis in Asia. Transmission is seasonal in some areas (e.g., May to September in northern Asia and monsoon related in India and Southeast Asia) but can occur year-round in other geographic regions (e.g., in Bali where rice paddies, pigs, and birds are abundant). JE has also been reported in the Torres Strait Islands in northern QLD, Australia. Country-specific information about transmission months can be found in the CDC Yellow Book.[1] JE infection is uncommon in tourists, with an estimated risk of one in 200,000 per week of exposure,[2] and <1% of infections result in symptomatic illness.[1] However, symptomatic cases are associated with significant morbidity related to acute encephalitis and present with a wide range of neurological symptoms. Case fatality rate of symptomatic cases is up to 30%. Of those who survive, 30%−50% report long-term neurological, psychological, and cognitive impairment.[1,2]

Travelers to JE-endemic areas should be advised to take precautions against mosquito bites, particularly from dusk to dawn. Vaccination should also be considered, and recommendations should take into account the risk of infection (country, urban vs. rural, farming areas, seasons, outdoor activities, trip duration, and repeated travel). The high risk of death and serious long-term sequelae from symptomatic infections and the cost of vaccines are other important considerations. As a general rule, the Advisory Committee on Immunization Practices recommends vaccination for travelers who plan to spend a total of ≥1 month in endemic areas during the transmission season. Given that some US cases occurred in short-term travelers, duration may not be the best factor in decision-making about vaccination against JE for an individual traveler to Asia. This disease is rare but has significant consequences. We offer JE vaccine for persons traveling outside of major urban areas. Those who plan to return to Asia will benefit from vaccination against the cumulative risk. Those traveling for <1 month should consider choosing vaccination if spending time in rural areas; taking part in high-risk activities (e.g., farming, outdoor sporting activities); staying in accommodations without screens, bed nets, or air conditioning; or traveling to outbreak areas.[1] Vaccination is strongly recommended for expatriates planning to live in Asia for more than 6−12 months, even in urban areas, because they often travel extensively throughout the region for work and vacations.[2]

Vaccine[1]: The only JE vaccine available in the USA is an inactivated Vero cell culture vaccine, Ixiaro (Valneva). In 2009 it was licensed for use in those aged ≥17 years, and in May 2013 the license was extended to children aged ≥2 months. Primary immunization consists of two IM doses given on days 0 and 28, completed at least a week before departure. Each dose is 0.25 mL for children aged <3 years and 0.5 mL for those aged ≥3 years. For adults with ongoing exposure to JE a booster dose is recommended 1−2 years after the primary course. There is currently limited evidence about the need for boosters for those aged <18 years. An accelerated scheduled—day 0 and day 7 with a booster in 1 year—has been shown to provide excellent protection and is approved for last-minute travelers to risk regions who are ages 18 to 65, weighing seasonal risk and planned outdoor activity.

Adverse reactions: Local reactions such as pain and swelling are reported in ~1% of vaccine recipients. Systemic reactions include headache, myalgia, fatigue, and fever.

Contraindications: Ixiaro is contraindicated in persons who have had serious adverse reactions from any JE vaccines or any of the vaccine components (including protamine sulfate or formaldehyde). No preservatives, stabilizers, or antibiotics are added to the formulation. For the manufacturing process Ixiaro also contains bovine serum albumin (not more than 100 ng/mL), Vero host cell DNA (not more than 200 pg/mL), sodium metabisulfite (not more than 200 ppm), and host cell protein (not more than 100 ng/mL). Safety data in pregnant women are currently lacking. The risk of vaccination to mother and fetus really cannot be defined, so this is an undefined situation in terms of making a decision based on risk. Ixiaro use should be avoided during pregnancy or breast feeding.

Other considerations:

- For travelers who have been vaccinated with the previously available mouse brain−derived JE vaccine (JE-Vax, Biken), there is currently insufficient evidence regarding the effectiveness and duration of protection from a single booster dose of Ixiaro. Until further data are available, these travelers should be given a primary two-dose course of Ixiaro.
- For adult travelers who do not have time to complete the two-dose primary course before departure, an accelerated course of two doses on days 0 and 7 may be considered.[3]
- In immunocompromised hosts the immune response to Ixiaro is not well documented.
- Vaccination is recommended for residents of the Torres Strait Islands in Australia, as well as those traveling to the area for a cumulative total of ≥30 days during the wet season (December to May).

Very few international tourists travel to the Torres Strait Islands, which are situated between the northern tip of Queensland and Papua New Guinea.

Vaccines available outside the USA: A live attenuated recombinant Vero cell vaccine (Imojev, Sanofi Aventis) is available in Australia and some countries in Asia including Thailand, Malaysia, Hong Kong, Singapore, and the Philippines.[4] The vaccine is licensed for use in those aged $\geq$ 9 months. A single dose of 0.5 mL subcutaneously provides long-term protection in adults, but a booster is recommended for those aged 9 months to 18 years. Imojev is a live attenuated vaccine and therefore contraindicated in pregnant women, breastfeeding mothers, and immunosuppressed hosts. In Australia and New Zealand, Ixiaro is marketed as JEspect. In some countries a mouse brain—derived vaccine, with a poorly understood and worrisome safety profile, and other live attenuated vaccines are also in use.[4]

RABIES VACCINE

Rabies is a fatal neurotropic infection caused by a *Lyssavirus*, transmitted to humans through mammal bites or scratches that penetrate the skin. Rarely, rabies is transmitted via inhalation (e.g., in bat-infested caves or laboratories) or through organ transplantation. After an incubation period that usually lasts a week to months (occasionally years), clinical presentations are variable but include pain and paresthesia at the wound, fever, and severe encephalopathy which is invariably fatal. Rabies occurs worldwide except for Antarctica and is estimated to cause at least 55,000 deaths annually, mostly in Asia and Africa. All mammals can potentially be infected, but dogs are responsible for ~98% of human rabies infections, and bats are particularly important reservoirs. Although deaths from rabies are rare in travelers, it is not uncommon for travelers to be bitten or scratched by animals in rabies-endemic areas. Children are at higher risk of rabies because they are usually attracted to animals and might not report minor bites. They are also less able to defend themselves from animal bites and more likely to sustain severe bites to high-risk parts of the body, especially the head and neck.

Travelers to rabies-endemic areas should be advised to avoid contact with mammals (especially dogs and bats), consider preexposure vaccination, and if bitten, seek urgent medical care and postexposure prophylaxis even if they have received preexposure vaccination. Preexposure vaccination should be considered especially for those traveling to areas with a high incidence of rabies and/or places where postexposure prophylaxis (PEP/rabies treatment) might be difficult to obtain; or if expecting to have contact with animals (e.g., veterinarians, animal workers, bat handlers, cavers); or planning extended and/or repeated travel to rabies-endemic areas. Cyclists are also often chased and bitten by dogs. Travelers should be advised that if bitten or scratched by an animal, they should wash the wound(s) thoroughly with soap, water, and povidone-iodine and seek rabies treatment as soon as possible.

Vaccines and rabies immunoglobulin[1–3]: Two inactivated cell culture rabies vaccines are available in the USA: (1) human diploid cell vaccine (HDCV)—Imovax (Sanofi)—and (2) purified chick embryo cell vaccine (PCECV)—RabAvert (Novartis). Both vaccines can be used for preexposure vaccination and PEP/rabies treatment and are clinically interchangeable.

For *preexposure vaccination*, both the Imovax and RabAvert vaccines are given as 1.0-mL IM injections on days 0, 7, and 21 or 28. Vaccination provides long-term protection, and boosters are not recommended except for those at very high risk (e.g., veterinarians, bat handlers, laboratory workers exposed to the virus). We strongly recommend rabies preexposure vaccination for travelers who plan long stays in countries with risk. All animal handlers or adventure travelers who may stay in remote regions without easy access to healthcare and adequate postexposure rabies treatment within 24—48 h after a rabies exposure should consider preexposure rabies vaccination. One of the barriers against preexposure rabies vaccination is the high cost of the vaccines. Intradermal vaccination that uses a fraction of the original dose is more affordable. It is currently off label in the USA but might be considered in some circumstances.[4]

Recommendations for *postexposure prophylaxis* (PEP) depend on whether the traveler has previously been vaccinated. For those who have previously completed a full-course rabies vaccination, PEP involves two 1.0-mL IM doses of rabies vaccines given on days 0 and 3, and rabies immunoglobulin (RIG) is not needed. For those who have never been vaccinated, PEP involves the administration of both (1) RIG (20 IU/kg for human RIG, 40 IU/kg for equine RIG), infiltrated into and around the wound as much as possible, and the remainder given IM; and (2) four doses of rabies vaccines on days 0, 3, 7, and 14. Immunocompromised persons should receive a fifth dose on day 28.

If possible, PEP should be commenced as soon as possible (preferably within 48 h) but should be given regardless of the time lapse since the bite or scratch because at times there is a very long incubation period.

It can be very difficult to access rabies vaccines in developing countries and even more difficult to access RIG.5 The worldwide shortage of RIG further adds to the difficulties. If RIG is unavailable, rabies vaccine should be started as soon as possible, and RIG is given up to 7 days later. After day 7 of the vaccine schedule, it is not necessary to give RIG because the vaccine-induced antibodies will have developed. Travelers sometimes need to be evacuated to another country or return home to receive appropriate PEP, resulting in significant stress and disruption of travel plans. Preexposure vaccination removes the need for RIG, reduces the urgency of PEP, and makes it easier for travelers to complete PEP in a timely manner.

Adverse reactions: Rabies vaccines are generally well tolerated. Common local reactions include pain, pruritus, redness, and swelling at the injection site. Systemic reactions include headache, myalgia, nausea, dizziness, and abdominal pain. Severe hypersensitivity reactions have been reported in ~5% of vaccine recipients 2–21 days after booster doses of HDCV and sometimes during the primary course.

Contraindications: Because rabies is fatal, there are no absolute contraindications for the use of vaccines or RIG in PEP. If there is a history of severe hypersensitivity to one vaccine, another vaccine should be used. For those with egg hypersensitivity, HDCV should be used instead of PCECV.

Other considerations:
- Pregnancy is not a contraindication to PEP.
- Immune response to rabies vaccines is reduced in immunocompromised persons, and postvaccination serology should be performed to confirm seroconversion. In previous studies all healthy persons tested 2–4 weeks after completion of preexposure and postexposure rabies virus prophylaxis demonstrated a significant antibody response to rabies virus. The best test for this purpose is the rapid fluorescent focus inhibition test (RFFIT), which is a rabies virus neutralization test performed in cell culture to determine the rabies virus–neutralizing antibody level in human or animal sera. Immunofluorescent staining of infected cells is used as an indicator of rabies virus replication. The RFFIT takes ~20 h and is both sensitive and specific in the hands of well-trained laboratory personnel.
- If intradermal vaccination is given, postvaccination serology is recommended after 3 weeks.
- Because rabies is invariably fatal, the full course of PEP vaccination should be completed unless adverse reactions are very severe.

Vaccines available outside the USA: Multiple cell culture vaccines are available around the world, and many can be considered interchangeable with Imovax and RabAvert, including (1) HDCV (e.g., Merieux, Rabivac), (2) PCECV (e.g., Rabipur), (3) purified Vero cell vaccine (e.g., Verorab), and (4) purified duck embryo vaccine (e.g., Lyssavac N). Nerve tissue vaccines are still used in some countries, particularly in Southeast Asia. These vaccines are less effective than cell culture vaccines, require large volumes of injections, and are associated with a high incidence of serious adverse effects including severe allergic encephalomyelitis. Travelers should be advised not to accept these vaccines and to seek PEP elsewhere.

POLIO VACCINE
Polio virus is an enterovirus typically spread via fecal-oral transmission and less frequently via oral-oral transmission. Most infections are asymptomatic or present as an undifferentiated and self-limited gastroenteritis. However, in <1% of cases of polio infection an acute and florid paralysis may occur. In most cases, paralysis involves the legs, but the upper extremities, throat, and diaphragm may also be affected. Complications can include respiratory failure. Depending on available supportive medical care, fatality rates range from 2% to 75%. Recovered patients usually have some form of residual neuromuscular sequelae. Humans are the only affected species, and no carrier state exists beyond the initial infection. For this reason, polio is amenable to eradication. Polio has been eradicated from the Americas since 1991, and many other countries of the world are currently free of polio. Wild-type polio infections continue to occur in Afghanistan, Pakistan, and Nigeria. A total of 37 cases of WPV occurred globally in 2016.

Infection may be caused by either wild polio virus (WPV) or by vaccine-derived polio virus (VDPV). The latter is derived from oral polio virus (OPV) vaccine and may result in vaccine-associated paralytic poliomyelitis (VAPP). Wild-type virus is divided into three serotypes. No cases of WPV 2 have occurred since 1999, and no cases of WPV 3 have occurred since 2012. The introduction of WPV into a previously polio-free country remains a risk. Information regarding the current risk of transmission of WPV can be obtained at the CDC Travelers' Health website (www.cdc.gov/travel). VDPV (usually type 2) may occur in an individual vaccinated with OPV, or in such a person's contacts, as a result of shedding. Information regarding current transmission or outbreaks of VDPV can be obtained from the Global Polio Eradication Initiative (www.polioeradication.org or www.polioeradication.org/dataandmonitoring/poliothisweek.aspx). No VDPV has occurred in the United States since a switch to the use of inactivated polio vaccine (IPV) in 2000. OPV vaccine is used in many developing countries of the world. Travelers may be at risk of acquiring infection from either WPV or VDPV. In 2005 an unvaccinated adult from the United States developed the VAPP syndrome while traveling after contact with a child who had recently received OPV.

Considerations: All children should receive a primary series of four doses of IPV beginning at an age of 2 months. Adults and older children who have received a primary series should receive a dose of IPV if traveling to a country in which WPV or VDPV transmission is active. Vaccine should be administered at least 4 weeks before departure. In certain cases, long-term travelers to countries that border countries with transmission of WPV or VDPV should also receive a primary series (if unvaccinated) or a booster of IPV, so should travelers involved in healthcare, work in refugee camps, or other types of activities involving humanitarian aid, war, or political, environmental, or social disruption.

Unvaccinated children can begin a primary series as young as 6 weeks of age and receive a second and third doses 4 weeks after the prior dose. A fourth dose should be administered 6 months after the third dose. Unvaccinated adults should receive a series of three doses of IPV. Doses should be administered at time 0, 1–2 months, and 6–12 months. If time allows, three doses can be given at time 1, 4, and 8 weeks to complete a primary series. A fourth dose should then be given more than 6 months after the previous dose.

Family and other caregivers of children who are adopted from countries that use OPV or where WPV transmission occurs should complete a primary series (if unvaccinated) or a booster dose of IPV or booster dose of IPV before the adoption.

Contraindications

Allergy: IPV contains formaldehyde and trace amounts of streptomycin, neomycin, and polymyxin B. Those with an allergy to any of these three antibiotics should not receive IPV.

Age: IPV may be administered to infants as young as 6 weeks of age. The primary series is usually initiated at an age of 2 months.

Pregnancy: IPV can be administered during pregnancy or while breastfeeding if indicated.

Compromised hosts: OPV should not be administered to individuals who are immunosuppressed including those with HIV infection, cancer, or primary immunodeficiencies, nor should OPV be administered to their close contacts. Immunosuppressed individuals

should avoid contact with anyone who has recently received OPV. IPV is generally safe in such individuals.

Shedding and transmission: There is no human-to-human transmission of IPV. There is significant shedding of OPV in the stool, and this can both result in extension of the effect of the immunization within a community and also cause VAPP. Shedding occurs for up to 6 weeks after vaccination.

Dosing: IPOL (Sanofi-Pasteur) is a trivalent IPV available in the United States. The dose of IPV for all ages is 0.5 mL. It may be given intramuscularly or subcutaneously. Several combination vaccines that incorporate IPV are available for use in children as part of a primary series.

TICK-BORNE ENCEPHALITIS VACCINE

Tick-borne encephalitis (TBE) is a viral infection of the central nervous system caused by TBE virus. Up to two-thirds of infections may be asymptomatic. There are three subtypes (European, Far Eastern, Siberian) endemic to Europe and northern Asia. Infection is transmitted through the bite of an infected *Ixodes* tick or, less commonly, the ingestion of unpasteurized milk from infected animals or even blood transfusion. The tick vector responsible for the transmission of TBE can also transmit *Borrelia*, *Anaplasma*, and Babesia infections. Transmission of TBE generally occurs from April to December.

Illness is typically biphasic with an initial flu-like syndrome developing approximately 7–28 days after infection. This is followed by a period of convalescence and then relapse characterized by headache, aseptic meningitis, cranial nerve palsies, seizures, encephalopathy, and muscular paralysis. Recovery, case fatality rates, and development of neurologic sequelae vary by subtype with the highest incidence of these complications caused by the Far Eastern subtype. Risk is greatest among travelers who engage in outdoor activities with significant exposure to ticks. Protective measures such as the use of DEET-containing insect repellants, inspection for attached ticks, and wearing long-sleeved shirts and long pants may reduce risk. Disease incidence and severity are highest among those older than 50 years.[1,2]

Considerations: There are no vaccines effective against TBE currently licensed in the United States. There are several inactivated vaccines available in Europe, Asia, and Australia. FSME-IMMUN (Baxter, Austria) and Encepur (Novartis, Germany) are available in Europe. Pediatric dosing and schedules are available for FSME-IMMUN and Encepur. TBE-Moscow

(Chumakov Institute, Russia) and EnceVir (Microgen) are available in Russia.[3,4]

All four vaccines provide protection against the three subtypes of virus. Vaccine efficacy is approximately 95%. Vaccine failure is possible in immunocompromised travelers and the elderly. Vaccination schedules vary by specific formulation, but generally initial vaccination is followed by booster doses at 1−3 and 9−12 months. An accelerated schedule with doses at 0, 7, and 21 days has been used with seroconversion rates similar to those obtained using longer recommended schedule. The accelerated schedule should be followed by a booster dose at 12−18 months.[5]

Owing to the time required for complete vaccination, even using the accelerated schedule, and the lack of availability of vaccine in the US, vaccination is not practical for most travelers. It may, however, be reasonable to vaccinate travelers undertaking more prolonged stays or residence in endemic areas particularly if engaging in high-risk activities.[6]

Contraindications

Allergy: Vaccines for TBE should not be administered to those with a history of severe allergic reaction such as anaphylaxis to any component of the vaccines. FSME-IMMUN, TBE-Moscow, and EnceVir contain human albumin as a stabilizer.[3]

Both FSME-IMMUN and Encepur are produced according to WHO manufacturing requirements. They are grown on chicken embryonic fibroblast cells, inactivated by formaldehyde, and use aluminum hydroxide as the adjuvant. The vaccines do not contain polygeline or thiomersal, but traces of formaldehyde (in FSME-Immun only), gentamicin, neomycin, and chlortetracycline (in Encepur only) may be found in the final products.

Pregnancy: Potential risks of administration of the vaccines during pregnancy or breastfeeding are unknown.

Compromised host: Active or unknown central nervous system disease, especially when associated with fever and immune suppression, are relative contraindications for vaccination with any of the formulations mentioned.

Dosing: All vaccines are given intramuscularly; the dose of each vaccine is 0.5 mL with the exception of the pediatric formulations of FSME-IMMUN Junior and Encepur-Children which are each given in a dose of 0.25 mL. FSME-IMMUN Junior is labeled for children aged 1−15 years; Encepur-Children is labeled for children aged 1−11 years. TBE-Moscow and EnceVir

are each labeled for adults and pediatric patients aged above 3 years.

Shedding and transmission: Transmission of virus-related vaccine or shedding have not been described.

Adverse reactions: In general, the FSME-IMMUN and Encepur are well tolerated. Pain and swelling at the site of injection are the most commonly reported side effects. Fever is relatively common in children and reported in as many as 30% of recipients by the manufacturer. Newer formulations of FSME-IMMUN and Encepur are reported to be less likely to cause fever. Neither vaccine has been commonly associated with severe adverse reactions. Booster doses are generally well tolerated and less likely to lead to adverse reactions than are the initial doses. Headache, nausea, insomnia, myalgia, fever, and malaise are reported in as many as 10% of healthy recipients particularly after the first dose. There are few published data regarding adverse reactions to the Russian manufactured formulations, but these appear to have similar side effects and safely profiles to the European formulations.

CONCLUSION

It is always a pleasure and a privilege to advise travelers with expansive journeys. This review should aid the primary care practitioner to vaccinate their traveling patients when possible and know when to refer those with complex itineraries—including travel to malaria-endemic regions—for further guidance by Travel Medicine experts.

ACKNOWLEDGMENTS

The authors would like to thank Frank J. Bia MD, MPH, Professor, Emeritus Internal Medicine [Infectious Diseases] Yale School of Medicine for his keen editorial guidance and insight into the field of Travel Medicine.

REFERENCES

Adult Immunizations and General Vaccine Recommendations
1. https://www.cdc.gov/mmwr/preview/mmwrhtml/rr6002a1.htm.
2. https://www.cdc.gov/vaccines/schedules/downloads/adult/adult-combined-schedule.pdf.

Hepatitis A
1. Fiore AE, Wasley A, Bell BP. Prevention of hepatitis A through active or passive immunization: recommendations of the Advisory Committee on Immunization Practices (ACIP). *Morb Mortal Wkly Rep Recomm Rep.* 2006;55(7): 1−CE.

2. Wu D, Guo C-Y. Epidemiology and prevention of hepatitis a in travelers. *J Travel Med.* 2013;20(6):394–399. https://doi.org/10.1111/jtm.12058.

3. Mayer CA, Neilson AA. Hepatitis A—prevention in travelers. *Aust Fam Physician.* 2010;39(12):924–928.

4. Van Damme P, Leroux-Roels G, Suryakiran P, Folschweiller N, Van Der MO. Persistence of antibodies 20 y after vaccination with a combined hepatitis A and B vaccine. *Hum Vaccine Immunother.* 2017;13(5):972–980. https://doi.org/10.1080/21645515.2016.1274473.

5. Kroger AT, Duchin J, Vázquez M. General best practice guidelines for immunization. *Best Pract Guid Advis Comm Immun Pract (ACIP).*

6. Nelson NP. Updated dosing instructions for immune globulin (human) GamaSTAN S/D for hepatitis a virus prophylaxis. *MMWR.* 2017;66:959–960.

7. Patel RR, Liang SY, Koolwal P, Kuhlmann FM. Travel advice for the immunocompromised traveler: prophylaxis, vaccination, and other preventive measures. *Ther Clin Risk Manag.* 2015;11:217–228.

Hepatitis B

1. Mast EE, Margolis HS, Fiore AE, et al. A comprehensive immunization strategy to eliminate transmission of hepatitis B virus infection in the United States. *MMWR.* 2005;54(16): 1–32.

2. *Global Hepatitis Report 2017.* Geneva: World Health Organization; 2017.

3. Wong J, Payne M, Hollenberg S. A double-dose hepatitis B vaccination schedule in travelers presenting for late consultation. *J Travel Med.* 2014;21(4):260–265. https://doi.org/10.1111/jtm.12123.

4. *Hepatitis B Vaccines: WHO Position Paper – No 27.* Vol 92. 2017:369–392.

5. *Dynavax Announces FDA Approval of HEPLISAV-B(TM) for Prevention of Hepatitis B in Adults [Press Release].* Berkley, California: Dynavax; November 9, 2017.

Typhoid

1. Basnyat B, Maskey AP, Zimmerman MD, Murdoch DR. Enteric (typhoid) fever in travelers. *Clin Infect Dis.* 2005; 41(10):1467–1472.

2. Updated recommendations for the use of typhoid vaccine— advisory Committee on immunization practices, United States 2015. *CDC MMWR.* 2015;64(11):305–308.

3. Wain J, Hendriksen RS, Mikoleit ML, Keddy KH, Ochiai RL. Typhoid fever. *Lancet.* 2015;385(9973):1136–1145.

4. Anwar E, Goldberg E, Fraser A, Acosta CJ, Paul M, Leibovici L. Vaccines for preventing typhoid fever. *Cochrane Database Syst Rev.* 2014;2(1):CD001261.

Yellow Fever

1. https://wwwnc.cdc.gov/travel/yellowbook/2018/infectious-diseases-related-to-travel/yellow-fever.

2. Mark D, Gershman MD, Staples JE. Centers for Disease Control and Prevention (CDC). Yellow Fever. Accessed 2/26/2018. https://wwwnc.cdc.gov/travel/yellowbook/2018/infectious-diseases-related-to-travel/yellow-fever.

3. https://wwwnc.cdc.gov/travel/yellow-fever-vaccination-clinics/search.

4. https://wwwnc.cdc.gov/travel/page/search-for-stamaril-clinics.

5. Gotuzzo E, Yactayo S, Gordova E. Efficacy and duration of immunity after yellow fever vaccination: systematic review on the need for a booster every 10 years. *Am J Trop Med Hyg.* 2013;89(3):434–444.

6. Staples JE, Gershman M, Fischer M, Centers for disease Control and prevention (CDC). Yellow fever vaccine: recommendations of the Advisory Committee on Immunization Practices (ACIP). *MMWR Recomm Rep.* 2010;59(RR-7): 1–27.

Meningococcal

1. Centers for Disease Control and Prevention: "Recommended Immunization Schedules for Adults." Accessed 10/1/2017. https://www.cdc.gov/vaccines/schedules/hcp/adult.html.

2. *Center for Disease Control and Prevention: "Recommended Immunization Schedule for Children and Adolescents Aged 18 Years or Younger, United States, 2017.* https://www.cdc.gov/vaccines/schedules/hcp/child-adolescent.html.

3. Wilder-Smith A. Meningococcal disease: risk for international travelers and vaccine strategies. *Travel Med Infect Dis.* 2008;6:182–186.

4. Crum-Cianflone N, Sullivan E. Meningococcal vaccinations. *Infect Dis Ther.* 2016;5:89–112.

5. Cramer JP, Wilder-Smith A. Meningococcal disease in travelers: update on vaccine options. *Curr Opin Infect Dis.* 2012;25:507–517.

6. CDC. *The Yellow Book. CDC Health Information for International Travel.* Oxford University Press; 2017.

Cholera

1. Fillion K, Mileno MD. Cholera in travelers: shifting tides in epidemiology, management, and prevention. *Curr Infect Dis Rep.* 2015;17(1):455.

2. Wong KK, Burdette E, Mahon BE, Mintz ED, Ryan ET, Reingold AL. Recommendations of the advisory committee on immunization practices for use of cholera vaccine. *MMWR Morb Mortal Wkly Rep.* 2017;66(18):482–485.

3. https://www.fda.gov/downloads/BiologicsBloodVaccines/Vaccines/ApprovedProducts/UCM506235.pdf.

4. Vaxchora Package Insert—PaxVax Connect. https://www.paxvaxconnect.com/PDF/Vaxchora_Prescribing_Information.pdf.

Japanese Encephalitis

1. Hills SL, Rabe IB, Fischer M. Japanese Encephalitis. CDC Yellow Book 2018—Health Information for International Travel. Available from: https://wwwnc.cdc.gov/travel/yellowbook/2018/infectious-diseases-related-to-travel/japanese-encephalitis.

2. Yung A, Leder K, Torresi J, et al. *Manual of Travel Medicine* Chapter 2.7 Japanese Encephalitis. 3rd ed. Victoria: IP Communications East Hawthorn; 2011.

3. Jelinek T, Burchard GD, Dieckmann S, et al. Short-Term immunogenicity and safety of an accelerated preexposure prophylaxis regimen with Japanese encephalitis vaccine in combination with a rabies vaccine: a phase III, multicenter, observer-blind study. *J Travel Med.* 2015;22(4):225–231.

4. Batchelor P, Petersen K. Japanese encephalitis: a review of clinical guidelines and vaccine availability in Asia. *Trop Dis Trav Med Vaccines*. 2015;1(11). https://doi.org/10.1186/s40794-015-0013-6.

Rabies

1. Petersen BW, Wallace RM, Schlim DR. Rabies. CDC Yellow Book 2018 — Health Information for International Travel. Available from: https://wwwnc.cdc.gov/travel/yellowbook/2018/infectious-diseases-related-to-travel/rabies.
2. World Health Organization. *Rabies Vaccines: WHO Position Paper. Weekly Epidemiological Record*; 2010. Available from: http://www.who.int/wer/2010/wer8532.pdf?ua=1.
3. Yung A, Leder K, Torresi J, et al. *Manual of travel medicine* Chapter 2.13 Rabies. 3rd ed. Victoria: IP Communications East Hawthorn; 2011.
4. Schlim DR. Perspectives: Intradermal Rabies Preexposure Immunization. Rabies. CDC Yellow Book 2018—Health Information for International Travel. Available from: https://wwwnc.cdc.gov/travel/yellowbook/2018/infectious-diseases-related-to-travel/perspectives-intradermal-rabies-preexposure-immunization.
5. Mills DJ, Lau CL, Weinstein P. Animal bites and rabies exposure in Australian travellers. *Med J Aust*. 2011;195:673–675.

Polio

,. .

Tick-borne Encephalitis

,. .

CHAPTER 11

Immunizations for Healthcare Personnel

DAVID J. WEBER, MD, MPH • EMILY E. SICKBERT-BENNETT, MS, PHD

Healthcare is the fastest growing sector of the US economy, employing over 18 million workers.[1] Healthcare personnel (HCP) are commonly exposed to vaccine-preventable infectious agents via sharps injuries (e.g., hepatitis B virus [HBV]) and via direct patient care for contact-transmitted diseases (e.g., herpes zoster), droplet spread diseases (e.g., influenza, pertussis), and airborne spread diseases (e.g., measles, varicella). The risks and methods of preventing occupational acquisition of infection by HCP have been reviewed.[2–4] The prevention of infectious disease acquisition and transmission among HCP and patients is an important component of safe healthcare delivery in all healthcare settings. A key component to protecting HCP and their patients is HCP immunity to vaccine-preventable diseases.[5–8] Other important recommended practices to minimize the risk of disease acquisition among HCP include: (1) proper training of HCP at initiation of healthcare practice and annually (e.g., infection control practices and sharps injury prevention); (2) evaluation of HCP who are exposed to communicable diseases for receipt of postexposure prophylaxis (PEP); (3) adherence to standard precautions when providing patient care, especially the performance of appropriate hand hygiene practices before and after patient care[4]; (4) rapid institution of appropriate isolation precautions for patients with a known or suspected communicable disease; and (5) proper use of personal protective equipment, such as masks, N-95 respirators, eye protection, and gowns, when caring for patients with potentially communicable diseases.[8] This chapter will focus on preventing infection in HCP using preexposure and postexposure immunization. Vaccines can be used to prevent infection or illness, provide PEP, and/or to aid in control of outbreaks (Table 11.1).

DEFINITIONS

HCP refer to all paid and unpaid persons serving in healthcare settings who have the potential for direct or indirect exposure to patients and/or infectious materials, including body substances, contaminated medical supplies and equipment, contaminated environmental surfaces, or contaminated air. These HCP may include but are not limited to emergency medical service personnel, nurses, nursing assistants, physicians, technicians, therapists, phlebotomists, pharmacists, students and trainees, contractual staff not employed by the healthcare facility, and persons (e.g., clerical, dietary, environmental services, laundry, security, engineering and facilities management, administrative, billing, and volunteer personnel) not directly involved in patient care but potentially exposed to infectious agents that can be transmitted among HCP and patients.[5] In general, HCP who have regular or frequent contact with patients, body fluids, or specimens have a higher risk of acquiring or transmitting infections than do HCP who have only brief contact with patients and their environment (e.g., beds, food trays, medical equipment). However, all HCP who work within the confines of a healthcare facility should be covered by the occupational health service and receive appropriate screening and preexposure prophylaxis for vaccine-preventable diseases, even if they do not provide direct patient care, as they frequently interact with HCP providing direct care and are therefore at risk for acquiring or transmitting infectious pathogens.

The term "healthcare settings" refers to places where healthcare is delivered and includes, but is not limited to, acute care facilities, long-term acute care facilities, long-term-care (LTC) facilities, assisted living facilities, rehabilitation facilities, psychiatric facilities, home healthcare settings, vehicles where healthcare is delivered (e.g., ambulances), and outpatient facilities, such as dialysis centers, physician offices, and others.

PREEXPOSURE IMMUNIZATIONS
General Recommendations

General recommendations regarding vaccination of HCP have been published by the Centers for Disease Control and Prevention (CDC),[2] the Advisory

Vaccinations. https://doi.org/10.1016/B978-0-323-55435-0.00011-2

TABLE 11.1
Vaccines Recommended for Healthcare Personnel

Vaccine	HCP Population	May Be Used For Postexposure Prophylaxis	May Be Useful In Controlling an Outbreak
Mumps (provided as MMR)	All	No	Yes
Measles (provided as MMR)	All	Yes	Yes
Rubella (provided as MMR)	All	No	Yes
Hepatitis B	Potential exposure to blood or OPIM	Yes	NR
Varicella	All	Yes	Yes
Influenza	All	No	Yes
Tdap	All	No	Yes (pertussis)
Meningococcal A,C,Y,W	Microbiologists	No	Yes
Meningococcal B	Microbiologists	No	Yes
Diphtheria	Special circumstances	No	Yes
Hepatitis A	Special circumstances	Yes	Yes

MMR, mumps, measles and rubella; *NR*, not relevant; *OPIM*, other potential infectious material (e.g., cerebrospinal fluid, joint fluid, pericardial fluid, peritoneal fluid); *Tdap*, tetanus-toxoid, diphtheria-toxoid, acellular pertussis.

Committee on Immunization Practices (ACIP),[5,9] the American Academy of Pediatrics [Red Book][10], and the Association for Professionals in Infection Control and Epidemiology (APIC).[7] The most recent ACIP-approved immunization schedule that summarizes their recommendations should always be consulted.[9] All HCP are recommended by CDC/ACIP to be immune to mumps, measles, rubella, varicella, pertussis, and influenza (Table 11.1). Additional vaccines, such as hepatitis B vaccine (HCP who might have contact with blood or body fluids) and meningococcal vaccines (microbiology personnel who might be spinning cerebrospinal fluid from patients with meningococcal meningitis), may be recommended for specific groups of HCP depending on their potential exposures (Table 11.1). In addition to vaccines specifically recommended for HCP, all HCP should receive the appropriate vaccines recommended for adults based on their age and underlying medical conditions, such as human papillomavirus, herpes zoster, and pneumococcal vaccines, or be referred to their local medical provider.[9,11,12]

Persons providing vaccines to HCP should be familiar with FDA-approved package inserts for the individual vaccines, the specific CDC/ACIP recommendations for each vaccine, and CDC's Best Practice Guidelines for Immunization.[12] Vaccines should be provided at the recommended dose intervals and by the recommended route; booster doses may be recommended (Table 11.2). Specifically, vaccine providers should adhere to the following CDC recommendations: (1) Administer vaccines at recommended ages and in accordance with recommended intervals between doses of multidose antigens to provide optimal protection; (2) Maintain records of all vaccines provided in the HCP's occupational health record including vaccine provided, date, dose, route, location, and lot number; and (3) Assess the HCP for precautions and contraindications before administering a vaccine. If such a condition is present, the risks and benefits of vaccination need to be carefully weighed by the occupational health provider and the HCP. The most common contraindication is a history of an anaphylactic reaction to a previous dose of the vaccine or to a vaccine component. Factors that are not contraindications to immunization include the following: (1) household contact with a pregnant woman; (2) breastfeeding; (3) reaction to a previous vaccination consisting only of mild-to-moderate local tenderness, swelling, or both or fever less than 40.5°C (105°F); (4) mild acute illness with or without low-grade fever; (5) current antimicrobial therapy except for certain live attenuated vaccines such as oral typhoid vaccine, live attenuated influenza vaccine (LAIV), and live attenuated varicella or zoster vaccines

TABLE 11.2
Administration of Vaccines Recommended for Healthcare Personnel

Vaccine	Administration	Boosters	Comments
Mumps (provided as MMR)	2 doses SC	No	A third dose may be recommended during an outbreak (see text)
Measles (provided at MMR)	2 doses SC	No	Avoid if immunocompromised, defer if pregnant
Rubella (provided as MMR)	1 dose SC	No	—
Hepatitis B	3 doses IM at 0, 1, and 6 mo	No	Additional doses may be indicated (see text)
Varicella	2 doses SC	No	Avoid if immunocompromised, defer if pregnant
Influenza	1 dose yearly (IM, ID)	No	—
Tdap	1 dose IM	No	One dose after age 11 is sufficient
Meningococcal A,C,Y,W-135	1 dose IM	Every 5 years if exposure continues	PEP with antibiotics still required even if immunized
Meningococcal B	2 doses IM	No	PEP with antibiotics still required even if immunized

ID, intradermal; *IM*, intramuscular; *SC*, subcutaneous.

or convalescence from a recent illness; (6) personal history of allergies except a history of an anaphylactic reaction to a previous vaccine dose or vaccine component; and (7) family history of allergies, serious adverse reactions to vaccination, or seizures. Although allergic reactions are a common concern for vaccine providers, these reactions are uncommon, and anaphylaxis after vaccines is rare, occurring at a rate of approximately one per million doses for many vaccines. However, epinephrine and equipment for managing an airway should be available for immediate use by vaccine providers.[12]

Vaccine providers need to be aware of several important general CDC recommendations for vaccine providers[12] (1) Vaccine providers should administer vaccines as close to the recommended intervals as possible. However, intervals between doses that are longer than recommended typically do not reduce final antibody concentrations, although protection may not be attained until the recommended number of doses has been administered[2]; (2) All inactivated vaccines indicated for HCP can be provided simultaneously; (3) measles, mumps, and rubella (MMR) and varicella vaccine can be administered simultaneously. However, if not administered simultaneously, they should be administered at least 1 month apart. LAIV plus simultaneous MMR or varicella has not been studied in adults; (4) It is preferred that doses of vaccine in a series come

from the same manufacturer; however, if this is not possible or if the manufacturer of doses given previously is unknown, providers should administer the vaccine that they have available; (5) With regard to vaccines recommended for HCP, providers should only accept written, dated records as evidence of vaccination (the CDC/ACIP recommend accepting a healthcare provider's statement of receipt of influenza vaccine, although many healthcare facilities will require written proof of immunization); (6) Vaccines can be safely administered to persons who have a mild illness. However, presence of a moderate or severe acute illness with or without a fever is a precaution to administration of all vaccines; (7) Routine physical examinations and procedures (e.g., measuring temperatures) are not prerequisites for vaccinating persons who appear to be healthy; and (8) All vaccines recommended for HCP can be provided regardless of where the HCP works in the healthcare facility except for LAIV (i.e., HCP receiving this vaccine should not interact with patients in a "protected environment" [i.e., hematopoietic stem cell transplant unit] until 7 days after immunization).

Depending on the vaccine-preventable disease, immunity may be assured by several different measures (Table 11.3). The CDC/ACIP states that the majority of persons born before 1957 are likely to have been infected naturally and may be presumed immune to measles, mumps, and rubella.[5,9] The strategy is supported by data demonstrating that HCP born before 1957 are highly likely to be immune to mumps, measles, and rubella.[13] For unvaccinated personnel born before 1957 who lack laboratory evidence of measles (also true for mumps and rubella) immunity or laboratory confirmation of disease, healthcare facilities should consider vaccinating personnel with 2 doses of MMR vaccine at the appropriate interval. For unvaccinated personnel born before 1957 who lack laboratory confirmation of physician-diagnosed disease or evidence of immunity to mumps, measles, or rubella, healthcare facilities should recommend 2 doses of MMR vaccine during an outbreak of mumps or measles or a single dose of MMR during an outbreak of rubella.[5] Regarding varicella, the CDC/ACIP state that the status of being "US-born before 1980 is evidence of immunity".[9] As with mumps, measles, and rubella, serologic studies of HCP have demonstrated that the great majority of HCP born before 1980 are, in fact, immune to varicella.[14] However, the CDC/ACIP recommends that all HCP who do not have other evidence of immunity to varicella should receive appropriate varicella immunization.

HCP who are not immune to vaccine-preventable diseases should receive appropriate immunization(s) (Table 11.1). However, it is important to note that even if HCP are considered immune via vaccination to a preventable disease transmitted by the droplet

(i.e., pertussis, invasive meningococcal infection, mumps, rubella) or airborne route (varicella), they should wear a mask (donned before entering the room) while providing care to a patient with one of these diseases because immunization is not 100% effective in preventing infection.[5] All HCP with potential exposure to blood or body fluids should be immune to hepatitis B.

Influenza vaccine should be offered to all HCP yearly. In the past few years, editorials and commentaries have recommended that yearly influenza immunization (unless contraindicated) should be a condition of employment for HCP.[15–17] In February 2012 the National Vaccine Advisory Committee issued recommendations on how to achieve the Healthy People 2020 seasonal influenza vaccine coverage target of 90% for HCP; for facilities that have implemented the recommended initial strategies but have "not consistently achieved the Healthy People target for vaccination coverage of HCP in an efficient and timely manner," it was recommended that they should "strongly consider an employer requirement for influenza immunization".[18]

Special Populations

In special circumstances, HCP, laboratory personnel, and researchers should be offered immunization with other vaccines such as polio,[19] rabies,[20] vaccinia (smallpox),[21] anthrax,[22] and meningococci (ACWY and B

TABLE 11.3
Methods of Demonstrating Proof of Immunity of Healthcare Personnel (HCP)[a]

Vaccine	Birth before 1957	Physician Diagnosis	Positive Serology	Self-Report	Documented Appropriate Vaccine Series[b]
Mumps (MMR)	Yes[c]	Yes[e]	Yes	No	Yes
Measles (MMR)	Yes[c]	Yes[e]	Yes	No	Yes
Rubella (MMR)	Yes[c,d]	No	Yes	No	Yes
Varicella	No	Yes	Yes	No	Yes
Hepatitis B	No	—	>10 mIU/mL[f]	No	Yes
Pertussis (Tdap)	No	No	No	No	Yes
Influenza	No	No	No	No	Yes

[a] Yes in any column is acceptable evidence of immunity.
[b] Written documentation required (i.e., signed by a healthcare provider).
[c] Consider immunization of HCP born before 1957; recommend during an outbreak.
[d] All HCP of childbearing potential should be immunized.
[e] Requires laboratory confirmation of infection.
[f] Obtain anti-HBs titer, 1–2 months after last vaccine dose; if immunization remote and anti-HBs titer not available, see text for management.
This table and been adapted from the study by Weber DJ, Rutala WA, Schaffner W. Lessons learned: protection of healthcare workers from infectious disease risks. Crit Care Med 2010;38(suppl.):S306–S314.

vaccines; as mentioned in the following). In addition, HCP who are traveling outside the United States for work-related activities should be evaluated and provided CDC-recommended immunizations such as hepatitis A, yellow fever, typhoid, cholera, and Japanese encephalitis.[23,24]

Immunocompromised HCP require special consideration in the provision of immunizations.[5,9,12,25] First, live attenuated virus vaccines (e.g., measles-mumps-rubella, varicella, live attenuated influenza) may be contraindicated depending on the nature of the immune compromise. Second, vaccines not routinely recommended may be indicated (e.g., pneumococcal, meningococcal, *Haemophilus influenzae* type b). Third, higher antigen doses (e.g., hepatitis B vaccine in people with end-stage renal disease), additional doses of vaccine (e.g., rabies vaccine in immunocompromised persons), or postimmunization serologic evaluation may be indicated (e.g., titer for antibodies against hepatitis B surface antigen [anti-HBs] after hepatitis B vaccine, antibody response to rabies vaccine) because immunization of immunocompromised people may elicit a lower antibody response. Finally, such personnel should be individually evaluated for reassignment (with the consent of the employee) depending on their job duties. Of importance, caring for an immunocompromised patient is not a contraindication to receipt of a live attenuated vaccine, although HCP receiving LAIV should not work in a protected environment (i.e., hematopoietic stem cell transplant unit) for 7 days after immunization.[26]

Pregnant HCP also require special consideration in the provision of immunizations. The risks from immunization during pregnancy are largely theoretical.[12] The benefit of immunization among pregnant women usually outweighs the potential risks for adverse reactions, especially when the risk for disease exposure is high, infection would pose a special risk to the mother or fetus, and the vaccine is unlikely to cause harm.[9,12,27,28] Furthermore, newer information continues to confirm the safety of vaccines given inadvertently during pregnancy. Ideally, women of childbearing age, including HCP, should have been immunized against vaccine-preventable diseases as recommended by the CDC and ACIP (e.g., measles, mumps, rubella, varicella, diphtheria, pertussis, and hepatitis B) as children or adolescents before becoming pregnant. However, because this may not have occurred, it is especially important that all pregnant HCP be screened for immunity to vaccine-preventable diseases. There is no convincing evidence of risk from immunizing pregnant women with inactivated viral or bacterial vaccines or toxoids. Women who are pregnant during respiratory virus season should receive inactivated influenza immunization.[9] In 2011 the ACIP recommended that healthcare providers implement a Tdap vaccination program for pregnant women who had not previously received Tdap. In 2012 ACIP updated its recommendations to indicate that healthcare providers should administer a single dose of Tdap during every pregnancy regardless of prior vaccination history preferably during 27–36 weeks gestation. If not administered during pregnancy, Tdap should be administered immediately postpartum.[29] Live attenuated vaccines should be provided only to nonpregnant HCP and deferred for pregnant women. Susceptible pregnant women at high risk for specific infections should receive, as indicated, the following vaccines: (1) hepatitis A, (2) hepatitis B, (3) pneumococcal polysaccharide, (4) meningococcal, (5) rabies, and (6) poliovirus (inactivated).[9,12] In spite of the lack of evidence of risk, HPV vaccine, an inactivated vaccine, is not recommended during pregnancy. Importantly, the indications for use of immunoglobulin (IG) preparations are the same in pregnant and nonpregnant women. Breastfeeding does not adversely affect the response to immunization and is not a contraindication for any of the current routinely recommended vaccines.

Measles, Mumps, and Rubella Vaccine

The incidence of measles, mumps, and rubella has decreased dramatically since the widespread use of MMR vaccine. Cases reported to the CDC in 2015 were as follows (cases per 100,000 population): (1) mumps, 1329 (0.41); (2) measles, 188 (0.06); (3) rubella, 5 (0); and (4) congenital rubella, 1 (0).[30] Since 2000 when measles was declared eliminated from the United States, the annual number of cases has ranged from a low of 37 in 2004 to a high of 667 in 2014.[31] During 2001–08, a total of 27 reported measles cases were transmitted in US healthcare facilities, accounting for 5% of all reported US measles cases.[5] In recent years, there has been an increase in the number of reported mumps cases, from 229 cases in 2012 to 6366 cases in 2016.[32] The recent increase has been mainly due to multiple mumps outbreaks reported across the country in settings where people often have close contact with one another, such as college campuses. Rubella remains rare in the United States.

Measles, mumps, and rubella represent important health hazards for HCP for the following reasons. First, all three are highly infectious and transmitted by the droplet route; measles is also highly infectious, but is transmitted by the airborne route. Second, in all three diseases, persons become infectious before developing a clinically recognizable illness. Third, measles is highly contagious. Transmission may occur for more than an hour after an infected person has left an enclosed area. Fourth, a history of prior disease may be unreliable for determining whether a healthcare provider actually suffered from measles, mumps, or rubella in the past. Hence many unimmunized healthcare providers may falsely believe themselves immune. Fifth, the cost of outbreaks for these diseases is high in both monetary terms and human suffering. Sixth, patients with congenital rubella are capable of transmitting rubella to susceptible adults.

All HCP should be immune to measles, mumps, and rubella. Immunity may be demonstrated by meeting one of the following criteria: (1) birth before 1957 (with the exception that women with childbearing potential should be immune to rubella), (2) laboratory evidence of immunity (persons with indeterminate levels of antibody to a specific vaccine-preventable disease such as measles are considered susceptible), (3) laboratory confirmation of disease, or[4] (4) evidence of appropriate immunizations (Table 11.3). Physician-diagnosed disease is no longer considered adequate evidence of immunity. Because of the excellent efficacy of MMR, written history of appropriate immunization is considered adequate evidence of immunity regardless of serologic results.[5]

Appropriate immunization consists of documented administration of two doses of live measles virus vaccine, two doses of live mumps virus vaccine, and one dose of live rubella virus vaccine (use of MMR vaccine is preferred). The American Academy of Pediatrics recommends that all susceptible HCP who may be exposed to patients with rubella or who take care of pregnant women should be immunized regardless of gender.[10] MMR vaccine is highly effective in preventing measles with a 1-dose vaccine effectiveness of 95% when administered on or after the age of 12 months and a 2-dose vaccine effectiveness of 99%. MMR vaccine has a 1-dose vaccine effectiveness in preventing mumps of 80%–85% (range: 75%–91%) and a 2-dose vaccine effectiveness of 79%–95%.[12] Vaccine effectiveness of the RA 27/3 rubella vaccine against clinical rubella is 95% (confidence interval [CI]: 85%–99%) and >99% for clinical laboratory–confirmed rubella.[12]

In response to the recent outbreaks of mumps, the CDC/ACIP recently recommended that "persons previously vaccinated with 2 doses of a mumps virus–containing vaccine who are identified by public health authorities as being part of a group or population at increased risk for acquiring mumps because of an outbreak should receive a third dose of a mumps virus–containing vaccine to improve protection against mumps disease and related complications".[33] The CDC noted that several studies found decreasing MMR vaccine effectiveness against mumps with increasing time after receipt of the second dose or reported increased risk for mumps with increasing time after receipt of the second dose. Limited laboratory data on immune response to mumps virus indicate both lower antibody titers and poorer antibody quality (e.g., lower avidity antibodies, failure to generate strong memory B cell responses) after either natural mumps infection or mumps vaccination than the responses to infection with or vaccination against measles and rubella. Both neutralizing and nonneutralizing mean mumps antibody titers decline over time in persons who have received 2 doses of MMR vaccine.[5] CDC also noted that since 2006 the predominant circulating mumps virus genotype in the United States has been genotype G. When studied 4–6 weeks and 10 years after receipt of the second MMR dose at the age of 4–6 years, all recipients had neutralizing antibody against genotype G mumps strain (predominant circulating strain); however, the geometric mean titers of antibodies were lower than those against the vaccine strain. Three epidemiologic studies[34–36] have reported lower attack rates among persons who received a third MMR vaccine dose during a mumps outbreak than those in persons who had received only 2 doses, but only one study[34] found a statistically significant risk ratio (6.7 vs. 14.5 per 1000 person-years; $P < .001$). Incremental vaccine effectiveness of the third versus the second MMR dose in these studies ranged from 61% to 88%, with one estimate being statistically significant (78.1%, 95% CI: 60.9%–87.8%).[34] This study also found that students who had received 2 doses of MMR vaccine ≥13 years before the outbreak had nine or more times the risk of contracting mumps than did those who had received the second vaccine dose within the 2 years preceding the outbreak. Multiple studies have demonstrated that a third dose of MMR vaccine is safe with mild adverse events reported at a low rate.[33]

Hepatitis B Virus Vaccine

The risk of HBV acquisition by HCP has declined dramatically over the years; the number of HBV infections among HCP declined by approximately 98% from an estimated 17,000 infections in 1983 to 263 acute HBV infections in 2010.[37] This decline was likely due to decreased exposure from improved work practice controls and preexposure HBV immunization of HCP. On the basis of national health survey data, approximately 850,000 persons are currently estimated to be living with HBV infection in the United States.[38] Studies based on data from countries of persons migrating to the United States and census data indicate that the total prevalence of chronic hepatitis B might be as high as 2.2 million persons, suggesting that the national health survey–based estimate might be conservative. Foreign-born persons account for approximately 95% of newly reported chronic infections in the United States; the prevalence of chronic HBV infection is approximately 3.5% among foreign-born persons, and the majority of chronic HBV infections in the United States are among Asians/Pacific Islanders.[38]

Hepatitis B acquisition represents a major hazard for HCP for several reasons. First, HCP have high rates of percutaneous blood contact. The 2015 EPINet Report from multiple hospitals noted that the percutaneous injury rate was 31.7 per 100 average daily census (ADC) with the rates in teaching hospitals being 38.5 per 100 ACI and nonteaching hospitals being 19.9 per 100 ADC.[39] Second, hepatitis B is highly infectious and can be transmitted in the absence of visible blood.[37] Third, HBV is relatively stable in the environment, as demonstrated by its survival after drying and storage at 25°C and 42% relative humidity for at least 1 week.[40] Fourth, HBV is more transmissible than either HIV or hepatitis C virus. In studies of HCP who sustained injuries from needles contaminated with blood containing HBV, the risk for developing clinical hepatitis if the blood was both hepatitis B surface antigen (HBsAg)-positive and HBeAg-positive was 22%–31%; the risk for developing serologic evidence of HBV infection was 37%–62%.[37] By comparison, the risk for developing clinical hepatitis from a needle contaminated with HBsAg-positive, HBeAg-negative blood was 1%–6%, and the risk for developing serologic evidence of HBV infection was 23%–37%.[37] The risks of disease transmission via mucosal contact or contact with nonintact skin have not been quantitated but appear to be much lower than those for percutaneous exposure. HBV infection has been acquired via ocular exposure[41] and has been transmitted to multiple patients while obtaining arterial blood gases by a respiratory therapist with severe exudative dermatitis.[42] The high frequency of hepatitis B among hospital personnel who did not recall a percutaneous exposure in the era before HBV vaccine has been attributed to inapparent inoculation through mucous membranes or small breaks in the skin.[43] Fifth, chronic hepatitis B remains common, and many patients are unaware of their infectious status. Finally, many HCP remain unimmunized. The CDC reported that in

2015 only 74.1% of HCP aged 19 years or older with direct care duties had received the full series of hepatitis B vaccine.[44] Transmission of hepatitis B via contaminated medical instruments and environmental surfaces is well described. Nosocomial outbreaks of HBV infection have been associated with a blood-contaminated jet gun injector, an endoscope, multidose medication vials, electroencephalography electrodes, finger-stick (i.e., capillary) blood-sampling devices, and reuse of needles and syringes.[45]

The key method of preventing healthcare-associated HBV infection among HCP is HBV immunization before beginning direct patient care of all HCP with potential blood or body fluid exposure. The Occupational Safety and Health Administration (OSHA) mandates that employers offer hepatitis B vaccination to all employees who have occupational risk and that PEP be available after an exposure.[46] For HCP immunized in training or at initiation of patient contact, an anti-HBs quantitative titer should be drawn 1–2 months after the last dose of vaccine. HCP with >10 mIU/mL anti-HBs are considered immune for life. HCP who do not respond adequately should be reimmunized with 3 additional doses of vaccine and tested for immunity 1–2 months after the last (i.e., sixth) dose. HCP who have not responded adequately (i.e., >10 mIU/mL anti-HBs) should be tested for HBsAg. Nonresponders to 6 doses of vaccine should be counseled to return to report any exposures to blood or body fluids as they may be prophylaxed with hepatitis B immune globulin (HBIG) (Table 11.4). HCP, especially trainees, with a remote history of hepatitis B vaccine should have their immunity to HBV assessed using the algorithm recommended by the CDC.[37]

As stated by the CDC/ACIP the 3-dose HBV vaccine series administered intramuscularly at 0, 1, and 6 months produces a protective antibody response in approximately 30%–55% of healthy adults aged ≤40 years after the first dose, 75% after the second dose, and >90% after the third dose.[5] After the age of 40 years, <90% of persons vaccinated with 3 doses have a protective antibody response, and by the age of 60 years, protective levels of antibody develop in approximately 75% of vaccinated persons. Smoking, obesity, genetic factors, and immune suppression are associated with diminished immune response to hepatitis B vaccination.[5] The vaccine should be administered in the deltoid, as buttock administration has been associated with a poorer antibody response.[47] Protection against symptomatic and chronic HBV infection has been documented to persist for >22 years in vaccine responders.[48]

TABLE 11.4
Postexposure Management of Healthcare Personnel after Occupational Percutaneous or Mucosal Exposure to Blood or Body Fluids by Healthcare Personnel Hepatitis B Vaccination and Response Status

HCP Status	Postexposure Testing		Postexposure Prophylaxis		
	Source patient (HBsAg)	HCP testing (anti-HBs)	HBIG[a]	Vaccination	Postvaccination serologic testing[b]
Documented responder[c] after complete series (≥3 doses)	No action needed				
Documented nonresponder[d] after two complete series	Positive/ unknown	—[e]	HBIG × 2 separated by 1 month	—	No applicable
	No action needed				
Response unknown after complete series	Positive/ unknown	<10 mIU/mL[e]	HBIG × 1	Initial revaccination	Yes
	Negative	<10 mIU/mL	None		
	Any result	≥10 mIU/mL	No action needed		
Unvaccinated/ incompletely vaccinated or vaccine refusers	Positive/ unknown	—[e]	HBIG × 1	Complete vaccination	Yes
	Negative	—	None	Complete vaccination	Yes

anti-HBs, antibody to hepatitis B surface antigen; *HBIG*, hepatitis B immune globulin; *HBsAg*, hepatitis B surface antigen; *HCP*, healthcare personnel.
[a] HBIG should be administered intramuscularly as soon as possible after exposure when indicated. The effectiveness of HBIG when administered >7 days after percutaneous, mucosal, or nonintact skin exposures is unknown. HBIG dosage is 0.06 mL/kg.
[b] Should be performed 1–2 months after the last dose of the HepB vaccine series (and 4–6 months after administration of HBIG to avoid detection of passively administered anti-HBs) using a quantitative method that allows detection of the protective concentration of anti-HBs (≥10 mIU/mL).
[c] A responder is defined as a person with anti-HBs ≥ 10 mIU/mL after ≥3 doses of HepB vaccine (complete series).
[d] A nonresponder is defined as a person with anti-HBs < 10 mIU/mL after ≥6 doses of HepB vaccine (2 complete series).
[e] HCP who have anti-HBs < 10 mIU/mL or who are unvaccinated or incompletely vaccinated and sustain an exposure to a source patient who is HBsAg-positive or has unknown HBsAg status should undergo baseline testing for HBV infection as soon as possible after exposure and follow-up testing approximately 6 months later. Initial baseline tests consist of total anti-HBc; testing at approximately 6 months consists of HBsAg and total anti-HBc.
This table and been adapted from the studies from Centers for Disease Control, Prevention Centers for Disease Control, Prevention. CDC guidance for evaluating health-care personnel for hepatitis B virus protection and for administering postexposure management. MMWR Recomm Rep 2013;62(RR-10):1–19; Centers for Disease Control and Prevention. Prevention of hepatitis B virus infection in the United States: recommendations of the Advisory Committee on Immunization Practices. MMWR Recomm Rep 2018;67(No. 1):1–31.

Varicella Vaccine

Before the introduction of the varicella vaccine in 1995, varicella was a common disease; an average of 4 million people got chickenpox, 10,500 to 13,000 were hospitalized, and 100 to 150 died each year.[49] Since the introduction of the varicella vaccine, there has been a dramatic decrease in the number of cases of varicella, hospitalizations, and deaths.[49] However, because varicella may be acquired from exposure to varicella or herpes zoster, exposure in healthcare settings will continue to occur. Multiple nosocomial outbreaks of varicella have been reported.[5] Varicella may be introduced into the hospital by infected patients, staff, or visitors. In several instances the source case for an outbreak was in the incubating phase of varicella.[50] Nosocomial transmission has been attributed to delays in the diagnosis or reporting of varicella or herpes zoster and in failures to implement control measures promptly. In hospitals and other healthcare settings, airborne transmission of varicella from patients with either varicella or herpes zoster has resulted in varicella in HCP and patients who had no direct contact with the index case patient.[50] Epidemiologic and tracer studies have confirmed relative airflow from rooms occupied by index cases as a major risk factor for the acquisition of varicella infection by susceptible hosts.[51] Varicella-zoster virus DNA has been detected by PCR 1.2–5.5 m from the beds of patients with varicella and from the room air of immunocompromised patients with herpes zoster.[52]

Although all susceptible patients in healthcare settings are at risk for severe varicella disease with complications, certain patients without evidence of immunity are at increased risk: (1) pregnant women, (2) premature infants born to susceptible mothers, (3) infants born at <28 weeks' gestation or who weigh ≤1000 g regardless of maternal immune status, and (4) immunocompromised persons of all ages (including persons who are undergoing immunosuppressive therapy, have malignant disease, or are immunodeficient).

The CDC/ACIP recommend that all HCP have evidence of immunity to varicella.[5] Evidence of immunity includes: (1) written documentation of vaccination with 2 doses of varicella vaccine at least 4 weeks apart; (2) laboratory evidence of varicella immunity or laboratory confirmation of disease; (3) diagnosis or verification of a history of varicella disease by a healthcare provider (when such documentation is lacking, persons should not be considered as having a valid history of disease because other diseases might mimic mild atypical varicella); or (4) diagnosis or verification of a history of herpes zoster by a healthcare provider.[5] HCP without evidence of immunity to varicella should receive 2 doses of varicella vaccine administered 4–8 weeks apart. If there is a >8 weeks elapse after the first dose, the second dose may be administered without restarting the schedule. Recently vaccinated HCP do not require any restriction in their work activities; however, HCP who develop a vaccine-related rash after vaccination should avoid contact with persons without evidence of immunity to varicella who are at risk for severe disease and complications until all lesions resolve (i.e., are crusted over) or, if they develop lesions that do not crust (macules and papules only), until no new lesions appear within a 24-h period. It is important to realize that commercial assays used to assess disease-induced immunity often lack sensitivity to detect vaccine-induced immunity (i.e., they might yield false-negative results).[5] Formal

studies to evaluate vaccine efficacy or effectiveness have not been performed in adults. Studies of varicella vaccine effectiveness performed among children indicated good performance of 1 dose for prevention of all varicella (80%–85%) and >95% effectiveness for prevention of moderate and severe disease.[5,53] A study of adults who received 2 doses of varicella vaccine 4 or 8 weeks apart and were exposed subsequently to varicella in the household estimated an 80% reduction in the expected number of cases.[5]

Influenza Vaccine

Protecting HCP and patients from acquiring influenza is a high public health priority.[54] Influenza occurs globally with an annual attack rate estimated at 5%–10% in adults and 20%–30% in children.[54] Infection may result in hospitalization and death, especially among high-risk groups. The CDC estimates that in the United States annually there are 9,200,000 to 35,600,000 cases that result in 140,000 to 710,000 hospitalizations and 12,000 to 56,000 deaths.[55] The World Health Organization (WHO) estimates that these annual epidemics result in 3–5 million cases of severe illness and about 290,000 to 650,000 respiratory deaths.[54] Several aspects of influenza epidemiology are important to remember: (1) influenza is easily spread from person to person; (2) it can affect anybody in any age group; (3) seasonal influenza is a serious public health problem that causes severe illness and death in high-risk populations; (4) prior influenza disease does not assure immunity because the virus frequently mutates from year to year (antigenic drift); (5) although antiviral drugs are available for treatment, influenza viruses can develop resistance to drugs; and (6) influenza vaccination is the most effective way to prevent influenza.[56]

Healthcare-associated influenza is a major worldwide problem for several reasons.[15,57,58] First, hospitals provide care to persons at high risk for morbidity and mortality if they acquire influenza, including neonates, older persons, those with chronic illnesses (e.g., diabetes, heart disease, asthma, lung disease), and immunocompromised persons. Second, nosocomial influenza outbreaks are frequent, and their control remains challenging. Third, the diagnosis of influenza is commonly missed because many infected and infectious persons are asymptomatic or mildly symptomatic, and the clinical signs and symptoms of influenza can be confused with similar respiratory illnesses caused by a variety of other pathogens. Furthermore, persons with influenza may be infectious before the onset of symptoms. Fourth, molecular analyses have revealed transmission from patients to HCP and from HCP to patients. HCP have served both as sources of nosocomial outbreaks and propagators of healthcare-associated outbreaks.[54]

As noted by the Society for Healthcare Epidemiology of America (SHEA), influenza vaccination of HCP serves several purposes: (1) to prevent transmission to patients, including those with a lower likelihood of vaccination response themselves; (2) to reduce the risk that the HCP will become infected with influenza; (3) to create "herd immunity" that protects both HCP and patients who are unable to receive vaccine or unlikely to respond with a sufficient antibody response; (4) to maintain a critical societal workforce during disease outbreaks; and[5] (5) to set an example concerning the importance of vaccination for every person.[15] Four cluster randomized trials and 4 observational studies conducted in LTC or hospital settings have demonstrated that immunization of HCP demonstrates a "significant protective association for influenza-like illness and laboratory-confirmed influenza".[59] For the reasons listed previously, influenza immunization annually of all HCP is recommended by the CDC,[5,9,57] WHO,[60] and many professional organizations. Nevertheless, attaining optimal influenza immunization of HCP is challenging for two key reasons: (1) the vaccine effectiveness varies year to year depending on how well the viral strains in the vaccine match with the circulating strains and (2) the vaccine must be provided each year. Furthermore, many HCP harbor misconceptions about the vaccine, including that one can acquire influenza from the vaccine.

The CDC assessed HCP immunization rates during the 2016−17 influenza season and reported that 78.6% of survey respondents reported receiving vaccination.[61] This was similar to the reported coverage in the previous three influenza seasons. Per the CDC report, vaccination coverage continued to be higher among HCP working in hospitals (92.3%) and lower among HCP working in ambulatory (76.1%) and LTC (68.0%) settings. As in previous seasons, coverage was highest among HCP who were required by their employer to be vaccinated (96.7%) and lowest among HCP working in settings where vaccination was not required, promoted, or offered on site (45.8%). Overall, vaccination coverage in 2016−17 was highest among physicians (95.8%), nurse practitioners and physician assistants (92.0%), nurses (92.6%), and pharmacists (93.7%) and lowest among other clinical HCP (80.0%), assistants and aides (69.1%), and nonclinical HCP (73.7%).[61] However, in hospital settings, vaccination coverage was approximately 90% or higher in all occupational groups, including assistants and aides and nonclinical personnel.

The barriers and solutions to achieving high coverage of influenza immunization among HCP have been reviewed and include: (1) inconvenient access to vaccine (solution: off-hours clinics, use of mobile vaccination carts, vaccination at staff and department meetings, and provision of adequate staff and resources)[2]; (2) cost (solution: provision of free vaccine); (3) concerns for vaccine adverse events (solution: targeted education including specific information to dispel vaccine myths); and (4) other (solution: strong and viable administrative leadership, visible vaccination of key leaders, active declination of HCP who do not wish or cannot be vaccinated, accurate tracking of individual HCP and unit-based compliance of HCP with vaccination, and surveillance for healthcare-associated influenza). Substantial additional research has been published on the effectiveness of different methods to improve influenza vaccine acceptance by HCP (Table 11.5).[15,54,62]

Several methods for increasing HCP compliance with influenza immunization deserve further discussion: (1) the use of declination forms, (2) the requirement that HCP who are unable or unwilling to receive influenza vaccine wear a surgical mask while providing patient care or while on a patient unit, and (3) mandatory influenza immunization.[54] The 2005 SHEA Guideline on influenza vaccination of HCP recommended the use of a declination form to be signed by HCP who were unwilling to accept vaccine as one modality to increase vaccine uptake.[62] This declination form described the risk to the HCP and their patients from the HCP refusing immunization. Subsequent research has demonstrated that the use of such forms was associated with only a modest increase in vaccine use by HCP, even when combined with other strategies to increase vaccine coverage. Multiple studies demonstrated that the introduction of declination forms continued to lead to vaccine coverage <80%[63−65] and often <70%.[66] The 2010 revised SHEA Guideline on influenza vaccination of HCP included the statement "the use of statements (i.e., declination forms) should not be viewed as the primary method for increasing vaccination rates".[15]

Another intervention that has been recommended is to require unvaccinated HCP to wear a surgical mask during the influenza season.[15] Several potential issues related to the masking requirement have been raised. First, implementation of such a policy is logistically challenging (i.e., developing methods to identify those HCP required to wear a mask during clinical care). Developing a simple method to identify such HCP without stigmatizing those HCP who chose not to be vaccinated or were unable to be vaccinated due to

TABLE 11.5

Interventions that Have Been Shown Alone or in Combination to Improve Influenza Vaccine Coverage for Healthcare Personnel

- Mobile carts
- Free vaccine
- Adequate staff resources for vaccine campaign
- Education on benefits and risks (or lack of risks) for immunization
- Incentives for immunization
- Immunizations available on nights and weekends
- Immunization available at convenient locations (e.g., meetings, common areas)
- Administrative support including visible vaccination of key personnel
- Tracing vaccination by individual healthcare providers and hospital units with regular feedback to healthcare providers and administrators
- Sanctions for failure to be immunized
- Employment conditional upon receipt of vaccine

This table and been adapted from the study by Weber DJ, Rutala WA, Schaffner W. Lessons learned: protection of healthcare workers from infectious disease risks. Crit Care Med 2010;38(suppl.):S306–S314.

vaccine contraindications has proved difficult. Second, the ability of policy of masking nonimmunized HCP to protect patients against acquisition of influenza has not been demonstrated. A review by Thomas reported that "none of four randomized clinical trials of HCP mask wearing (two directly observed and two not) showed an effect because they were underpowered either due to small sample size or low circulation of influenza.[67] Third, although a review of methods of preventing nosocomial influenza in a single US state revealed that many facilities required nonimmunized HCP to wear a mask, there was poor consistency on required locations for mask use (i.e., while in the facility, while on the patient care unit, or while providing clinical care [i.e., within 6 feet]), and actual compliance with the policy and frequency of penalties for noncompliance were not assessed.[68]

The most successful strategy to improve HCP influenza vaccine coverage has been to make receipt of vaccine a condition of employment (i.e., "mandatory" immunizations). Hospitals using this strategy exempt HCP with a medical contraindication to immunization and some also exempt HCP with a religious objection. Multiple reports from hospitals that use this strategy have reported vaccination coverage rates >95%.[66,69–72] Increasing numbers of hospitals in the United States now require receipt of influenza vaccine as a condition of employment.[61] Concern has been raised about the ethics of "mandatory" immunization of HCP. However, multiple professional societies have endorsed that employment as HCP should be

conditional on willingness to receive influenza vaccine, as vaccination protects both HCP and their patients.[54,62]

In conclusion, influenza causes substantial morbidity and mortality worldwide each year, and healthcare-associated influenza is a frequent event. HCP may be the source for infecting patients and may propagate nosocomial outbreaks. All HCP should receive a dose of influenza vaccine each year to protect themselves and others. Multiple methods have been used by healthcare facilities to improve influenza vaccine coverage among HCP, with varying rates of success; most of these methods were more effective when used in combination with each other (Table 11.5). The only proven method to reliably achieve a coverage level >95% among HCP is to require influenza immunization as a condition of employment.

Pertussis Vaccine

In the United States, the highest recorded annual incidence of pertussis occurred in 1934, when more than 260,000 cases were reported.[73] After the introduction of pertussis vaccines in the 1940s when case counts frequently exceeded 100,000 cases per year, reports declined dramatically to fewer than 10,000 by 1965. During the 1980s pertussis case reports began increasing gradually, and by 2015 more than 20,000 cases were reported nationwide. Possible explanations for this increase in disease and failure of current pertussis-containing vaccines include the following: (1) decay in antibody over time; (2) a T helper (Th)

1/Th2 versus a Th1/Th17 cellular response; (3) incomplete antigen package; (4) incorrect balance of antigens in the vaccine; (5) linked epitope suppression; and (6) the occurrence of pertactin-deficient *Bordetella pertussis* strains.[74–77]

CDC has noted that pertussis is a common (endemic) disease in the United States, with peaks in reported disease every few years and frequent outbreaks.[78] In 2012, the most recent peak year, states reported 48,277 cases of pertussis, and many more cases go unreported. At the University of North Carolina Hospitals, pertussis is now the most common source of infectious disease exposure evaluations (Weber, unpublished data, 1994–2015). Multiple nosocomial outbreaks of pertussis have been reported, including outbreaks in which an infected HCP was the source.[79] Nosocomial outbreaks have occurred for several reasons: (1) failure to immunize all HCP with Tdap vaccine; (2) failure to recognize and appropriately isolate infected patients, (3) failure to provide antibiotic prophylaxis to exposed staff, and (4) failure to furlough symptomatic staff.[79]

In 2006 CDC recommended that hospitals and ambulatory-care facilities should provide Tdap vaccination to HCP and use approaches that maximize vaccination rates (e.g., education about the benefits of vaccination, convenient access, and the provision of Tdap at no charge).[80] CDC also stated that because Tdap is not licensed for multiple administrations, after receipt of Tdap, HCP should receive Td or tetanus toxoid for booster immunization against tetanus and diphtheria according to previously published guidelines.[80] In the 2018 Immunization Schedule for Adults, the CDC clarified what constitutes receipt of Tdap as an "adult" as follows: "Administer to adults who previously did not receive a dose of tetanus toxoid, reduced diphtheria toxoid, and acellular pertussis vaccine (Tdap) as an adult or child (routinely recommended at age 11–12 years) 1 dose of Tdap, followed by a dose of tetanus and diphtheria toxoids (Td) booster every 10 years".[9] Thus adult HCP who received Tdap as an adolescent would not receive any additional Tdap doses even if they become a healthcare provider in later life. Pregnant HCP should be referred to their primary care provider as a dose of Tdap vaccine is recommended during each pregnancy to protect the women's newborn child against pertussis.[29,81]

The duration of protection against pertussis afforded by Tdap vaccine wanes with time.[82–84] Because current CDC/ACIP guidelines for HCP recommend only a single Tdap even if the Tdap was provided to an adolescent (i.e., ages of 11–12 years), it is likely that the majority of HCP will have inadequate vaccine-induced long-term protection against pertussis.

Neisseria meningitidis Vaccines

Rates of invasive meningococcal disease are at historic lows in the United States and have been declining in the United States since the late 1990s.[85] In 2016 there were about 370 total cases of meningococcal disease reported to CDC.

Currently there are two types of meningococcal vaccines in the United States: (1) quadrivalent meningococcal conjugate vaccine, which provides protection against serogroups A, C, W, and Y, and (2) serogroup B meningococcal vaccine.[86] Although meningococcal vaccines are not routinely recommended for HCP, they are recommended for microbiologists who are routinely exposed to *N. meningitidis* such as by spinning cerebrospinal fluid.[5] Specifically, microbiologists should receive both the meningococcal conjugate vaccine and the serogroup B meningococcal vaccine.[87,88] Immunization for microbiologists is recommended because of multiple reports of the acquisition of invasive meningococcal disease from exposures in the clinical microbiology laboratory.[89–91] Sejvar et al. reviewed the literature from 1985 to 2001 and identified 16 cases of laboratory-acquired meningococcal disease of which 8 cases (50%) were fatal.[90] They calculated an attack rate of 13 in 100,000 microbiologists between 1996 and 2001, compared with 0.2 in 100,000 among US adults in general. Currently microbiologists at continued risk for exposure to *N. meningitidis* should receive a booster dose of meningococcal conjugate vaccine every 5 years; there is no current recommendation for a booster dose of serogroup B meningococcal vaccine.

POSTEXPOSURE PROPHYLAXIS
General Recommendations

General guidelines on PEP are available from CDC,[2] the ACIP,[5] the American Academy of Pediatrics,[10] and the American Public Health Association.[92] All HCP should be educated at their initiation of employment or service about when and how to report a potential infectious disease exposure. In general, HCP should complete an incident form, have it signed by their supervisor, and then report to the Occupational Health Clinic. Occupational health evaluation should be available 24/7 for exposed HCP. The incident form should be reviewed by Occupational Health Clinic and communicated to the Worker's Compensation Department. HCP with serious or life-threatening injuries or exposures should be referred to an emergency department or specialty clinic as appropriate. If patient or visitor exposures also occurred, the Infection Prevention Department should be notified.

A well-defined protocol should be in place that details the steps in evaluation and management of HCP potentially exposed to an infectious agent. Proper counseling of the exposed healthcare provider is critical. Appropriate first aid should be provided, including proper care of any sharps injury or mucosal membrane exposure (e.g., copious rinsing of eyes in the case of splash to eyes). A proper evaluation of the source case should also be conducted to confirm the report by the exposed HCP that the source patient does indeed have a communicable disease. For blood and body fluid exposures, appropriate laboratory tests should be obtained from the source patient to determine if the source patient can transmit HIV, HBV, or HCV.

PEP is available for many infectious diseases including but not limited to diphtheria, hepatitis A and B, HIV, influenza, measles, invasive meningococcal infection, pertussis, rabies, and varicella/herpes zoster (Table 11.6). Unfortunately, PEP is not currently available for exposure to hepatitis C, mumps, and rubella. PEP may consist of antivirals, antibiotics, IG preparations, and/or vaccines. IG preparations may be indicated as part of PEP for exposure to hepatitis A (IG), hepatitis B (HBIG), measles (IG), rabies (rabies immune globulin [RIG]), tetanus (tetanus immune globulin [TIG]), varicella and potentially zoster (i.e., disseminated herpes zoster or localized zoster in an immunocompromised patient) (varicella-zoster immune globulin [VariZIG]), and vaccinia (vaccinia immune globulin [VIG]). Importantly, preexposure prophylaxis with recommended immunizations is not considered sufficient protection after an exposure to the diseases such as pertussis, meningococcal infection, and diphtheria, and postexposure antimicrobial prophylaxis is still recommended. More than one PEP modality may be recommended for disease exposures; this section will focus on the use of vaccines for PEP of HCP.

Measles

Patients with measles should be placed on airborne precautions (i.e., placed in a single room with negative pressure, >12 air exchanges per hour, and the air is

TABLE 11.6
Recommendations for Postexposure Prophylaxis (PEP) of Healthcare Providers Exposed to a Vaccine-Preventable Disease

Disease	Vaccine PEP	Immunoglobulins for PEP	Antiinfectives
Measles	Yes, provide within 72 hours	Yes, provide within 6 days; 0.25 mL/kg (40 mg IgG/kg) (CDC) or 0.50 mL/kg (AAP)	—
Hepatitis B	Yes, provide within 7 days. See Table 11.4.	Yes, See Table 11.4.	—
Varicella	Yes, ideally provide within 3–5 days (see text)	Yes, VariZIG (see text)	—
Influenza	No	No	Antivirals may be used for postexposure prophylaxis (see text)
Pertussis	No	No	Antibiotics may be used for postexposure prophylaxis (see text)
Neisseria meningitidis	No	No	Antibiotics may be used for postexposure prophylaxis (see text)
Hepatitis A	Yes, within 14 days	Yes	—
Rabies	Yes, as soon as possible (see text)	Yes, as soon as possible (see text)	—
Diphtheria	Yes (see text)	No	Yes (see text)

AAP, American Academy of Pediatrics [Red Book], 2015; CDC, Centers for Disease Control and Prevention, 2011.

directly exhausted out or recirculated through a HEPA filter before return).[93] Because of the possibility, albeit low (~ 1%), of measles vaccine failure in HCP exposed to infected patients, all HCP including those previously vaccinated should observe airborne precautions in caring for patients with measles.[5] If measles exposures occur in a healthcare facility, all nonprotected HCP should be evaluated immediately for presumptive evidence of measles immunity.[5,8] HCP without evidence of immunity should be offered the first dose of MMR vaccine and excluded from work from day 5–21 after exposure.[5,8] Available data suggest that live virus measles vaccine, if administered within 72 h of measles exposure, will prevent or modify disease. Even if it is too late to provide effective PEP by administering MMR vaccine, the vaccine can provide protection against future exposure to all three infections. HCP without evidence of immunity who are not vaccinated after exposure should be removed from all patient contact and excluded from the facility from day 5 after their first exposure through day 21 after the last exposure, even if they have received postexposure intramuscular immune globulin (IGIM). Recommendations for providing immune globulin (i.e., indications, dose) have been provided by the CDC[5] and American Academy of Pediatrics.[10] Those with documentation of 1 MMR vaccine dose may remain at work and should receive a second dose of MMR. IG PEP is especially recommended for serosusceptible pregnant women and severely immunocompromised persons within 6 days of exposure to prevent or modify disease. If IG is administered to an exposed person, observations should continue for signs and symptoms of measles for 28 days rather than 21 days after exposure because IG might prolong the incubation period.

Hepatitis B

HCP exposed to an HBsAg-positive patient should be evaluated for prophylaxis per the recommended CDC algorithm (Table 11.4).[94] Exposure consists of a percutaneous injury or mucosal or nonintact skin exposure to blood or certain internal body fluids (e.g., peritoneal, pleural, cerebrospinal, pericardial, joint).[8] Contact with a patient's blood or a body fluid with the healthcare provider's intact skin is not considered an exposure. Unless visibly contaminated with blood, the following fluids do not constitute an exposure requiring consideration for hepatitis B PEP: (1) sweat, (2) tears, (3) saliva, (4) urine, (5) vomitus, (6) sputum, and (7) stool.[8] The following paragraphs in this section were excerpted

from the CDC/ACIP recommendations for the prevention of Hepatitis B transmission in the United States.[94]

Vaccinated HCP: For vaccinated HCP (who have written documentation of a complete HepB vaccine series) with subsequent documented anti-HBs ≥ 10 mIU/mL, testing the source patient for HBsAg is unnecessary. No PEP for HBV is necessary, regardless of the source patient's HBsAg status.[94] For vaccinated HCP (who have written documentation of a complete HepB vaccine series) without previous anti-HBs testing, the healthcare provider should be tested for anti-HBs, and the source patient (if known) should be tested for HBsAg as soon as possible after the exposure. Anti-HBs testing should be performed using a method that allows detection of the protective concentration of anti-HBs (≥10 mIU/mL). Testing the source patient and the healthcare provider should occur simultaneously; testing the source patient should not be delayed while waiting for the healthcare provider's anti-HBs test results, and likewise, testing the healthcare provider should not be delayed while waiting for the source patient's HBsAg results.[94]

If the healthcare provider has anti-HBs < 10 mIU/mL and the source patient is HBsAg-positive or has an unknown HBsAg status, the healthcare provider should receive 1 dose of HBIG and be revaccinated as soon as possible after the exposure. HepB vaccine may be administered simultaneously with HBIG at a separate anatomical injection site (e.g., separate limb). The healthcare provider should then receive the subsequent 2 doses of HepB vaccine to complete the second series (likely 6 doses total when accounting for the original series) according to the vaccination schedule. So the healthcare provider's vaccine response status can be documented for future exposures, and anti-HBs testing should be performed 1–2 months after the final vaccine dose.

If the healthcare provider has anti-HBs < 10 mIU/mL and the source patient is HBsAg-negative, the healthcare provider should receive an additional single HepB vaccine dose, followed by repeat anti-HBs testing 1–2 months later. HCP whose anti-HBs remains <10 mIU/mL should undergo revaccination with two more doses (likely 6 doses total when accounting for the original series). So the healthcare provider's vaccine response status can be documented for future exposures, and anti-HBs testing should be performed 1–2 months after the final dose of vaccine.

If the healthcare provider has anti-HBs ≥ 10 mIU/mL at the time of the exposure, no postexposure HBV management is necessary, regardless of the source patient's HBsAg status.

For vaccinated HCP with anti-HBs < 10 mIU/mL after two complete HepB vaccine series, the source patient should be tested for HBsAg as soon as possible after the exposure. If the source patient is HBsAg-positive or has unknown HBsAg status, the healthcare provider should receive 2 doses of HBIG. The first dose should be administered as soon as possible after the exposure, and the second dose should be administered 1 month later. HepB vaccine is not recommended for the exposed healthcare provider who has previously completed two HepB vaccine series. If the source patient is HBsAg-negative, neither HBIG nor HepB vaccine is necessary (Table 11.4).

Unvaccinated HCP: For unvaccinated or incompletely vaccinated HCP, the source patient should be tested for HBsAg as soon as possible after the exposure. Testing unvaccinated or incompletely vaccinated HCP for anti-HBs is not necessary and is potentially misleading because anti-HBs ≥ 10 mIU/mL as a correlate of vaccine-induced protection has only been determined for persons who have completed an approved vaccination series. If the source patient is HBsAg-positive or has an unknown HBsAg status, the healthcare provider should receive 1 dose of HBIG and 1 dose of HepB vaccine administered as soon as possible after the exposure. HepB vaccine may be administered simultaneously with HBIG at a separate anatomical injection site (e.g., separate limb). The healthcare provider should complete the HepB vaccine series according to the vaccination schedule. To document the healthcare provider's vaccine response status for future exposures, anti-HBs testing should be performed approximately 1−2 months after the final vaccine dose. Anti-HBs testing should be performed using a method that allows detection of the protective concentration of anti-HBs (≥10 mIU/mL). Because anti-HBs testing of HCP who received HBIG should be performed after anti-HBs from HBIG is no longer detectable (6 months after administration), it might be necessary to defer anti-HBs testing for a period longer than 1−2 months after the last vaccine dose in these situations (Table 11.4).

If the source patient is HBsAg-negative, the HCP should complete the HepB vaccine series according to the vaccination schedule. So the healthcare provider's vaccine response status can be documented for future exposures, and anti-HBs testing should be performed approximately 1−2 months after the final vaccine dose (Table 11.4).

PEP should be provided as soon as possible but always within 7 days of exposure. HCP who have anti-HBs < 10 mIU/mL (or who are unvaccinated or incompletely vaccinated) and sustain an exposure to a source patient who is HBsAg-positive or has an unknown HBsAg status should undergo baseline testing for HBV infection as soon as possible after the exposure and follow-up testing approximately 6 months later. Testing immediately after the exposure should consist of total antibodies to hepatitis B core antigen (anti-HBc), and follow-up testing approximately 6 months later should consist of HBsAg and total anti-HBc.[94] HCP exposed to a source patient who is HBsAg-positive or has an unknown HBsAg status do not need to take special precautions to prevent secondary transmission during the follow-up period; however, they should refrain from donating blood, plasma, organs, tissue, or semen. The exposed healthcare provider does not need to modify sexual practices or refrain from becoming pregnant. If an exposed healthcare provider is breastfeeding, she does not need to discontinue. No modifications to an exposed healthcare provider's patient care responsibilities are necessary to prevent transmission to patients based solely on exposure to a source patient who is HBsAg-positive or has an unknown HBsAg status.[94]

Varicella/Zoster

Guidelines for PEP after unprotected exposure by HCP to a patient with varicella or zoster are available from the CDC,[2] ACIP,[5] American Academy of Pediatrics,[10] and the American Public Health Association.[90] Exposure to VZV is defined as close contact with an infectious person, such as close indoor contact (e.g., in the same room) or face-to-face contact. Experts differ regarding the duration of contact, that is, some suggest 5 minutes and others up to 1 hour.[5] All agree that it does not include transitory contact.[10] PEP with varicella vaccination or VariZIG depends on immune status of the exposed HCP. HCP who have received 2 doses of vaccine and who are exposed to VZV (from varicella, disseminated herpes zoster, or uncovered lesions of a localized herpes zoster) should be monitored daily during days 8−21 after exposure for fever, skin lesions, and systemic symptoms suggestive of varicella. HCP can be monitored directly by their occupational health program or infection preventionists or instructed to report fever, headache, or other constitutional symptoms and any atypical skin lesions immediately. HCP should be excluded from a work facility immediately if symptoms occur.[5] HCP who have received 1 dose of vaccine and who are exposed to VZV should receive the second dose within 3−5 days after exposure to rash (provided 4 weeks have elapsed after the first dose). After vaccination, management is similar to that of 2-dose vaccine recipients. Those who did not receive a second dose or who received the second dose >5 days after exposure should be excluded from work for 8–21 days after exposure (see work restrictions mentioned in the following). Unvaccinated HCP who have no other evidence of immunity and who are exposed to VZV (from varicella, disseminated herpes zoster, or uncovered lesions of a localized herpes zoster) are potentially infective from days 8–21 after exposure and should be furloughed during this period. They should also receive postexposure vaccination as soon as possible. Vaccination within 3–5 days of exposure to rash might modify the disease if infection occurred. Vaccination >5 days after exposure is still indicated because it induces protection against subsequent exposures (if the current exposure did not cause infection).

For HCP at risk for severe disease and for whom varicella vaccination is contraindicated (e.g., pregnant or immunocompromised HCP without evidence of immunity), VariZIG after exposure is recommended. The VariZIG product currently used in the United States is VariZIG (Cangene Corporation, Winnipeg, Canada).[93] VariZIG, if indicated, should be administered as soon as possible after varicella-zoster virus exposure, ideally within 96 hours for greatest effectiveness but always within 10 days. VariZIG is supplied in 125-IU vials and should be administered intramuscularly; the recommended dose is 125 IU/10 kg of body weight, up to a maximum of 625 IU (five vials). If VariZIG is not available, intravenous immune globulin (IGIV) can be used.[10] This recommendation for use of IGIV is based on the "best judgment of experts" and is supported by reports comparing VZV IgG antibody titers measured in licensed IGIV preparations and patients given VariZIG. No clinical data demonstrating effectiveness of IGIV for PEP of varicella are available.[10] The recommended dose for IGIV PEP of varicella is 400 mg/kg, administered once intravenously.[10] Importantly, VariZIG might prolong the incubation period by a week, thus extending the time during which personnel should not work from 21 to 28 days.

If VariZIG is indicated but not available or >10 days have elapsed since the exposure, some experts recommend that PEP can be provided with oral acyclovir (20 mg/kg per dose administered 4 times per day; maximum daily dose 3200 mg) or oral valacyclovir (20 mg/kg per dose administered 3 times per day; maximum daily dose 3000 mg) beginning on day 8 (7–10 days) after exposure and continuing for 7–14 days for immunocompromised patients without evidence of immunity.[10]

Influenza

Influenza immunization is not effective when used as PEP due to the short incubation period of influenza. This explanation is provided on the CDC website: "Because multiple exposures to influenza are likely during influenza season, routine antiviral prophylaxis is not recommended. CDC does not recommend widespread or routine use of antiviral medications for chemoprophylaxis except as one of multiple interventions to control institutional influenza outbreaks".[95] However, antiviral medications can be considered for chemoprophylaxis to prevent influenza in certain situations, such as the following examples: (1) prevention of influenza in persons at high risk of influenza complications during the first 2 weeks after vaccination after exposure to a person with influenza; (2) prevention for people at high risk for complications from influenza who cannot receive influenza vaccine due to a contraindication after exposure to a person with influenza; and (3) prevention for people with severe immune deficiencies or others who might not respond to influenza vaccination, such as persons receiving immunosuppressive medications, after exposure to a person with influenza.[95] To be effective as chemoprophylaxis, an antiviral medication must be taken each day for the duration of potential exposure to a person with influenza and continued for 7 days after the last known exposure. For persons taking antiviral chemoprophylaxis after inactivated influenza vaccination, the recommended duration is until immunity after vaccination develops (antibody development after vaccination takes about 2 weeks in adults and can take longer in children depending on age and vaccination history).

Use of antiviral chemoprophylaxis to control outbreaks among high-risk persons in institutional settings, such as long-term-care facilities, is recommended only for unvaccinated HCP. For newly vaccinated staff, antiviral chemoprophylaxis can be offered for up to 2 weeks (the time needed for antibody development) after influenza vaccination. Chemoprophylaxis can also be offered for all employees, regardless of their influenza vaccination status, if the outbreak is caused by a strain of influenza virus that is not well matched by the vaccine. As noted previously, an emphasis on close monitoring for signs and symptoms of influenza and initiation of early antiviral treatment is an alternative to chemoprophylaxis for HCP.[4] For institutional outbreak management, antiviral chemoprophylaxis should be administered for a minimum of 2 weeks and continued for at least 7 days after the last known case was identified.[95] Antiviral agents and doses are available from the CDC.[95]

Pertussis

Prevention of pertussis transmission in healthcare settings involves diagnosis and early treatment of clinical cases, droplet isolation of infectious patients, exclusion from work of HCP who are infectious, and PEP.[5] Guidelines for postexposure management of HCP exposed to pertussis have been published by the CDC,[5] American Academy of Pediatrics,[10] and the American Public Health Association.[92] Exposure is defined as close contact (i.e., face-to-face exposure within 3 feet or direct contact with respiratory, nasal, or oral secretions) with a symptomatic patient.[10]

Data on the need for PEP in Tdap-vaccinated HCP are inconclusive; Tdap might not preclude the need for PEP.[96] Per CDC/ACIP, postexposure antimicrobial prophylaxis is recommended for all HCP who have unprotected exposure to pertussis and are likely to expose a patient at risk for severe pertussis (e.g., hospitalized neonates and pregnant women). Other HCP should either receive postexposure antimicrobial prophylaxis or be monitored daily for 21 days after pertussis exposure and treated at the onset of signs and symptoms of pertussis.[5] Tdap is not considered useful for PEP in exposed unvaccinated HCP.

Bordetella pertussis is highly susceptible in vitro to erythromycin and the newer macrolides, azithromycin, and clarithromycin. It is also susceptible to trimethoprim-sulfamethoxazole. Azithromycin has been demonstrated to be effective in the prophylaxis and treatment of pertussis. It is now the preferred agent because compared with erythromycin, it requires a short period of PEP or therapy (5 vs. 7—14 days), reduced dosing frequency (1 vs. 4 times per day), and is less likely to result in gastrointestinal distress.[10] Trimethoprim-sulfamethoxazole is the recommended alternative for treatment and for chemoprophylaxis of individuals intolerant to a macrolide, although its efficacy as a chemoprophylactic agent has not been evaluated.[10]

Invasive *N. meningitidis*

Chemoprophylaxis is advised for all exposed HCP who have had intensive, unprotected contact (i.e., without wearing a mask) with patients with invasive meningococcal disease, e.g., via mouth-to-mouth resuscitation, endotracheal intubation, or endotracheal tube management. Chemoprophylaxis for HCP should be recommended even if the healthcare provider has been vaccinated with either the meningococcal conjugate or polysaccharide vaccine.[5] Because the rate of secondary disease for close contacts is highest immediately after onset of disease in the index patient, antimicrobial chemoprophylaxis should be administered as soon as possible (ideally <24 h after identification of the index patient). Conversely, chemoprophylaxis administered >14 days after exposure to the index patient is probably of limited or no value. Oropharyngeal or nasopharyngeal cultures are not helpful in determining the need for chemoprophylaxis and might unnecessarily delay institution of this preventive measure.

There is strong evidence that several antibiotics (i.e., rifampin, ciprofloxacin, ceftriaxone) and moderate evidence that other antibiotics (i.e., azithromycin, cefixime) are highly effective in eradication of meningococcal carriage (i.e., 90%—95%). A 5-day course of azithromycin is the first-line choice for treatment and PEP.[10] Resistance to macrolide antibiotics has been rarely reported. The preferred agent in pregnant women is ceftriaxone (250 mg intramuscularly, 1 dose; diluted with 1% lidocaine to decrease pain at the injection site).[10] Although sporadic resistance to rifampin and ciprofloxacin have been reported worldwide, meningococcal resistance to chemoprophylaxis antibiotics remains rare in the United States.

Special Use Vaccine: Rabies

Rabies is primarily a disease of animals.[97] Human-to-human transmission has been rarely reported.[97] Human rabies cases in the United States are rare, with only 1 to 3 cases reported annually.[98]

Rabies prophylaxis may occasionally need to be provided to HCP who work out of doors (e.g., maintenance workers, personnel who care for grounds) and suffer a bite from a wild animal that could potentially transmit rabies (e.g., fox, raccoon, and so forth) or have bat exposure. Concern about rabies transmission is frequent among HCP who have cared for human patients with rabies, especially since fluids from the upper and lower respiratory tracts of humans frequently test positive for rabies virus. One review paper reported that ∼30% of HCP who provided direct care for a patient with rabies were provided PEP.[99] The CDC recommends that patients with possible or known rabies be cared for using standard precautions.[94] However, given HCP concerns and the rare possible risk of rabies transmission, HCP might opt to use personal protective equipment to prevent contact with the patient's saliva and respiratory secretions (i.e., gown, gloves, face shield or mask with eye protection). Unvaccinated HCP with mucous membrane or percutaneous skin exposure to a potentially rabid animal or human should receive postexposure rabies vaccine and RIG as recommended by the CDC.[100]

Special Use Vaccine: Hepatitis A

Occasional outbreaks of hepatitis A virus (HAV) have been reported in hospitals.[101] Risk factors for HAV transmission to HCP have included activities that increase the risk of fecal–oral contamination, including caring for a person with unrecognized hepatitis A infection; sharing food, beverages, or cigarettes with patients, their families, or the staff; nail biting; handling bile without proper precautions; and not washing hands or wearing gloves when providing care to infected patients.[101] However, routine immunization of HCP with hepatitis A vaccine is not recommended as seroprevalence studies have not demonstrated that HCP are at increased risk for HAV infection because of occupational exposure.[5,101] Maintenance workers who might be exposed to sewage are also not at increased risk for acquisition of hepatitis A and do not need to be vaccinated.

The American Academy of Pediatrics states that hepatitis A vaccine or IG may be used for control of nosocomial outbreaks and PEP for HCP in close contact with infected patients.[10] In these cases only monovalent hepatitis A vaccine should be used and should be administered within 14 days of exposure. For PEP, immune globulin (0.02 mL/kg intramuscularly) also can be used.[102] For healthy adults 40 years or younger, hepatitis A vaccine is the preferred PEP, whereas for HCP older than 40 year of age, IGIM is preferred because of the absence of data regarding vaccine performance in this age group.[10] The efficacy of hepatitis A vaccine and immune globulin for PEP when administered more than 2 weeks after exposure has not been established.

Special Use Vaccine: Diphtheria

Although diphtheria was a widespread disease in the United States before the use of vaccines, it is now a rare disease. In the past decade, there were less than five cases of diphtheria in the United States reported to CDC, although the disease continues to cause illness globally.[103] Importantly, the case-fatality rate is still ~10%, even with treatment.[104] HCP are not at greater risk for diphtheria than the general population.[5] For HCP exposed to nasopharyngeal secretions of a patient known or suspected to have diphtheria, the following postexposure measures should be taken regardless of their immunization status: (1) surveillance for 7 days for evidence of disease, (2) culture for *C. diphtheriae*, and (3) antimicrobial prophylaxis with erythromycin (1 gm orally for 7–10 days) or a single injection of penicillin G benzathine (1.2 million

U intramuscularly × 1 dose).[10] Asymptomatic exposed HCP should also receive a booster dose of Td, if they have not received a booster dose of a diphtheria toxoid–containing vaccine within 5 years (Tdap is preferred if the HCP has not received a dose of Tdap previously as an adolescent or an adult).[10] Exposed HCP should not receive equine diphtheria antitoxin as there is no evidence that antitoxin provides additional benefits for contacts who have received antimicrobial prophylaxis.

ACKNOWLEDGMENTS

The authors wish to thank Drs. Emily Ciccone and Joseph D. Tucker for editorial assistance. This chapter includes material that was previously included in previous papers by Weber and Rutala. However, text and references have been updated to include all new and revised CDC/ACIP recommendations as well as present new material.

REFERENCES

1. Centers for Disease Control and Prevention. Workplace safety & health topics. Healthcare workers. http://www.cdc.gov/niosh/topics/healthcare/.
2. Bolyard EA, Tablan OC, Williams WW, et al. Guideline for infection control in health care personnel. *Am J Infect Control.* 1998;26:289–354.
3. Weber DJ, Rutala WA, Schaffner W. Lessons learned: protection of healthcare workers from infectious disease risks. *Crit Care Med.* 2010;38(suppl):S306–S314.
4. Sebazco S. Occupational health. In: *APIC Text of Infection Control and Epidemiology.* 4 ed. Washington, DC: Association for Professionals in Infection Control and Epidemiology; 2014:100.1–16.
5. Centers for Disease Control and Prevention. Immunization of health-care personnel: Recommendations of the Advisory Committee on Immunization Practices (ACIP). *MMWR Recomm Rep.* 2011;60(RR-7):1–45.
6. Talbot TR. Update on immunizations for healthcare personnel in the United States. *Vaccine.* 2014;32: 4869–4875.
7. Sparks V. Immunization of healthcare personnel. In: *APIC Text of Infection Control and Epidemiology.* 4 ed. Washington, DC: Association for Professionals in Infection Control and Epidemiology; 2014:103.1–36.
8. Weber DJ, Rutala WA. Occupational health update: focus on preventing the acquisition of infections with preexposure prophylaxis and postexposure prophylaxis. *Infect Dis Clin North Am.* 2016;30:729–757.
9. Centers for Disease Control and Prevention. Recommended Immunization Schedule for Adults Aged 19 Years or Older, United States 2018. https://www.cdc.gov/vaccines/schedules/hcp/adult.html.

10. American Academy of Pediatrics. Immunization in health care personnel. In: Kimberlin DW, Brady MT, Jackson MS, Long SS, eds. *Red Book: 2015 Report of Communicable Diseases.* 30th ed. Elk Grove Village, IL: American Academy of Pediatrics; 2015:95−98.

11. Centers for Disease Control, Prevention. *Epidemiology and Prevention of Vaccine-preventable Diseases. The Pink Book: Course Textbook.* 13th ed. 2015. https://www.cdc.gov/vaccines/pubs/pinkbook/index.html.

12. Kroger AT, Duchin J, Vazquez M. General Best Practice Guidelines for Immunization.Best Practices Guidance of the Advisory Committee on Immunization Practices (ACIP). https://www.cdc.gov/vaccines/hcp/acip-recs/general-recs/index.html.

13. Weber DJ, Consoli S, Sickbert-Bennett E, Miller MB, Rutala WA. Susceptibility to measles, mumps, and rubella in newly hired (2006−2008) healthcare workers born before 1957. *Infect Control Hosp Epidemiol.* 2010; 31:655−657.

14. Troiani L, Hill 3rd JJ, Consoli S, Weber DJ. Varicella-zoster immunity in US healthcare personnel with self-reported history of disease. *Infect Control Hosp Epidemiol.* 2015;36:1467−1468.

15. Talbot TR, Babcock H, Caplan AL, et al. Revised SHEA position paper: influenza vaccination of healthcare personnel. *Infect Control Hosp Epidemiol.* 2010;31:987−995.

16. Lee LM. Adding justice to the clinical and public health ethics arguments for mandatory seasonal influenza immunization for healthcare workers. *J Med Ethics.* 2015; 41:682−686.

17. Maltezou HC, Poland GA. Immunization of health-care providers: necessity and public health policies. *Healthc (Basel).* 2016;4(3).

18. National Vaccine Advisory Committee. Recommendations on strategies to achieve the Healthy People 2020 annual vaccine coverage goal for health care personnel. nvac_adult_immunization_work_group.pdf.

19. Centers for Disease Control, Prevention. Poliomyelitis prevention in the United States: updated recommendations of the Advisory Committee on Immunization Practices (ACIP). *MMWR Recomm Rep.* 2000;49(RR05):1−22.

20. Manning SE, Rupprecht CE, Fishbein D, et al. Human rabies prevention −- United States, 2008: recommendations of the Advisory Committee on Immunization Practices. *MMWR.* 2008;57(RR03):1−26, 28.

21. Petersen BW, Harms TJ, Reynolds MG, et al. Use of vaccinia virus smallpox vaccine in laboratory and health care personnel at risk for occupational exposure to ortho-poxviruses — recommendations of the Advisory Committee on Immunization Practices (ACIP), 2015. *MMWR.* 2016;65(10):257−262.

22. Wright JG, Quinn CP, Shadomy S, et al. Use of anthrax vaccine in the United States: recommendations of the Advisory Committee on Immunization Practices (ACIP), 2009. *MMWR.* 2010;59(RR06):1−30.

23. Centers for Disease Control and Prevention. Traveler's Health: Vaccines, medicines, advice. https://wwwnc.cdc.gov/travel.

24. Centers for Disease Control, Prevention. *CDC Health Information for International Travel (Yellow Book)*; 2018. https://wwwnc.cdc.gov/travel/page/yellowbook-home/.

25. Rubin LG, Levin MJ, Ljungman P, et al. 2013 IDSA clinical practice guideline for vaccination of the immunocompromised host. *Clin Infect Dis.* 2014;58: 309−318.

26. Talbot TR, Babcock H, Cotton D, et al. The use of live attenuated influenza vaccine (LAIV) in healthcare personnel (HCP): guidance from the Society for Healthcare Epidemiology of America (SHEA). *Infect Control Hosp Epidemiol.* 2012;33:981−983.

27. Bazan JA, Mangino JE. Infection control and postexposure prophylaxis for the pregnant healthcare worker. *Clin Obstet Gynecol.* 2012;55:571−588.

28. Lynch L, Spivak ES. The pregnant healthcare worker: fact and fiction. *Curr Opin Infect Dis.* 2015;28:362−368.

29. Centers for Disease Control and Prevention. Updated recommendations for use of tetanus toxoid, reduced diphtheria toxoid, and acellular pertussis vaccine (Tdap) in pregnant women — Advisory Committee on Immunization Practices (ACIP), 2012. *MMWR Recomm Rep.* 2013; 62(07):131−135.

30. Centers for Disease Control and Prevention. Summary of notifiable infectious diseases and conditions — United States, 2015. *MMWR Notif Dis.* 2017;64(53):1−143.

31. Centers for Disease Control and Prevention. Measles. https://www.cdc.gov/measles/hcp/index.html.

32. Centers for Disease Control and Prevention. Mump cases and outbreaks. https://www.cdc.gov/mumps/outbreaks.html.

33. Centers for Disease Control, Prevention. Recommendation of the Advisory Committee on Immunization Practices for use of a third dose of mumps virus−containing vaccine in persons at increased risk for mumps during an outbreak. *MMWR.* 2018;67:33−38.

34. Cardemil CV, Dahl RM, James L, et al. Effectiveness of a third dose of MMR vaccine for mumps outbreak control. *N Engl J Med.* 2017;377:947−956.

35. Nelson GE, Aguon A, Valencia E, et al. Epidemiology of a mumps outbreak in a highly vaccinated island population and use of a third dose of measles-mumps-rubella vaccine for outbreak control−Guam 2009 to 2010. *Pediatr Infect Dis J.* 2013;32(4):374−380.

36. Ogbuanu IU, Kutty PK, Hudson JM, et al. Impact of a third dose of measles-mumps-rubella vaccine on a mumps outbreak. *Pediatrics.* 2012;130(6):e1567−e1574.

37. Centers for Disease Control, Prevention. CDC guidance for evaluating health-care personnel for hepatitis B virus protection and for administering postexposure management. *MMWR Recomm Rep.* 2013;62(RR-10):1−19.

38. Centers for Disease Control and Prevention. Prevention of hepatitis B virus infection in the United States: recommendations of the Advisory Committee on Immunization Practices. *MMWR Recomm Rep.* 2018;67(No. 1):1−31.

39. International Safety Center. *EPINet Report for Needlestick and Sharp Object Injuries*; 2015. https://international safetycenter.org/exposure-reports/.

40. Bond WW, Favero MS, Petersen NJ, Gravelle CR, Ebert JW, Maynard JE. Survival of hepatitis B virus after drying and storage for one week. *Lancet.* 1981;1(8219):550–551.

41. Kew MC. Possible transmission of serum (Australia-antigen-positive) hepatitis via the conjunctiva. *Infect Immun.* 1973;7:823–824.

42. Snydman DR, Hindman SH, Wineland MD, Bryan JA, Maynard JE. Nosocomial viral hepatitis B. A cluster among staff with subsequent transmission to patients. *Ann Intern Med.* 1976;85:573–577.

43. Ingerslev J, Mortensen E, Rasmussen K, Jørgensen J, Skinhøj P. Silent hepatitis-B immunization in laboratory technicians. *Scand J Clin Lab Invest.* 1988;48:333–336.

44. Centers for Disease Control, Prevention. Surveillance of vaccination coverage among adult populations - United States, 2015. *MMWR.* 2017;66(No. 11):1–28.

45. Weber DJ, Hoffmann KK, Rutala WA. Management of the healthcare worker infected with human immunodeficiency virus: lessons from nosocomial transmission of hepatitis B virus. *Infect Control Hosp Epidemiol.* 1991;12:625–630.

46. US Department of Labor. Occupational Safety and Health Administration. OSHA Law and Regulations. https://www.osha.gov/law-regs.html.

47. Lemon SM, Weber DJ. Immunogenicity of plasma-derived hepatitis B vaccine: relationship to site of injection and obesity. *J Gen Intern Med.* 1986;1:199–201.

48. McMahon BJ, Dentinger CM, Bruden D, et al. Antibody levels and protection after hepatitis B vaccine: results of a 22-year follow-up study and response to a booster dose. *J Infect Dis.* 2009;200:1390–1396.

49. Centers for Disease Control and Prevention. Monitoring the Impact of Varicella Vaccination. https://www.cdc.gov/chickenpox/surveillance/monitoring-varicella.html.

50. Weber DJ, Rutala WA, Hamilton H. Prevention and control of varicella-zoster infections in healthcare facilities. *Infect Control Hosp Epidemiol.* 1996;17:694–705.

51. Josephson A, Gombert ME. Airborne transmission of nosocomial varicella from localized zoster. *J Infect Dis.* 1988;158:238–241.

52. Sawyer MH, Chamberlin CJ, Wu YN, Aintablian N, Wallace MR. Detection of varicella-zoster virus DNA in air samples from hospital rooms. *J Infect Dis.* 1994;169:91–94.

53. Seward JF, Marin M, Vázquez M. Varicella vaccine effectiveness in the US vaccination program: a review. *J Infect Dis.* 2008;197(suppl 2):S82–S89.

54. Weber DJ, Orenstein W, Rutala WA. How to improve influenza vaccine coverage of healthcare personnel. *Isr J Health Policy Res.* 2016;5:61.

55. Centers for Disease Control and Prevention. Disease Burden of Influenza. https://www.cdc.gov/flu/about/disease/burden.htm.

56. World Health Organization. Influenza (seasonal). http://www.who.int/mediacentre/factsheets/fs211/en/.

57. Centers for Disease Control and Prevention. Influenza vaccination of health-care personnel: recommendations of the Healthcare Infection Control Practices Advisory Committee (HICPAC) and the Advisory Committee on Immunization Practices (ACIP). *MMWR Recomm Rep.* 2006;55(RR02):1–16.

58. Vanhems P, Bénet T, Munier-Marion E. Nosocomial influenza: encouraging insights and future challenges. *Curr Opin Infect Dis.* 2016;29:366–372.

59. Ahmed F, Lindley MC, Allred N, Weinbaum CM, Grohskopf L. Effect of influenza vaccination of healthcare personnel on morbidity and mortality among patients: systematic review and grading of evidence. *Clin Infect Dis.* 2014;58:50–57.

60. World Health Organization. WHO recommendations for routine immunization – summary tables. Table 4, vaccination of health care workers. http://www.who.int/immunization/policy/immunization_tables/en/.

61. Centers for Disease Control and Prevention. Influenza vaccination coverage among health care personnel - United States, 2016–17 influenza season. *MMWR.* 2017;66:1009–1015.

62. Talbot TR, Bradley SE, Cosgrove SE, Ruef C, Siegel JD, Weber DJ. Influenza vaccination of healthcare workers and vaccine allocation for healthcare workers during vaccine shortages. *Infect Control Hosp Epidemiol.* 2005;26:882–890.

63. LaVela SL, Hill JN, Smith BM, Evans CT, Goldstein B, Martinello R. Healthcare worker influenza declination form program. *Am J Infect Control.* 2015;43:624–628.

64. Ajenjo MC, Woeltje KF, Babcock HM, Gemeinhart N, Jones M, Fraser VJ. Influenza vaccination among healthcare workers: ten-year experience of a large healthcare organization. *Infect Control Hosp Epidemiol.* 2010;31:233–240.

65. Ribner BS, Hall C, Steinberg JP, et al. Use of a mandatory declination form in a program for influenza vaccination of healthcare workers. *Infect Control Hosp Epidemiol.* 2008;29:302–308.

66. Talbot TR. Do declination statements increase health care worker influenza vaccination rates? *Clin Infect Dis.* 2009;49:773–779.

67. Thomas RE. Do we have enough evidence how seasonal influenza is transmitted and can be prevented in hospitals to implement a comprehensive policy? *Vaccine.* 2016;34:3014–3021.

68. Kim H, Lindley MC, Dube D, Kalayil EJ, Paiva KA, Raymond P. Evaluation of the impact of the 2012 Rhode Island health care worker influenza vaccination regulations: implementation process and vaccination coverage. *J Public Health Manag Pract.* 2015;21(3):E1–E9.

69. Fricke KL, Gastañaduy MM, Klos R, Bégué RE. Correlates of improved influenza vaccination of healthcare personnel: a survey of hospitals in Louisiana. *Infect Control Hosp Epidemiol.* 2013;34:723–729.

70. Miller BL, Ahmed F, Lindley MC, Wortley PM. Institutional requirements for influenza vaccination of healthcare personnel: results from a nationally representative

survey of acute care hospitals—United States, 2011. *Clin Infect Dis.* 2011;53:1051—1059.

71. Pitts S, Maruthur NM, Millar KR, Perl TM, Segal J. A systematic review of mandatory influenza vaccination in healthcare personnel. *Am J Prev Med.* 2014;47:330—340.

72. Johnson JG, Talbot TR. New approaches for influenza vaccination of healthcare workers. *Curr Opin Infect Dis.* 2011;24:363—369.

73. Centers for Disease Control and Prevention. Pertussis (whooping cough): Surveillance and Reporting. https://www.cdc.gov/pertussis/surv-reporting.html.

74. Cherry JD. Epidemic pertussis and acellular pertussis vaccine failure in the 21st century. *Pediatrics.* 2015;135:1130—1132.

75. Cherry JD. Pertussis: challenges today and for the future. *PLoS Pathog.* 2013;9(7):e1003418. *N Engl J Med.* 2012;367:785—787.

76. Cherry JD. Epidemic pertussis in 2012—the resurgence of a vaccine-preventable disease. *Pediatrics.* 2015;135:1130—1132.

77. Cherry JD. Why do pertussis vaccines fail? *Pediatrics.* 2012;129:968—970.

78. Centers for Disease Control and Prevention. Pertussis (whooping cough): About Pertussis Outbreaks. https://www.cdc.gov/pertussis/outbreaks/about.html. Access 15 January 2015.

79. Sydnor E, Perl TM. Healthcare providers as sources of vaccine-preventable diseases. *Vaccine.* 2014;32:4814—4822.

80. Centers for Disease Control, Prevention. Preventing tetanus, diphtheria, and pertussis among adults: use of tetanus toxoid, reduced diphtheria toxoid and acellular pertussis vaccine recommendations of the Advisory Committee on Immunization Practices (ACIP) and recommendation of ACIP, supported by the Healthcare Infection Control Practices Advisory Committee (HICPAC), for use of Tdap among health-care personnel. *MMWR Recomm Rep.* 2006;55(RR-17):1—42.

81. Liang JL, Tiwari T, Moro P, et al. Prevention of pertussis, tetanus, and diphtheria with vaccines in the United States: recommendations of the Advisory Committee on Immunization Practices (ACIP). *MMWR Recomm Rep.* 2018;67(2):1—44.

82. Skoff TH, Martin SW. Impact of tetanus toxoid, reduced diphtheria toxoid, and acellular pertussis vaccinations on reported pertussis cases among those 11 to 18 years of age in an era of waning pertussis immunity: a follow-up analysis. *JAMA Pediatr.* 2016;170:453—458.

83. Sanstead E, Kenyon C, Rowley S, et al. Understanding trends in pertussis incidence: an agent-based model approach. *Am J Public Health.* 2015;105:e42—e47.

84. Koepke R, Eickhoff JC, Ayele RA, et al. Estimating the effectiveness of tetanus-diphtheria-acellular pertussis vaccine (Tdap) for preventing pertussis: evidence of rapidly waning immunity and difference in effectiveness by Tdap brand. *J Infect Dis.* 2014;210:942—953.

85. Centers for Disease Control and Prevention. Meningococcal disease: Surveillance. https://www.cdc.gov/meningococcal/surveillance/index.html.

86. Centers for Disease Control and Prevention. Meningococcal Vaccination: What Everyone Should Know. https://www.cdc.gov/vaccines/vpd/mening/public/index.html#should.

87. Centers for Disease Control and Prevention. Prevention and control of meningococcal disease: recommendations of the Advisory Committee on Immunization Practices (ACIP). *MMWR Recomm Rep.* 2013;62(No. 2):1—28.

88. Centers for Disease Control and Prevention. Updated recommendations for use of MenB-FHbp serogroup B meningococcal vaccine - Advisory Committee on Immunization Practices, 2016. *MMWR.* 2017;66:509—513.

89. Centers for Disease Control and Prevention. Laboratory-acquired meningococcal disease—United States, 2000. *MMWR.* 2002;51:141—144.

90. Sejvar JJ, Johnson D, Popovic T, et al. Assessing the risk of laboratory-acquired meningococcal disease. *J Clin Microbiol.* 2005;43:4811—4844.

91. Ricco M, Vezzosi L, Signorelli C. Invasive meningococcal disease on the workplaces: a systematic review. *Acta Biomed.* 2017;88:337—351.

92. Heymann DL. *Control of Communicable Diseases.* 20th ed. Washington, DC: American Public Health Association; 2015.

93. Seigel JD, Rhinehart E, Jackson M, Chiarello L and the Healthcare Infection Control Practices Advisory Committee, 2007 Guideline for Isolation Precautions: Preventing Transmission of Infectious Agents in Healthcare Settings https://www.cdc.gov/infectioncontrol/guidelines/isolation/index.html. Access 15 January 2018.

94. Siegel JD, Rhinehart E, Jackson M, Chiarello L. 2007 Guideline for Isolation Precautions: Preventing Transmission of Infectious Agents in Healthcare Settings. https://www.cdc.gov/infectioncontrol/guidelines/isolation/index.html.

95. Centers for Disease Control and Prevention. Influenza Antiviral Medications: Summary for Clinicians. https://www.cdc.gov/flu/professionals/antivirals/summary-clinicians.htm.

96. Goins WP, Edwards KM, Vnencak-Jones CL, et al. A comparison of 2 strategies to prevent infection following pertussis exposure in vaccinated healthcare personnel. *Clin Infect Dis.* 2012;54:938—945.

97. Weber DJ, Rutala WA. Risks and prevention of nosocomial transmission of rare zoonotic diseases. *Clin Infect Dis.* 2001;32:446—456.

98. Centers for Disease Control and Prevention. Rabies: Human rabies. http://www.cdc.gov/rabies/location/usa/surveillance/human_rabies.html.

99. Helmick CG, Tauxe RV, Vernon AA. Is there a risk to contacts of patients with rabies? *Rev Infect Dis.* 1987;9:511—518.

100. Centers for Disease Control, Prevention. Use of a reduced (4-dose) vaccine schedule for postexposure prophylaxis to prevent human rabies: recommendations of the Advisory Committee on Immunization Practices. *MMWR Recomm Rep.* 2010;59(RR02):1—9.

101. Weber DJ, Rutala WA, Weigle K. Selection and use of vaccines for healthcare workers. *Infect Control Hosp Epidemiol.* 1997;18:682.

102. Centers for Disease Control, Prevention. Prevention of hepatitis a through active or passive immunization recommendations of the Advisory Committee on Immunization Practices (ACIP). *MMWR Recomm Rep.* 2006; 55(RR-7):1−23.

103. Centers for Disease Control and Prevention. About Diphtheria. https://www.cdc.gov/diphtheria/about/index.html.

104. Centers for Disease Control and Prevention. Diphtheria: Complications. https://www.cdc.gov/diphtheria/about/complications.html.

FURTHER READING

1. Weber DJ, Rutala WA. Pertussis: an underappreciated risk for nosocomial outbreaks. *Infect Control Hosp Epidemiol.* 1998;19:825−828.

2. Centers for Disease Control, Prevention. Updated recommendations for use of VariZIG — United States, 2013. *MMWR.* 2013;62:574−576.

CHAPTER 12

Pneumococcal Vaccines in Adults: Who, What, When?

SRINIVAS ACHARYA NANDURI, MD, MPH • TAMARA PILISHVILI, PHD, MPH •
NANCY M. BENNETT, MD, MS

BACKGROUND

Streptococcus pneumoniae, also known as pneumococcus, is one of the leading infectious causes of disease and significant mortality among adults in the United States. Among the elderly, pneumococcal infections lead to thousands of hospitalizations and emergency department and outpatient visits, accruing billions of dollars in direct medical costs.[1] Pneumococcus normally colonizes the nasopharynx, with colonization rates of 2%–10% among healthy adults and 20%–40% among children.[2–8] Pneumococcal colonization does not necessarily lead to infection but is thought to be a precursor of infection. Pneumococcal colonization causes infection either by direct aspiration from the nasopharynx to a contiguous anatomic site such as the upper or lower respiratory tract or by hematogenous spread to sites such as joints and heart valves. Pneumococcal pneumonia is common among elderly persons with impaired swallowing and cough reflexes, likely associated with aspiration of nasopharyngeal secretions.[9]

Infections caused by pneumococci can be categorized as either noninvasive or invasive. The most common noninvasive presentation is sinusitis among adults and otitis media among children. Invasive pneumococcal disease (IPD) is defined as the isolation of pneumococci from a normally sterile site such as blood, cerebrospinal fluid (CSF), pleural fluid, or synovial fluid. Clinical presentations of IPD include pneumonia, meningitis, bacteremia, septic arthritis, and peritonitis. Pneumococcal pneumonia can be either bacteremic or nonbacteremic. Challenges in the collection of lower respiratory tract specimens adequate for diagnostic purposes contribute to underrecognition of nonbacteremic pneumococcal pneumonia. In addition, most burden studies consider only bacteremic pneumonia, further contributing to underestimation of pneumococcal disease burden.[10]

More than 90 serotypes of pneumococci are recognized based on antigenic differences in the capsular polysaccharide. Pneumococcal serotypes differ in their propensity to colonize the nasopharynx and their invasive potential.[11–13] Protective immunity to pneumococci is mediated in large part through capsular antibodies and is serotype specific.[14–16] Since the last quarter of the 20th century, pneumococcal vaccines have been routinely used to prevent disease among adults. These vaccines contain the capsular polysaccharide antigen and therefore provide serotype-specific immunity. The first vaccine with widespread use was the 23-valent pneumococcal polysaccharide vaccine (PPSV23) directed against the 23 most common serotypes. Because this vaccine was not immunogenic when administered to children aged <2 years, protein-conjugated polysaccharide vaccines were developed. The 7-valent pneumococcal conjugate vaccine (PCV7), introduced in 2000 for infants and young children, was highly effective against both invasive disease and pneumonia and was included in immunization schedules in many countries. Efforts continued to develop higher valency conjugate vaccines with coverage for a larger number of serotypes. Currently a 10-valent pneumococcal conjugate vaccine (PCV10) and a 13-valent pneumococcal conjugate vaccine (PCV13) are available in the global market. However, only PCV13 is licensed and available in the United States. PPSV23 contains 12 serotypes in common with PCV13 and 11 additional serotypes (Table 12.1). Because immunity is serotype specific, for the rest of the chapter, we will refer to groups of serotypes as PCV7, PCV13, or PPSV23 type while describing their epidemiology.

In this chapter we describe the epidemiology of pneumococcal disease among adults in the United States and available pneumococcal vaccines, supporting evidence and current Advisory Committee on

Vaccinations. https://doi.org/10.1016/B978-0-323-55435-0.00012-4

TABLE 12.1
Pneumococcal Vaccine Formulations

VACCINE	SEROTYPE																							
	1	2	3	4	5	6A	6B	7F	8	9N	9V	10A	11A	12F	14	15B	17F	18C	19A	19F	20	22F	23F	33F
PPSV23*	●	●	●	●	●		●	●	●	●	●	●	●	●	●	●	●	●	●	●	●	●	●	●
PCV7				●			●				●				●			●		●			●	
PCV10	●			●	●		●	●			●				●			●		●			●	
PCV13*	●		●	●	●	●	●	●			●				●			●	●	●			●	

*Vaccines currently licensed and available in the United States. Green shaded boxes indicate inclusion of serotype in the particular vaccine.

Immunization Practices (ACIP) recommendations regarding their use among adults.

EPIDEMIOLOGY OF PNEUMOCOCCAL DISEASE AMONG ADULTS

Asymptomatic human hosts colonized in their nasopharynx with pneumococci are likely the reservoir and source of transmission. Children play an important role because 20%–40% are carriers at any given time in the United States and similar settings.[4,7] Person-to-person transmission occurs via respiratory droplets; infection can also occur as a result of autoinoculation in persons carrying the bacteria in their upper respiratory tract.[17] The rate of transmission increases with crowding, presence of young children in the household, and concurrent viral respiratory tract infections.[18] Similar to other respiratory diseases, pneumococcal infections are more prevalent during the winter and in early spring. Studies have shown clear midwinter peaks and midsummer nadirs for IPD among adults.[19,20] Only a small fraction of individuals who become colonized will develop disease; factors related to the progression of colonization to disease are not well understood.

Given the difficulties in obtaining a specific diagnosis in cases of suspected bacterial pneumonia, pneumococcal pneumonia is likely underdiagnosed.[10] Laboratory-based surveillance data on IPD is available but do not capture nonbacteremic pneumococcal pneumonia and thus underestimates the true burden of pneumococcal disease among adults; for example, a review of studies using various diagnostic methods, including culture and urine antigen tests, estimated that only around 25% of pneumococcal pneumonia cases were bacteremic.[10]

Before conjugate vaccines were introduced, the incidence of severe pneumococcal disease followed a bimodal age distribution, being more common in young children and adults aged ≥65 years. Since the introduction of pneumococcal conjugate vaccines, vaccine-type IPD rates among young children have declined by approximately 90%.[21,22] There has been a concomitant dramatic decline in vaccine-type invasive infections in older adults attributed to indirect, "herd" effects of the conjugate vaccines.[21,22] Data from the Active Bacterial Core surveillance (ABCs), an active population- and laboratory-based surveillance system at 10 sites across the United States which is a component of the Centers for Disease Control and Prevention's Emerging Infections Program, indicated that after the introduction of PCV7 among children in 2000, dramatic reductions occurred in incidence of IPD among

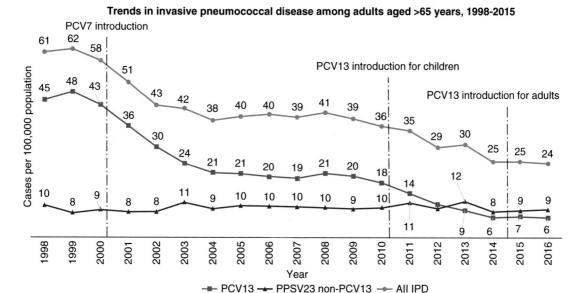

Trends in invasive pneumococcal disease among adults aged >65 years, 1998-2015

FIG. 12.1 **Trends in Invasive Pneumococcal Disease Among Adults Aged ≥65 years, 1998–2015.** This figure shows changes in the incidence of invasive pneumococcal disease (IPD) among adults aged 65 years or above from 1998 through 2015 in the United States. Rates of IPD expressed as cases per 100,000 population are shown on the y-axis and calendar year of surveillance on the x-axis. The green line represents the incidence rate of IPD due to all serotypes, the red line represents rate of IPD due to serotypes contained in PCV13, and the blue line represents the rate of IPD due to the 11 serotypes unique to PPSV23. The rates of IPD due to serotypes contained in PCV13 declined as a result of indirect effects from vaccination of children, whereas the rates of IPD due to serotypes that are unique to PPSV23 and not present in PCV13 did not change.

both children (direct effects) and adults of all ages (indirect effects).[22] Additional declines in disease incidence were observed after PCV13 introduction in 2010.[21] These trends were driven by reductions in disease caused by serotypes included in PCV7 and PCV13. Among adults aged ≥65 years there was a decline in IPD rate from 58 per 100,000 population in 2000 (before PCV7 introduction) to 24 per 100,000 population in 2016 (6 years after PCV13 introduction) (Fig. 12.1). However, despite these reductions caused by indirect PCV effects, there is still a significant burden of IPD among adults. In 2015 based on data from ABCs, the estimated incidence rate of IPD among adults aged ≥65 years was 25/100,000 population. This was 2.5 times more than the rate of 9/100,000 among children aged <5 years. Among persons aged ≥65 years, incidence rates increased with increasing age, ranging from 18.2/100,000 among persons aged 65–74 years to 45.3/100,000 among persons aged ≥85 years.[23] Approximately 40% of IPD among adults aged ≥65 years is caused by serotypes unique to PPSV23 and around 25% by serotypes included in PCV13.[24,25]

Pneumococcal disease is more common and more severe among persons with certain underlying conditions. A retrospective cohort study using data from 2006 to 2010 from three large healthcare claim repositories found 2.8–3.2 times higher rates of all-cause pneumonia, pneumococcal pneumonia, and IPD among those with underlying conditions than among healthy adults without these conditions. The highest rates seen in this study were among those with functional/anatomic asplenia, diseases of white blood cells, and congenital immunodeficiencies.[26] Rates of IPD among adults with underlying conditions were even higher before the introduction of PCV among children. A study using data from ABCs from 1999 to 2000 estimated that compared to healthy adults aged ≥18 years, the incidence of IPD was 3.4 times higher among adults with diabetes, 5.6 times higher among those with chronic lung disease, 6.4 times higher among those with chronic heart disease, and 11.4 times higher among those with current or recent history of alcohol abuse.[27]

PNEUMOCOCCAL VACCINES FOR ADULTS
Pneumococcal Polysaccharide Vaccine
History and development
Attempts at development of vaccines against pneumococcal disease began around the turn of the 20th century. Early pneumococcal vaccines were whole-cell heat-killed pneumococcal formulations; however, as understanding of the antigenicity of the capsular polysaccharide and serotype-specific nature of immunity to pneumococci evolved, polysaccharide vaccines containing 2–8 capsular polysaccharides were developed. These vaccines were evaluated since the Second World War but were not widely adopted. The current PPSV23 was licensed in 1983.[28] Since 1983, PPSV23 has been recommended for adults aged ≥65 years and for persons aged ≥2 years with underlying medical conditions.[25]

Immunogenicity
As with other purified polysaccharide vaccines, the immune response to PPSV23 is T-cell independent and leads to antibody production from B-cells without the involvement of T-helper cells. In addition to being nonimmunogenic among children aged <2 years, the immune response is not long-lasting and fails to elicit a reliable booster response on repeat doses.[25] Furthermore, there is no mucosal immunity induced, and consequently nasopharyngeal carriage is not affected. Immune response to pneumococcal vaccines is evaluated primarily using two parameters—serotype-specific anticapsular immunoglobulin G (IgG) antibody concentrations, as measured by enzyme-linked immunosorbent assay, and functional activity, as measured by an opsonophagocytic assay (OPA). However, there are no established levels of these parameters that correlate with protection against pneumococcal disease after vaccination among adults. Among generally healthy adults, PPSV23 induces both serotype-specific anticapsular antibody and OPA responses. PPSV23 induces an antibody response in older adults, whereas both anticapsular antibody titers and OPA titers are lower in younger adults.[29,30] Studies have shown that anticapsular antibodies generated in response to PPSV23 decline with time after vaccination and for some serotypes, decline to prevaccine levels 5–7 years after vaccination.[29,31,32]

Efficacy and effectiveness
Clinical trials and observational studies have demonstrated efficacy and effectiveness of PPSV23 against IPD, especially bacteremia and meningitis. A Cochrane review including data from 11 randomized controlled trials (RCTs) involving 36,489 participants found vaccine efficacy of 74% against IPD.[33] However, the reviewers did not find evidence of PPSV23 efficacy against IPD among adults with chronic diseases. The pooled estimate of efficacy against all-cause pneumonia in the aforementioned metaanalysis was 28%; however, there was substantial variability in the data from the 16 RCTs that were considered.[33] Although an efficacy of 73% against vaccine-type presumptive pneumococcal pneumonia defined as clinically and radiologically confirmed pneumonia with isolation of *S. pneumoniae* from a culture of sputum or nasal swab was reported, only one of the studies that contributed to this estimate used the current formulation of PPSV23.[34–37] Although some metaanalyses support the finding of protective efficacy of PPSV23 against pneumococcal pneumonia, others have concluded that vaccination with PPSV23 is not protective.[38–40] The protective efficacy of PPSV23 against pneumonia among adults, especially the elderly, remains controversial, with most metaanalyses considering the same studies but differing on assessment of study quality, taking into consideration enrollment and, more importantly, endpoints and diagnostic methods used.[33,38–41]

Although PPSV23 confers individual-level protection against invasive disease, it does not reduce acquisition of nasopharyngeal carriage with pneumococci and therefore does not contribute to herd protection. Despite recommendations since 1983 for use of PPSV23, no measurable impact on IPD caused by serotypes unique to PPSV23 has ever been demonstrated at the population level.

Numerous observational studies have been carried out to assess effectiveness of PPSV23 against endpoints of IPD, nonbacteremic pneumococcal pneumonia, and all-cause pneumonia. There is evidence from observational studies supporting a protective effect of PPSV23 against IPD among both healthy adults and those with underlying conditions.[42–45] However, the results of studies on effectiveness against pneumonia are not consistent, with some finding no protection and others finding a reduced risk of pneumonia with PPSV23 vaccination.[46–51]

Safety
The most common adverse events after vaccination with PPSV23 are injection-site reactions. These are generally mild and short-lived, resolving spontaneously in 1–2 days.[52,53] Although very infrequent, cellulitis was noted as a serious adverse event in postmarketing surveillance and is listed on the package insert.[54] A recent study looked at all reports to the Vaccine Adverse Event

Reporting System for 1990–2013 for possible adverse events after vaccination with PPSV23. Injection-site erythema, injection-site pain, and injection-site swelling were the most common nonserious adverse events in adults. Although quite rare, among serious adverse events reported, cellulitis was the most common.[55]

To address the time-limited immune response to vaccination with PPSV23, periodic revaccination with PPSV23 was suggested as a strategy in the 1980s. However, there were safety concerns based on findings of an increased frequency of induration, erythema, and other injection-site reactions in initial studies from the 1970s.[56–58] Since then, multiple studies have evaluated safety of revaccination in healthy adults as well as older adults and found the vaccine to be tolerated well on repeat doses, albeit with a higher frequency of local reactions.[52,53,59]

Administration

The polysaccharide vaccine currently available in the United States (Pneumovax 23, Merck) contains 25 mcg of each antigen per dose and contains 0.25% phenol as a preservative. The vaccine is available in a single-dose vial or syringe and in a five-dose vial, given by injection and may be administered intramuscularly.

Pneumococcal Conjugate Vaccine
History and development

Given the inability of polysaccharide vaccines to protect children aged <2 years, the focus shifted to the development of pneumococcal conjugate vaccines, after the remarkable success of *Haemophilus influenzae* type b (Hib) conjugate vaccines at preventing severe Hib disease. The conjugation of the capsular polysaccharide with the protein moiety modifies the nature of the immune response from T cell independent to T cell dependent. This is important for infants because a T-helper cell response leads to a better primary response and a strong booster response at reexposure.[25]

The first licensed conjugate vaccine, a PCV7, was highly effective against IPD, pneumonia, and otitis media among infants.[60–65] In late 2000s, PCV7 was licensed and recommended for routine use in US infants and young children. Postlicensure observational studies have demonstrated its effectiveness against both invasive and noninvasive pneumococcal disease as well as acquisition of nasopharyngeal carriage with the serotypes contained in the vaccine. Reduction in nasopharyngeal carriage among children was associated with declines in burden of disease due to the vaccine serotypes in unvaccinated populations (older children and adults) comparable to the decline observed in the vaccine target age group.

Efforts to expand coverage to include other common serotypes in addition to those already in PCV7 led to the development of higher valency vaccines with two formulations currently available globally—PCV10 and PCV13. PCV10 was never licensed in the United States. PCV13 includes 13 purified capsular polysaccharides coupled with a nontoxic variant of diphtheria toxin, CRM197. PCV13 was licensed in 2010 based on immunogenicity studies demonstrating a noninferior response to the serotypes it had in common with PCV7 and replaced PCV7 as the recommended vaccine for children in the United States. PCV13 was licensed for use among adults aged ≥50 years under the Food and Drug Administration's accelerated approval pathway based on noninferior immunogenicity compared to PPSV23.[25]

Immunogenicity

The immunogenicity of PCV13 in adults was investigated in two randomized, multicenter, immunogenicity studies conducted in the United States and Europe. In these trials, adults aged ≥50 years received a single dose of PCV13 or PPSV23, and their immune responses were evaluated. The OPA geometric mean antibody titers (GMTs) to the 12 serotypes common to both vaccines were equivalent or higher in adults aged 60–64 years naïve to pneumococcal vaccines who were vaccinated with PCV13 when compared with those vaccinated with PPSV23.[66] In adults aged ≥70 years who previously had been immunized with a single dose of PPSV23 at least 5 years before enrollment, the PCV13 responses were significantly greater than the PPSV23 responses for 10 of the 12 serotypes.[67]

Among HIV-infected adults, PCV7 immunogenicity has been shown to be noninferior or superior to PPSV23 in four studies from the United States and Europe.[68–71] A similar result was obtained when comparing responses to PCV13 and PPSV23 in HIV-infected adults.[88]

Efficacy and effectiveness

PCV7 was 75% efficacious in preventing IPD among immunocompromised adults in a trial among HIV-infected adults in Malawi. This trial did not find any protection against all-cause pneumonia.[72]

To date, only one randomized trial evaluating efficacy of PCV13 among adults has been reported. The Community-Acquired Pneumonia Immunization (CAPiTA) trial was a parallel-group, randomized, placebo-controlled, double blind trial carried out in the Netherlands among approximately 85,000 adults aged ≥65 years conducted during 2008–2013. The primary objective of the study was to evaluate efficacy of

PCV13 in preventing pneumococcal pneumonia. The results of the CAPiTA trial demonstrated 45.6% (95% confidence interval [CI] = 21.8%−62.5%) efficacy of PCV13 against all vaccine-type pneumococcal pneumonia, 45.0% (CI = 14.2%−65.3%) efficacy against vaccine-type nonbacteremic pneumococcal pneumonia, and 75.0% (CI = 41.4%−90.8%) efficacy against vaccine-type IPD among adults aged ≥65 years.[73−75] However, the study did not find statistically significant protection against all-cause community-acquired pneumonia. Subsequent supplementary analyses of the study data suggested that the protective efficacy of the vaccine declined with increasing age and that there might have been no protection afforded to those aged ≥85 years.[76]

Observational studies evaluating effectiveness of PCV13 among adults and impact of PCV13 use at the population level among adults are ongoing. However, significant declines in IPD caused by PCV13 types among adults have occurred through indirect protection due to routine PCV use among children in the United States.[21,22]

Safety

Both PCV7 and PCV13 were found to be safe for use in adults in numerous carefully conducted randomized pre-licensure studies, both in adults not previously vaccinated with PPSV23 and in those who had previously received PPSV23. Common adverse events noted were mild and included mild local tenderness and fever.[66,77−82] There were no excess serious adverse events associated with vaccination with PCV13 in the CAPiTA trial, although there were higher minor systemic and local adverse events in the vaccinated group. These included marginally higher local redness, swelling, or pain, fever, generalized muscle pain, and fatigue.[74]

Rationale for use of PCV13 and PPSV23 in series. Although PPSV23 is effective against IPD, there is no consensus about its effectiveness in preventing pneumococcal pneumonia, and population-level impacts on pneumonia and IPD have not been observed despite modest increases in coverage. The CAPiTA trial showed that PCV13 was effective in preventing vaccine-type nonbacteremic pneumococcal pneumonia. Although indirect effects of PCV7 and then PCV13 have led to remarkable declines in vaccine-type disease among adults aged ≥65 years, there is a remaining burden of disease due to these serotypes. Furthermore, the serotypes unique to PPSV23 contribute significantly to IPD burden in this age group.[83] Thus there was interest in evaluating

administration of both PCV13 and PPSV23 to eligible adults, adding protection against pneumonia at the same time as retaining protection against the PPSV23 unique serotypes. A mathematical model estimating the expected impact of various policy options using PCV13 and/or PPSV23 showed that adding a dose of PCV13 to PPSV23 would lead to additional prevention of morbidity and mortality due to the vaccine types.[84] Several immunogenicity studies among healthy adults, as well as adults with HIV infection, have demonstrated an improved immune response when PCV7 or PCV13 was administered first, followed by PPSV23, versus the other way around.[80,85−87] One of the studies also showed lower GMTs as measured by the OPA when PPSV23 was followed by PCV13, as compared to the reverse order.[80] Intervals longer than a year between PCV13 dose followed by PPSV23 led to a higher immune response against serotypes that were in both PCV13 and PPSV23 compared to a single dose of either of the vaccines.[24] These data suggest that administering both the vaccines, with PCV13 first in the series followed by PPSV23 separated at least by a year, would provide additional protection to vaccinated adults.

VACCINATION SCHEDULE AND USE/RECOMMENDATIONS

History

The ACIP first published its recommendations regarding the use of PPSV23 among adults in 1984, subsequent to licensure of the vaccine in 1983.[88] These recommendations were updated in 1989, 1997, and 2010, on each occasion adding to the indications by expanding the list of underlying conditions for which PPSV23 is recommended for adults aged <65 years.[89−91] In 2012 the ACIP first recommended the use of PCV13 among adults belonging to groups at increased risk for pneumococcal disease including those who are immunocompromised.[92] This was followed in 2014 with recommendations to use PCV13 in series with PPSV23 in all adults aged ≥65 years. In 2015 an update to these recommendations adjusted the recommended intervals between the two vaccines.[24,83]

Current Recommendations

Currently, the ACIP recommendations for adult pneumococcal vaccination cover the following two categories of individuals:

1. all adults aged ≥65 years
2. adults aged ≥19 years with certain medical conditions (Table 12.2)

TABLE 12.2

Medical Conditions for Which Advisory Committee for Immunization Practices (ACIP) recommends Pneumococcal Vaccination Among Adults Aged 19–64 Years, by Risk Group[92]

Underlying Medical Conditions

IMMUNOCOMPETENT PERSONS

- Chronic heart disease—including congestive heart failure and cardiomyopathies and excluding hypertension.
- Chronic lung disease—including chronic obstructive pulmonary disease, emphysema, and asthma.
- Diabetes mellitus
- Cerebrospinal fluid leak
- Cochlear implant
- Alcoholism
- Chronic liver disease and cirrhosis
- Cigarette smoking

PERSONS WITH FUNCTIONAL OR ANATOMIC ASPLENIA

- Sickle cell disease/other hemoglobinopathy
- Congenital or acquired asplenia

IMMUNOCOMPROMISED PERSONS

- Congenital or acquired immunodeficiency—includes B- (humoral) or T-lymphocyte deficiency, complement deficiencies (particularly C1, C2, C3, and C4 deficiencies), and phagocytic disorders (excluding chronic granulomatous disease).
- Human immunodeficiency virus infection
- Chronic renal failure
- Nephrotic syndrome
- Leukemia
- Lymphoma
- Hodgkin disease
- Generalized malignancy
- Iatrogenic immunosuppression
- Solid organ transplant
- Multiple myeloma

Recommendations for PPSV23 and PCV13 for use in adults older than or equal to 65 years

The ACIP recommends that both PCV13 and PPSV23 be administered in series to all adults aged ≥65 years. A dose of PCV13 should be administered first if it was not received previously. This should be followed by a dose of PPSV23 at least 1 year later. Both vaccines should not be administered during the same office visit. In case PPSV23 is administered earlier than the recommended window of at least 1 year, the dose should not be repeated. If PPSV23 has been previously administered, PCV13 should be administered at least 1 year after PPSV23 administration. No additional doses of PPSV23 are indicated for adults vaccinated with PPSV23 at age ≥65 years.

The recommendation for an interval of at least 1 year between the PCV13 and PPSV23 doses is supported by the immunogenicity data discussed in the section on rationale for use of PCV13 and PPSV23 in series for adults. Furthermore, data from the 2012 National Health Interview Survey showed that >93% of adults aged 65 years or above reported at least one encounter with a health professional in the preceding year.[93] Thus the 1-year interval offered sufficient opportunity for most adults aged 65 years or above to receive the vaccinations without requiring extra visits to their healthcare providers.[24] This also aligned with the recently revised Centers for Medicare & Medicaid Services regulations allowing for Medicare coverage of a second, different pneumococcal vaccine at least a year after the first one.[24]

Recommendations for adults aged 19 years and above with certain medical conditions

Adults aged 19–64 years with chronic heart disease including congestive heart failure and cardiomyopathies (excluding hypertension); chronic lung disease including chronic obstructive lung disease, emphysema, and asthma; chronic liver disease including cirrhosis; alcoholism; or diabetes mellitus or who smoke cigarettes should receive PPSV23. At age ≥ 65 years, they should be administered PCV13 and another dose of PPSV23 ≥ 1 year after PCV13 and ≥ 5 years after the most recent dose of PPSV23.

Adults aged ≥ 19 years with immunocompromising conditions (Table 12.2) or anatomical or functional asplenia should receive PCV13 and a dose of PPSV23 ≥ 8 weeks after PCV13, followed by a second dose of PPSV23 ≥ 5 years after the first dose of PPSV23. Adults aged ≥ 19 years with CSF leaks or cochlear implants should receive PCV13 followed by PPSV23 ≥ 8 weeks after PCV13. For both these groups, if the most recent dose of PPSV23 was administered at age <65 years, at age ≥ 65 years, another dose of PPSV23 should be administered ≥ 8 weeks after PCV13 and ≥ 5 years after the most recent dose of PPSV23.[24] Studies among HIV-positive adults had previously shown improved antibody response when PPSV23 was administered 4 or 8 weeks after PCV7 compared with just the administration of PPSV23.[69,70] The recommended 8-week interval minimizes the risk window for IPD due to serotypes unique to PPSV23 in these highly vulnerable groups. For those who receive a dose of PPSV23 first, a dose of PCV13 is recommended to be administered after at least 1 year of the PPSV23 dose.

PUBLIC HEALTH CONSIDERATIONS

While there have been recommendations for administering PPSV23 to all adults aged ≥ 65 years for many years, vaccine coverage in this age group is less than satisfactory. Coverage with pneumococcal vaccine by vaccine type, PCV13 or PPSV23, was not measured in the recent adult National Health Information Survey in 2016. Overall pneumococcal vaccine coverage (including both PCV13 and PPSV23) among adults aged 19–64 years with pneumococcal vaccine indications was around 24% and that among adults aged ≥ 65 years was around 67% in 2016.[94] Both these parameters were well below the Healthy People 2020 targets—60% for adults aged 19–64 years at increased risk and 90% for adults aged ≥ 65 years.[95] The low pneumococcal vaccination rates among adults are similar to the lower coverage seen for most routinely recommended adult vaccines, which can be attributed to both patient- and provider-level barriers.[96,97] A recent provider survey identified the complexity of pneumococcal vaccine recommendations and difficulty determining prior vaccination history as major

barriers to implementation of current ACIP recommendations for pneumococcal vaccine use among adults.[98] It has been suggested that rapid uptake and improved vaccine coverage in the early years postrecommendation would be key to maximize the impact of PCV13 use among adults and that the largest impact would be in the short term.[99] However, in the long term, if, as expected, there is continued decline of vaccine-type disease among adults due to indirect protection from use of PCV13 among children, the benefit of vaccinating adults with PCV13 will be reduced substantially. Considering this, the ACIP recommended a reevaluation of the 2014 recommendations in 2018. At the time of writing of this chapter, multiple studies are ongoing to generate postlicensure data on the impact of the new recommendations on pneumococcal disease among adults aged 65 years or above. The results of these studies will inform the ACIP on whether revisions to the recommendations are needed. In addition, higher valency formulations of pneumococcal conjugate vaccines are in various stages of development[100–102]; licensure of conjugate vaccines covering a greater number of serotypes, with effectiveness against both IPD and pneumonia, could simplify pneumococcal recommendations for adults and lead to additional health benefits.

DISCLAIMER

The findings and conclusions in this chapter are those of the authors and do not necessarily represent the official position of the Centers for Disease Control and Prevention.

REFERENCES

1. Huang SS, Johnson KM, Ray GT, et al. Healthcare utilization and cost of pneumococcal disease in the United States. *Vaccine.* 2011;29:3398–3412.
2. Almeida ST, Nunes S, Santos Paulo AC, et al. Low prevalence of pneumococcal carriage and high serotype and genotype diversity among adults over 60 years of age living in Portugal. *PLoS One.* 2014;9(3):e90974.
3. Flamaing J, Peetermans WE, Vandeven J, Verhaegen J. Pneumococcal colonization in older persons in a non-outbreak setting. *J Am Geriatr Soc.* 2010;58:396–398.
4. Hamaluba M, Kandasamy R, Ndimah S, et al. A cross-sectional observational study of pneumococcal carriage in children, their parents, and older adults following the introduction of the 7-valent pneumococcal conjugate vaccine. *Med Baltim.* 2015;94:e335.
5. Krone CL, Wyllie AL, van Beek J, et al. Carriage of Streptococcus pneumoniae in aged adults with influenza-like-illness. *PLoS One.* 2015;10(3):e0119875.

6. Palmu AA, Kaijalainen T, Saukkoriipi A, Leinonen M, Kilpi TM. Nasopharyngeal carriage of Streptococcus pneumoniae and pneumococcal urine antigen test in healthy elderly subjects. *Scand J Infect Dis.* 2012;44: 433–438.
7. Regev-Yochay G, Raz M, Dagan R, et al. Nasopharyngeal carriage of Streptococcus pneumoniae by adults and children in community and family settings. *Clin Infect Dis.* 2004;38:632–639.
8. Ridda I, Macintyre CR, Lindley R, et al. Lack of pneumococcal carriage in the hospitalised elderly. *Vaccine.* 2010; 28:3902–3904.
9. Janoff EN, Musher DM. Streptococcus pneumoniae. In: Bennett JE, Dolin R, Blaser MJ, eds. *Mandell, Douglas, and Bennett's Principles and Practice of Infectious Diseases.* Vol. 2. Philadelphia: Elsevier Saunders; 2015: 2310–2327.
10. Said MA, Johnson HL, Nonyane BA, et al. Estimating the burden of pneumococcal pneumonia among adults: a systematic review and meta-analysis of diagnostic techniques. *PLoS One.* 2013;8(4):e60273.
11. Brueggemann AB, Griffiths DT, Meats E, Peto T, Crook DW, Spratt BG. Clonal relationships between invasive and carriage Streptococcus pneumoniae and serotype- and clone-specific differences in invasive disease potential. *J Infect Dis.* 2003;187(9):1424–1432. Epub 2003 Apr 1424.
12. Crook DW. Capsular type and the pneumococcal human host-parasite relationship. *Clin Infect Dis.* 2006;42: 460–462.
13. Hausdorff WP, Bryant J, Paradiso PR, Siber GR. Which pneumococcal serogroups cause the most invasive disease: implications for conjugate vaccine formulation and use, part I. *Clin Infect Dis.* 2000;30:100–121.
14. Shurin PA, Rehmus JM, Johnson CE, et al. Bacterial polysaccharide immune globulin for prophylaxis of acute otitis media in high-risk children. *J Pediatr.* 1993;123: 801–810.
15. Siber GR, Thompson C, Reid GR, et al. Evaluation of bacterial polysaccharide immune globulin for the treatment or prevention of Haemophilus influenzae type b and pneumococcal disease. *J Infect Dis.* 1992;165: S129–S133.
16. Musher DM, Chapman AJ, Goree A, Jonsson S, Briles D, Baughn RE. Natural and vaccine-related immunity to Streptococcus pneumoniae. *J Infect Dis.* 1986;154: 245–256.
17. Bogaert D, De Groot R, Hermans PW. Streptococcus pneumoniae colonisation: the key to pneumococcal disease. *Lancet Infect Dis.* 2004;4:144–154.
18. Musher DM. How contagious are common respiratory tract infections? *N Engl J Med.* 2003;348(13):1256–1266.
19. Kim PE, Musher DM, Glezen WP, Rodriguez-Barradas MC, Nahm WK, Wright CE. Association of invasive pneumococcal disease with season, atmospheric conditions, air pollution, and the isolation of respiratory viruses. *Clin Infect Dis.* 1996;22:100–106.
20. Dowell SF, Whitney CG, Wright C, Rose Jr CE, Schuchat A. Seasonal patterns of invasive pneumococcal disease. *Emerg Infect Dis.* 2003;9:573–579.
21. Moore MR, Link-Gelles R, Schaffner W, et al. Effect of use of 13-valent pneumococcal conjugate vaccine in children on invasive pneumococcal disease in children and adults in the USA: analysis of multisite, population-based surveillance. *Lancet Infect Dis.* 2015. https://doi.org/10.1016/s1473-3099(1014) 71081-71083.
22. Pilishvili T, Lexau C, Farley MM, et al. Sustained reductions in invasive pneumococcal disease in the era of conjugate vaccine. *J Infect Dis.* 2010;201(1):32–41.
23. Centers for Disease Control, Prevention. Active bacterial Core surveillance report, emerging infections program network. *Streptococcus Pneumoniae*; 2015. https://www.cdc.gov/abcs/reports-findings/survreports/spneu15.html.
24. Kobayashi M, Bennett NM, Gierke R, et al. Intervals between PCV13 and PPSV23 vaccines: recommendations of the Advisory Committee on Immunization Practices (ACIP). *MMWR Morb Mortal Wkly Rep.* 2015;64: 944–947.
25. Pilishvili T, Bennett NM. Pneumococcal disease prevention among adults: strategies for the use of pneumococcal vaccines. *Vaccine.* 2015;33:D60–D65.
26. Shea KM, Edelsberg J, Weycker D, Farkouh RA, Strutton DR, Pelton SI. Rates of pneumococcal disease in adults with chronic medical conditions. *Open Forum Infect Dis.* 2014;1:ofu024.
27. Kyaw MH, Rose Jr CE, Fry AM, et al. The influence of chronic illnesses on the incidence of invasive pneumococcal disease in adults. *J Infect Dis.* 2005;192:377–386.
28. Grabenstein JD, Klugman KP. A century of pneumococcal vaccination research in humans. *Clin Microbiol Infect.* 2012;18:15–24.
29. Artz AS, Ershler WB, Longo DL. Pneumococcal vaccination and revaccination of older adults. *Clin Microbiol Rev.* 2003;16:308–318.
30. Romero-Steiner S, Musher DM, Cetron MS, et al. Reduction in functional antibody activity against Streptococcus pneumoniae in vaccinated elderly individuals highly correlates with decreased IgG antibody avidity. *Clin Infect Dis.* 1999;29:281–288.
31. Davidson M, Bulkow LR, Grabman J, et al. Immunogenicity of pneumococcal revaccination in patients with chronic disease. *Arch Intern Med.* 1994;154:2209–2214.
32. Hedlund J, Ortqvist A, Konradsen HB, Kalin M. Recurrence of pneumonia in relation to the antibody response after pneumococcal vaccination in middle-aged and elderly adults. *Scand J Infect Dis.* 2000;32(3): 281–286.
33. Moberley S, Holden J, Tatham DP, Andrews RM. Vaccines for preventing pneumococcal infection in adults. *Cochrane Database Syst Rev.* 2013:CD000422.
34. Kaufman P. Pneumonia in old age: active immunization against pneumonia with pneumococcus polysaccharide; results of a six year study. *Archives Intern Med.* 1947; 79(5):518–531.

35. Ortqvist A, Grepe A, Julander I, Kalin M. Bacteremic pneumococcal pneumonia in Sweden: clinical course and outcome and comparison with non-bacteremic pneumococcal and mycoplasmal pneumonias. *Scand J Infect Dis.* 1988;20(2):163–171.

36. Simberkoff MS, Cross AP, Al-Ibrahim M, et al. Efficacy of pneumococcal vaccine in high-risk patients. Results of a veterans administration cooperative study. *N Engl J Med.* 1986;315(21):1318–1327.

37. Smit P, Oberholzer D, Hayden-Smith S, Koornhof HJ, Hilleman MR. Protective efficacy of pneumococcal polysaccharide vaccines. *JAMA.* 1977;238(24):2613–2616.

38. Huss A, Scott P, Stuck AE, Trotter C, Egger M. Efficacy of pneumococcal vaccination in adults: a meta-analysis. *CMAJ.* 2009;180:48–58.

39. Schiffner-Rohe J, Witt A, Hemmerling J, von Eiff C, Leverkus FW. Efficacy of PPV23 in preventing pneumococcal pneumonia in adults at increased risk—a systematic review and meta-analysis. *PLoS One.* 2016;11(1):e0146338.

40. Falkenhorst G, Remschmidt C, Harder T, Hummers-Pradier E, Wichmann O, Bogdan C. Effectiveness of the 23-valent pneumococcal polysaccharide vaccine (PPV23) against pneumococcal disease in the elderly: systematic review and meta-analysis. *PLoS One.* 2017;12(1):e0169368.

41. Kraicer-Melamed H, O'Donnell S, Quach C. The effectiveness of pneumococcal polysaccharide vaccine 23 (PPV23) in the general population of 50 years of age and older: a systematic review and meta-analysis. *Vaccine.* 2016;34:1540–1550.

42. Moberley S, Krause V, Cook H, et al. Failure to vaccinate or failure of vaccine? Effectiveness of the 23-valent pneumococcal polysaccharide vaccine program in Indigenous adults in the Northern Territory of Australia. *Vaccine.* 2010;28:2296–2301.

43. Mooney JD, Weir A, McMenamin J, et al. The impact and effectiveness of pneumococcal vaccination in Scotland for those aged 65 and over during winter 2003/2004. *BMC Infect Dis.* 2008;8:53.

44. Singleton RJ, Butler JC, Bulkow LR, et al. Invasive pneumococcal disease epidemiology and effectiveness of 23-valent pneumococcal polysaccharide vaccine in Alaska native adults. *Vaccine.* 2007;25(12):2288–2295.

45. Vila-Corcoles A, Ochoa-Gondar O, Guzman JA, et al. Effectiveness of the 23-valent polysaccharide pneumococcal vaccine against invasive pneumococcal disease in people 60 years or older. *BMC Infect Dis.* 2010;10:73.

46. Jackson LA, Neuzil KM, Yu O, et al. Effectiveness of pneumococcal polysaccharide vaccine in older adults. *N Engl J Med.* 2003;348:1747–1755.

47. Nichol KL. The additive benefits of influenza and pneumococcal vaccinations during influenza seasons among elderly persons with chronic lung disease. *Vaccine.* 1999;17:S91–S93.

48. Skull SA, Andrews RM, Byrnes GB, et al. Prevention of community-acquired pneumonia among a cohort of hospitalized elderly: benefit due to influenza and pneumococcal vaccination not demonstrated. *Vaccine.* 2007;25: 4631–4640.

49. Suzuki M, Dhoubhadel BG, Ishifuji T, et al. Serotype-specific effectiveness of 23-valent pneumococcal polysaccharide vaccine against pneumococcal pneumonia in adults aged 65 years or older: a multicentre, prospective, test-negative design study. *The Lancet Infect Dis.* 2017; 17(3):313–321.

50. Vila-Corcoles A, Ochoa-Gondar O, Hospital I, et al. Protective effects of the 23-valent pneumococcal polysaccharide vaccine in the elderly population: the EVAN-65 study. *Clin Infect Dis.* 2006;43:860–868.

51. Ochoa-Gondar O, Vila-Corcoles A, Rodriguez-Blanco T, et al. Effectiveness of the 23-valent pneumococcal polysaccharide vaccine against community-acquired pneumonia in the general population aged >/= 60 years: 3 years of follow-up in the CAPAMIS study. *Clin Infect Dis.* 2014;58:909–917.

52. Grabenstein JD, Manoff SB. Pneumococcal polysaccharide 23-valent vaccine: long-term persistence of circulating antibody and immunogenicity and safety after revaccination in adults. *Vaccine.* 2012;30:4435–4444.

53. Musher DM, Manof SB, Liss C, et al. Safety and antibody response, including antibody persistence for 5 years, after primary vaccination or revaccination with pneumococcal polysaccharide vaccine in middle-aged and older adults. *J Infect Dis.* 2010;201(4):516–524.

54. Ito M, Nakano T, Kamiya T, et al. Activation of lymphocytes by varicella-zoster virus (VZV): expression of interleukin-2 receptors on lymphocytes cultured with VZV antigen. *J Infect Dis.* 1992;165:158–161.

55. Miller ER, Moro PL, Cano M, Lewis P, Bryant-Genevier M, Shimabukuro TT. Post-licensure safety surveillance of 23-valent pneumococcal polysaccharide vaccine in the vaccine adverse event reporting system (VAERS), 1990–2013. *Vaccine.* 2016;34:2841–2846.

56. Borgono JM, McLean AA, Vella PP, et al. Vaccination and revaccination with polyvalent pneumococcal polysaccharide vaccines in adults and infants. *Proc Soc Exp Biol Med.* 1978;157:148–154.

57. Carlson AJ, Davidson WL, McLean AA, et al. Pneumococcal vaccine: dose, revaccination, and coadministration with influenza vaccine. *Proc Soc Exp Biol Med.* 1979;161:558–563.

58. Hilleman MR, Carlson Jr AJ, McLean AA, Vella PP, Weibel RE, Woodhour AF. Streptococcus pneumoniae polysaccharide vaccine: age and dose responses, safety, persistence of antibody, revaccination, and simultaneous administration of pneumococcal and influenza vaccines. *Rev Infect Dis.* 1981;3:S31–S42.

59. Jackson LA, Benson P, Sneller VP, et al. Safety of revaccination with pneumococcal polysaccharide vaccine. *JAMA.* 1999;281:243–248.

60. Black S, Shinefield H, Fireman B, et al. Efficacy, safety and immunogenicity of heptavalent pneumococcal conjugate vaccine in children. Northern California Kaiser Permanente Vaccine Study Center Group. *Pediatr Infect Dis J.* 2000;19:187–195.

61. Black SB, Shinefield HR, Ling S, et al. Effectiveness of heptavalent pneumococcal conjugate vaccine in children younger than five years of age for prevention of pneumonia. *Pediatr Infect Dis J.* 2002;21:810–815.

62. Eskola J, Kilpi T, Palmu A, et al. Efficacy of a pneumococcal conjugate vaccine against acute otitis media. *N Engl J Med*. 2001;344:403–409.

63. Fireman B, Black SB, Shinefield HR, Lee J, Lewis E, Ray P. Impact of the pneumococcal conjugate vaccine on otitis media. *Pediatr Infect Dis J*. 2003;22:10–16.

64. O'Brien KL, Moulton LH, Reid R, et al. Efficacy and safety of seven-valent conjugate pneumococcal vaccine in American Indian children: group randomised trial. *Lancet*. 2003;362(9381):355–361.

65. Simonsen L, Taylor RJ, Young-Xu Y, Haber M, May L, Klugman KP. Impact of pneumococcal conjugate vaccination of infants on pneumonia and influenza hospitalization and mortality in all age groups in the United States. *MBio*. 2011;2:e00309–00310.

66. Jackson LA, Gurtman A, van Cleeff M, et al. Immunogenicity and safety of a 13-valent pneumococcal conjugate vaccine compared to a 23-valent pneumococcal polysaccharide vaccine in pneumococcal vaccine-naive adults. *Vaccine*. 2013;31:3577–3584.

67. Jackson LA, Gurtman A, Rice K, et al. Immunogenicity and safety of a 13-valent pneumococcal conjugate vaccine in adults 70 years of age and older previously vaccinated with 23-valent pneumococcal polysaccharide vaccine. *Vaccine*. 2013;31:3585–3593.

68. Crum-Cianflone NF, Huppler Hullsiek K, Roediger M, et al. A randomized clinical trial comparing revaccination with pneumococcal conjugate vaccine to polysaccharide vaccine among HIV-infected adults. *J Infect Dis*. 2010; 202:1114–1125.

69. Feikin DR, Elie CM, Goetz MB, et al. Randomized trial of the quantitative and functional antibody responses to a 7-valent pneumococcal conjugate vaccine and/or 23-valent polysaccharide vaccine among HIV-infected adults. *Vaccine*. 2002;20:545–553.

70. Lesprit P, Pedrono G, Molina JM, et al. Immunological efficacy of a prime-boost pneumococcal vaccination in HIV-infected adults. *AIDS*. 2007;21:2425–2434.

71. Penaranda M, Payeras A, Cambra A, Mila J, Riera M. Majorcan Pneumococcal Study G. Conjugate and polysaccharide pneumococcal vaccines do not improve initial response of the polysaccharide vaccine in HIV-infected adults. *AIDS*. 2010;24:1226–1228.

72. French N, Gordon SB, Mwalukomo T, et al. A trial of a 7-valent pneumococcal conjugate vaccine in HIV-infected adults. *N Engl J Med*. 2010;362:812–822.

73. Bonten M, Bolkenbaas M, Huijts S, et al. Community-acquired pneumonia immunisation trial in adults (CAPITA). *Pneumonia*. 2014;2014:95.

74. Bonten MJ, Huijts SM, Bolkenbaas M, et al. Polysaccharide conjugate vaccine against pneumococcal pneumonia in adults. *N Engl J Med*. 2015;372:1114–1125.

75. Hak E, Grobbee DE, Sanders EA, et al. Rationale and design of CAPITA: a RCT of 13-valent conjugated pneumococcal vaccine efficacy among older adults. *The Neth J Medicine*. 2008;66:378–383.

76. van Werkhoven CH, Huijts SM, Bolkenbaas M, Grobbee DE, Bonten MJ. The impact of age on the efficacy of 13-valent pneumococcal conjugate vaccine in elderly. *Clin Infect Dis*. 2015;61:1835–1838.

77. de Roux A, Schmole-Thoma B, Siber GR, et al. Comparison of pneumococcal conjugate polysaccharide and free polysaccharide vaccines in elderly adults: conjugate vaccine elicits improved antibacterial immune responses and immunological memory. *Clin Infect Dis*. 2008;46: 1015–1023.

78. Jackson LA, Neuzil KM, Whitney CG, et al. Safety of varying dosages of 7-valent pneumococcal protein conjugate vaccine in seniors previously vaccinated with 23-valent pneumococcal polysaccharide vaccine. *Vaccine*. 2005; 23:3697–3703.

79. Scott DA, Komjathy SF, Hu BT, et al. Phase 1 trial of a 13-valent pneumococcal conjugate vaccine in healthy adults. *Vaccine*. 2007;25:6164–6166.

80. Greenberg RN, Gurtman A, Frenck RW, et al. Sequential administration of 13-valent pneumococcal conjugate vaccine and 23-valent pneumococcal polysaccharide vaccine in pneumococcal vaccine–naïve adults 60–64 years of age. *Vaccine*. 2014;32:2364–2374.

81. Shiramoto M, Hanada R, Juergens C, et al. Immunogenicity and safety of the 13-valent pneumococcal conjugate vaccine compared to the 23-valent pneumococcal polysaccharide vaccine in elderly Japanese adults. *Hum Vaccin Immunother*. 2015;11(9):2198–2206.

82. Tinoco JC, Juergens C, Ruiz Palacios GM, et al. Open-label trial of immunogenicity and safety of a 13-valent pneumococcal conjugate vaccine in adults >/= 50 years of age in Mexico. *Clin Vaccine Immunol*. 2015;22: 185–192.

83. Tomczyk S, Bennett NM, Stoecker C, et al. Use of 13-valent pneumococcal conjugate vaccine and 23-valent pneumococcal polysaccharide vaccine among adults aged >65 Years: recommendations of the Advisory Committee on Immunization Practices (ACIP). *MMWR Morb Mortal Wkly Rep*. 2014;63:822–825.

84. Stoecker C, Kim L, Gierke R, Pilishvili T. Incremental cost-effectiveness of 13-valent pneumococcal conjugate vaccine for adults age 50 years and older in the United States. *J Gen Intern Med*. 2016;31:901–908.

85. Goldblatt D, Southern J, Andrews N, et al. The immunogenicity of 7-valent pneumococcal conjugate vaccine versus 23-valent polysaccharide vaccine in adults aged 50–80 years. *Clin Infect Dis*. 2009;49:1318–1325.

86. Jackson LA, Gurtman A, van Cleeff M, et al. Influence of initial vaccination with 13-valent pneumococcal conjugate vaccine or 23-valent pneumococcal polysaccharide vaccine on anti-pneumococcal responses following subsequent pneumococcal vaccination in adults 50 years and older. *Vaccine*. 2013;31:3594–3602.

87. Glesby MJ, Watson W, Brinson C, et al. Immunogenicity and safety of 13-valent pneumococcal conjugate vaccine in HIV-infected adults previously vaccinated with

pneumococcal polysaccharide vaccine. *J Infect Dis.* 2015; 212:18−27.

88. Centers for Disease C. Update: pneumococcal polysaccharide vaccine usage−United States. *MMWR Morb Mortal Wkly Rep.* 1984;33:273−276.

89. Prevention of pneumococcal disease. Recommendations of the Advisory Committee on Immunization Practices (ACIP). *MMWR Recomm Rep.* 1997;46(RR-8):1−24.

90. Centers for Disease C. Pneumococcal polysaccharide vaccine. *MMWR Morb Mortal Wkly Rep.* 1989;38:64−68.

91. Centers for Disease C. Prevention, Advisory Committee on Immunization P. Updated recommendations for prevention of invasive pneumococcal disease among adults using the 23-valent pneumococcal polysaccharide vaccine (PPSV23). *MMWR Morb Mortal Wkly Rep.* 2010;59: 1102−1106.

92. Centers for Disease C. Prevention. Use of 13-valent pneumococcal conjugate vaccine and 23-valent pneumococcal polysaccharide vaccine for adults with immunocompromising conditions: recommendations of the Advisory Committee on Immunization Practices (ACIP). *MMWR Morb Mortal Wkly Rep.* 2012;61:816−819.

93. Blackwell DL, Lucas JW, Clarke TC. Summary health statistics for U.S. adults: national health interview survey, 2012. *Vital Health Stat.* 2014;10:1−161.

94. Hung M, Williams WW, Lu PJ, et al. *Vaccination Coverage Among Adults in the United States.* National Health Interview Survey; 2016. https://www.cdc.gov/vaccines/imz-managers/coverage/adultvaxview/NHIS-2016.html#pneumo.

95. Williams WW, Lu PJ, O'Halloran A, et al. Surveillance of vaccination coverage among adult populations - United States, 2015. *MMWR Surveill Summ.* 2017;66:1−28.

96. Albright K, Hurley LP, Lockhart S, et al. Attitudes about adult vaccines and reminder/recall in a safety net population. *Vaccine.* 2017;35:7292−7296.

97. Hurley LP, Bridges CB, Harpaz R, et al. Physician Attitudes toward adult vaccines and other preventive Practices, United States, 2012. *Public Health Rep.* 2016;131:320−330.

98. Hurley LP, Allison MA, Pilishvili T, et al. Primary care physicians' struggle with current adult pneumococcal vaccine recommendations. *J Am Board Fam Med.* 2018; 31:94−104.

99. Pilishvili T, Gierke R, Kim L, Stoecker C. Potential public health impact of 13-valent pneumococcal conjugate vaccine use among adults 65 years of age or older. In: *Paper Presented at: IDWeek.* 2014. Philadelphia, PA.

100. Parham P. Flying the first class flag. *Nature.* 1992;357: 193−194.

101. Carrington M, Colonna M, Spies T, Stephens JC, Mann DL. Haplotypic variation of the transporter associated with antigen processing (TAP) genes and their extension of HLA class II region haplotypes. *Immunogenetics.* 1993;37:266−273.

102. Yewdell JW, Esquivel F, Arnold D, Spies T, Eisenlohr LC, Bennink JR. Presentation of numerous viral peptides to mouse major histocompatibility complex (MHC) class I-restricted T lymphocytes is mediated by the human MHC-encoded transporter or by a hybrid mouse-human transporter. *J Exp Med.* 1993;177:1785−1790.

Index

Note: Page numbers followed by "f" indicate figures and "t" indicate tables.

Printed in the United States
By Bookmasters